# Current Progress in Molecular Cytogenetics

# Current Progress in Molecular Cytogenetics

Edited by Camila Blair

AMERICAN
MEDICAL PUBLISHERS
www.americanmedicalpublishers.com

American Medical Publishers,
41 Flatbush Avenue,
1st Floor, New York,
NY 11217, USA

Visit us on the World Wide Web at:
www.americanmedicalpublishers.com



ISBN: 978-1-63927-246-4



**Cataloging-in-Publication Data**

Current progress in molecular cytogenetics / edited by Camila Blair.
p. cm.
Includes bibliographical references and index.
ISBN 978-1-63927-246-4
1. Cytogenetics. 2. Molecular genetics. 3. Chromosomes. I. Blair, Camila.

QH441.5 .C87 2022

611.018 16--dc23

# Table of Contents

# Preface

In my initial years as a student, I used to run to the library at every possible instance to grab a book and learn something new. Books were my primary source of knowledge and I would not have come such a long way without all that I learnt from them. Thus, when I was approached to edit this book; I became understandably nostalgic. It was an absolute honor to be considered worthy of guiding the current generation as well as those to come. I put all my knowledge and hard work into making this book most beneficial for its readers.

Molecular cytogenetics is a combination of molecular biology and cytogenetics. Molecular biology is a subset of biology that is concerned with the molecular basis of biological activity which occurs between biomolecules in numerous systems of a cell. Cytogenetics, on the other hand, is a field of genetics that deals with how the chromosomes are related to cell behavior during mitosis and meiosis. The aim of molecular cytogenetics is to distinguish between normal and cancer-causing cells using various substances. It is a useful tool for the diagnosis and treatment of various malignancies like haematological malignancies, brain tumors, etc. It uses the techniques of fluorescent in situ hybridization and comparative genomic hybridization. This book unravels the recent studies in the field of molecular cytogenetics. It strives to provide a fair idea about this discipline and to help develop a better understanding of the latest advances within this field. Students, researchers, experts and all associated with molecular cytogenetics will benefit alike from this book.

I wish to thank my publisher for supporting me at every step. I would also like to thank all the authors who have contributed their researches in this book. I hope this book will be a valuable contribution to the progress of the field.

**Editor**

1

# Interstitial 6q21q23 duplication - variant of variable phenotype and incomplete penetrance or benign duplication?

Malgorzata I. Srebniak[1*], Laura J. C. M. van Zutven[1], Florence Petit[2], Sonia Bouquillon[3], Ilse P. J. van Heel[1], Maarten F. C. M. Knapen[4,5], Jerome M. J. Cornette[4], Andreas Kremer[6], Diane Van Opstal[1] and Karin E. M. Diderich[1]

**Abstract**

**Background:** Chromosome 6q duplication syndrome is a chromosome abnormality associated with characteristic phenotypic features such as intellectual disability (ID), short stature, feeding difficulties, microcephaly, dysmorphic features (prominent forehead, downslanting palpebral fissures, flat nasal bridge, tented upper lip, micrognathia, short webbed neck) and joint contractures. Only a few cases of pure partial 6q trisomy have been published and the severity of the phenotype seems to depend on the breakpoint position. Unfortunately, most of these cases were identified using karyotyping or FISH, so breakpoints at the molecular level and thus gene content are not known.

**Cases presentation:** We report the first two families with an interstitial 6q duplication identified by karyotyping where the gene content and breakpoints were characterized with microarray. In family 1, the 6q22.1q23.2 duplication was detected in a female patient with ID. In family 2, the 6q21q22.33 duplication was identified in a male fetus with multiple congenital malformations. In both families, the duplication seems to show phenotypic heterogeneity and in family 1 also incomplete penetrance suggesting the co-existence of an "additional hit" in affected patients. This "additional hit" was identified in the first family to be a microduplication in 16p11.2, a known susceptibility locus (SL) for neurodevelopmental disorders, that co-segregated with an abnormal phenotype in the affected family members.

**Conclusions:** Our study shows that interstitial 6q21q23 duplication may represent a private variant that is benign, but may also contribute to developmental disorders of variable expressivity in a "multi-hit" model. Finding the "additional hit" within the family is therefore very important for genetic counseling and assessment of the CNV penetrance within the particular family.

**Keywords:** Interstitial 6q22.1q23.2 duplication, Interstitial duplication 6q21q22.33, 16p11.2 microduplication, Susceptibility locus, Second hit hypothesis

## Background

The chromosome 6q duplication syndrome is a known chromosome abnormality associated with characteristic phenotypic features such as severe intellectual disability (ID), short stature, feeding difficulties, microcephaly, dysmorphic features (prominent forehead, downslanting palpebral fissures, flat nasal bridge, tented upper lip, micrognathia, short webbed neck) and joint contractures [1–5]. Most reported patients carry unbalanced translocations leading to a partial trisomy 6q and a partial monosomy of another chromosome. In these cases the monosomic region of another chromosome is also of great influence on the patient's phenotype. There are only several cases of pure partial 6q trisomy and the severity of the phenotype seems to depend on the breakpoint position. In general, terminal duplications with co-existing monosomy of another chromosome region cause severe phenotypes whereas patients with pure

* Correspondence: m.srebniak@erasmusmc.nl
[1]Department of Clinical Genetics, Erasmus MC, Ee2475, Wytemaweg 80, 3015 CN Rotterdam, The Netherlands
Full list of author information is available at the end of the article

interstitial duplications seem to be only mildly affected [6–8]. Unfortunately the breakpoints of the majority of published cases were assessed with karyotyping or FISH, which hampers finding critical regions for ID and other features [9] so the genotype-phenotype studies in cases characterized by microarray are of great value [10].

We report on two families with an interstitial imbalance involving region 6q21q23: a familial duplication of 6q22.1q23.2 and one of 6q21q22.33. This is the first report where the gene content and breakpoints of a microscopically visible interstitial 6q duplication was characterized with microarray. In these families, some individuals carrying the imbalance did not show any structural anomalies or ID associated with trisomy 6q as described before, suggesting incomplete penetrance.

## Case presentation

### Family 1

A 23 year-old pregnant woman was referred to the department of Clinical Genetics due to isolated ID and a familial interstitial duplication on chromosome 6 characterized by karyotyping in the past. This duplication was discovered in 1983 in a family member that was known to suffer from ID, developmental delay (DD) and seizures. The observed ID in this family varied from very mild (low degrees and learning problems) to more severe (accompanied by DD and seizures).

The partner of the pregnant patient was known to have ID as well. He was an adopted child. His biological brother was said to have ID as well. Neither further family history, nor parental samples were available. Because of the pregnancy, our patient and her partner were investigated with genomic SNP array (Illumina HumanCytoSNP-12) to study their chromosomal constitution.

The pregnant patient carried an interstitial ~16.1 Mb 6q duplication and the array testing additionally revealed a susceptibility locus (SL) for neurodevelopmental disorders: a ~580 kb 16p11.2 microduplication (arr[hg19] 6q22.1q23.2(116,411,005-132,541,408)x3,16 p11.2(29,595,483-30,174,926)x3). The partner of the pregnant patient was shown to carry another SL for neurodevelopmental disorders, a ~806 kb 16p11.2 microdeletion (arr[hg19] 16p11.2(28,475,873-29,282,147)x1).

Because both partners had abnormal array results, prenatal diagnosis was advised. Amniocentesis was performed at 15 5/7 weeks of gestation and diagnostic array testing on uncultured amniotic fluid cells showed only the interstitial 6q duplication (Fig. 1). In order to enable clinical interpretation of this result, 4 other family members of the pregnant woman, two healthy and two affected (one mild and the other severe (the one that was karyotyped in 1983, see above)), were tested with SNP array. Two healthy relatives turned out to carry only the 6q duplication, whereas the two affected relatives carried both the 6q duplication and the 16p11.2 microduplication.

As the fetus inherited only the 6q duplication, in the absence of SL, the prognosis of the fetal phenotype may be favorable. The second trimester fetal ultrasound investigations showed no structural anomalies. A healthy baby boy without any dysmorphic features was born and there were no developmental abnormalities noted so far (follow up at the age of 1 year).

### Family 2

A 34 year-old pregnant woman was referred to a clinical geneticist after suspicion of fetal esophageal atresia at third trimester ultrasound investigations, based on polyhydramnios and lack of visualization of the stomach. This was the first pregnancy of non-consanguineous parents. Fetal karyotype (amniotic fluid) revealed an interstitial duplication on chromosome 6. SNP-array (Affymetrix CytoScan HD) was performed, showing a 15.3 Mb duplication (arr[hg19]6q21q22.33(113,465,762-128,774,807)x3) (Fig. 2). Given the combination of the duplication along with fetal structural abnormalities, the parents opted for termination of pregnancy at 33 weeks gestational age. The male fetus had normal biometry: weight 2593 g, height 49 cm, occipitofrontal circumference (OFC) 29 cm. Dysmorphic facial features were noted: short nose with anteverted nares and long eyelashes. Fetal autopsy confirmed the esophageal atresia and revealed additional structural abnormalities: an abnormal pulmonary lobulation (2 lobes on right lung and 1 lobe on left lung), a Meckel's diverticulum, bilateral hydronephrosis, pancreatic ectopia, and neuronal heterotopia of the cerebellum located on the dentate nuclei.

Familial studies revealed that the mother was carrier of the same interstitial duplication on chromosome 6 (karyotyping and Oligo aCGH Agilent 60 K), while her parents had normal karyotypes. No additional copy number variation was found in both the mother and the fetus. The mother had previously experienced learning difficulties, dyslexia and was known with a scoliosis. Cardiac ultrasound showed no abnormalities. No cerebral or abdominal imaging was performed. She works as a nurse assistant in a hospital.

## Discussion

In many laboratories over the world, genomic array testing is now a first-tier cytogenetic test. The interpretation of array results is mainly based on comparisons to CNVs in control and patient populations [11]. Comparison to previously reported cases with microscopically visible chromosome anomalies, however, is problematic. The breakpoints of the majority of published cases were assessed with karyotyping or FISH, which hampers the genotype-phenotype correlation studies as these breakpoints often are not

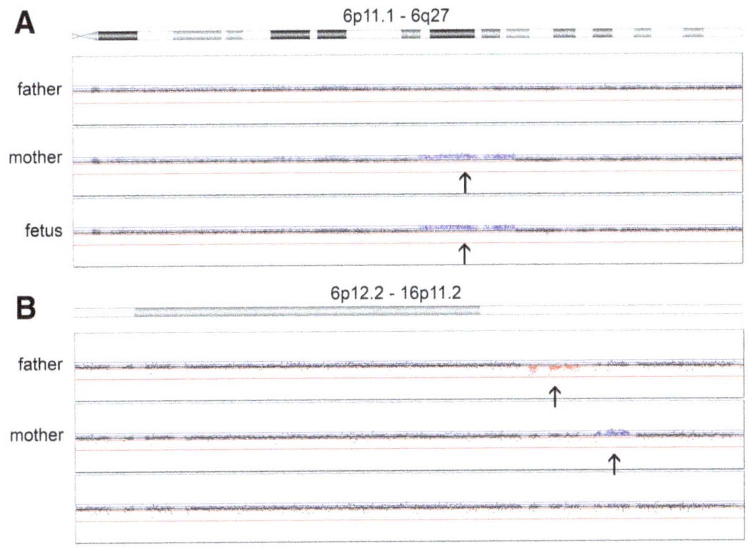


**Fig. 1** Family 1: Log Ratio plots of Illumina CytoSNP-12: **a** – partial chromosome 6q plot showing the 6q duplication in family 1: the mother and the fetus carry a 6q22q23 duplication. The arrows indicate the duplicated region. **b** - partial chromosome 16p plot showing the imbalances in 16p11: the father carries 16p11 microdeletion, the mother 16p11 microduplication, whereas the fetal array profile is normal for both 16p regions. The arrows indicate the imbalances in parental samples

accurate enough to compare them with array results [9]. In the karyotyping era a *de novo* unbalanced euchromatic chromosome aberration used to be almost always interpreted as pathogenic, however rare inherited variants were assumed to be benign and interpreted as unbalanced euchromatic abnormalities without phenotypic consequences (if inherited from a normal parent) [12–17]. At that time susceptibility CNVs (variants of variable expressivity and phenotypic heterogeneity) [18, 19], which expression seems to depend on other (genetic and/or environmental) factors, were less commonly known.

#### Phenotypes of 6q21q23 duplication carriers

The literature searched showed only 12 cases of interstitial duplications in chromosome region 6q21-6q23 (Table 1, Fig. 3) [7, 20–26]. The phenotype show variability and as shown in Fig. 3 not all duplication cases overlap with the families presented here. Congenital malformations seem to be infrequent, with only few patients reported to have variable cardiac anomalies (right ventricular hypertrophy, cardiomegaly, ventricular septal defect, pulmonary stenosis) [24, 25], and one suspicion of a corpus callosum agenesis [24]. The 6q duplications in the current families seem to overlap with the ISCA

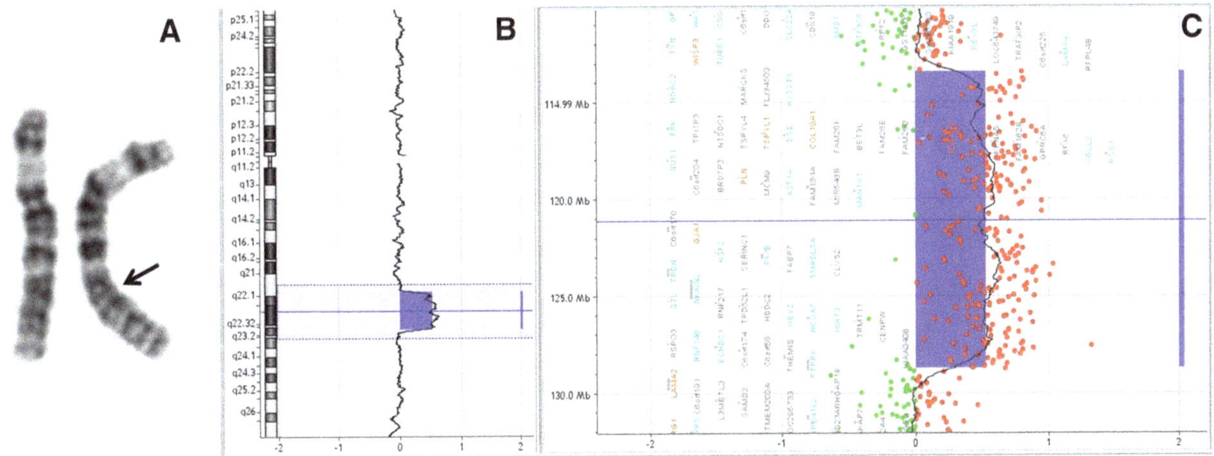


**Fig. 2** Family 2: **a** -Karyotype in standard resolution for chromosome 6, showing the interstitial duplication (arrow). **b** -array results (Oligo aCGH Agilent 60 K) for chromosome 6 in family 2 showing duplication of 6q present in family 2. **c**- The duplicated region and its gene content

**Table 1** Cases of interstitial duplications in chromosome region 6q21-6q23

| | Cytogenetic results | Molecular testing | Minimal duplication region according to molecular tests | Molecular breakpoints[a] in GRCh37/hg19 | Phenotype of the proband |
|---|---|---|---|---|---|
| Temple et al. 1996 | 46,XX, der(2) ins(2;6) (2pter-2p22.2::6q?22.32-?6q?23.1::2p22.2–2qter)pat[b] | Markers analysis | dup(6)(q23.3q24.1) (between markers D6S292 and D6S308) | chr6: 136315214-141256931 | small at birth, neonatal diabetes, microcephaly, myoclonic seizures, no DD (the insertion is resulting in partial trisomy: dup(6)(6q22.33–q23.3)) |
| Arthur et al. 1997 | 46,XX, inv dup(6)(q22q23)pat | Markers analysis | invdup(6) (q23.2q24.1) (between markers D6S270 and D6S310 | chr6: 134654821- 142102601 | transient neonatal diabetes mellitus, minor dysmorphic features |
| Henegariu et al.1997 | 46,XX,dir dup(6) (q23.3q25.3)[c] | FISH with painting probe for chr6 | ukn | ukn | dolichocephaly, dyspmorphic features, long fingers, bilateral single palmar creases, contractures at the wrists, long fingers, dorsiflexion of the first toes, mild syndactyly of toes 2–3, bradycardia, mild tricuspid insufficiency, a small patent ductus arteriosus, and small atrial septal defect, moderate cardiomegaly, short neck but not webbed, umbilical hernia, and mild generalized hypertonia |
| Pratt et al. 1998 (2 cases) | Case 1: 46,XY,dup(6) (q21q23.3)dn<br>Case 2: 46,XX,dup(6) (q21.15q23.3)dn | FISH with painting probe for chr6 | ukn | ukn | Case 1: dysmorphic features, bilateral clubfoot, ulnar deviation of hands, decreased muscle tone, decreased subcutaneous fat, brain anomalies, a thickened tricuspid valve, bilateral transverse palmar creases, ulnar deviation of the hands, club feet, and small hands and feet<br>Case 2: DD/ID (IQ 63), attention deficit disorder with hyperactivity, and coördination difficulties. Dysmorphic features, ventricular septal defect and pulmonic valvular stenosis, clinodactyly of the 5th finger, and thickened nails of the 5th toes, increased reflexes and ankle clonus. |
| Zneimer et al. 1998 | 46,XX,dup(6)(q21q23)dn | FISH with painting probe for chr6 | ukn<br>Possibly dup(6)(q22q24) ivm neonatal diabetes mellitus[d] | ukn | born with umbilical hernia and transient insulin dependent diabetes until 7 months, delayed development and speech (receives speech therapy), dysmorphic features, cardiomegaly of unknown etiology |
| Goh et al. 2000 | der(7)ins(7;6)(q21.11;q22.1q23.3)mat resulting in partial trisomy of 6q22.1q23.3 | N.D. | ukn | ukn | Case 1: obesity, brachycephaly, dysmorphic features, bilateral clinodactyly, DD, ID with IQ of 50.8, obstructive sleep apnoea<br>Case 2: (older sister of case 1) brachycephaly, dysmorphic features, bilateral clinodactyly, mild DD, no formal IQ test, but left school without academic credits. |
| Causio et al. 2001 | 46, XY, dup(6)(q23q23)dn | FISH with YAC probes | dup(6)(q23.2q24.1) according to minimal duplication breakpoints using YAC probes (970A12-949D3) | chr6: 132138813-142077202 | plagiocephaly, DD, ID, hiatus hernia (corrected surgically), acrocephaly, dysmorphic features, short hands with clinodactyly of fifth finger, joint contractures. Nuclear cataract in OD and rotating nystagmus in OO, bicuspid aortic valve with moderate failure, psychotic behavior and neurological tics. |
| Pazooki et al. 2007 (mother and child) | 46,XXdup(6)(q21q22.1)mat | FISH with BAC probes | dup(6)(q21q22.1) according to minimal breakpoints using BAC probes (RP11-428 F8 and RP1-64I15) | chr6: 111498415- 116048892 | Child: DD, stridor, nutritional problems, obesity, intention tremor, dysmorphic features (anteverted nares, depressed nasal bridge, hypertelorism, short fingers). |

**Table 1** Cases of interstitial duplications in chromosome region 6q21-6q23 *(Continued)*

| | | | | | |
|---|---|---|---|---|---|
| | | | | | Mother: cognitive difficulties, obesity, intermittent tremor. |
| ISCA nssv 1495729 | arr[hg19] 6q22.1q22.32(117,928,310-127,021,125)x3dn | Oligo aCGH | dup(6) (q22.1q22.32) | chr6: 117928310-127021125 | DD and/or other significant developmental or morphological phenotypes |
| Current family 1 | arr[hg19] 6q22.1q23.2(116,411,005-132,541,408)x3mat | Illumina Human CytoSNP-12 | dup(6)(q22.1q23.2) | chr6: 116411005-132541408 | -normal phenotype in 6q duplication carriers, -variable phenotype (from learning problem to developmental delay and intellectual disability) in carriers of both 6q duplication and 16p11.2 microduplication. |
| Current family 2 | arr[hg19] 6q21q22.33(113,464,340-128,801,386)x3mat | Affymetrix SNP CytoScan HD | dup(6)(q21q22.33) | chr6: 113464340-128801386 | Fetus: dysmorphic features (anteverted nares, short nose, long eyelashes), esophageal atresia, pulmonary lobulation anomaly, meckel diverticulum, bilateral hydronephrosis, pancreatic ectopia, neuronal heterotopia of the cerebellum (dentate nucleus). Termination of pregnancy at 33WG. |
| | arr[hg19] 6q21q22.33(113,465,762-128,774,807)x3dn | Oligo aCGH Agilent 60 K | dup(6)(q21q22.33) | chr6: 113465762-128774807 | Mother: learning difficulties, dyslexia, scoliosis. |

*N.D.* not done, *dn* de novo, *mat* maternal, *pat* paternal, *DD* developmental delay, *ID* intellectual disability, *ukn* unknown

[a]The molecular breakpoint were either given by the authors or translated from molecular markers/FISH probes and show minimal region of imbalance

[b] Father and grandfather had duplicated 6q, but no abnormal features or neonatal diabetes

[c] Not maternal, father not tested, if including band 6q24 probably *de novo* on maternal chromosome as neonatal diabetes mellitus was not stated

[d] The work of Docherty and colleagues proved that neonatal diabetes mellitus is associated with 6q24 (Docherty, Poole et al. 2010), it may be assumed that the actual duplicated region does not contain bands q21q23, but more distal region on the long arm of chromosome 6 including 6q22q24

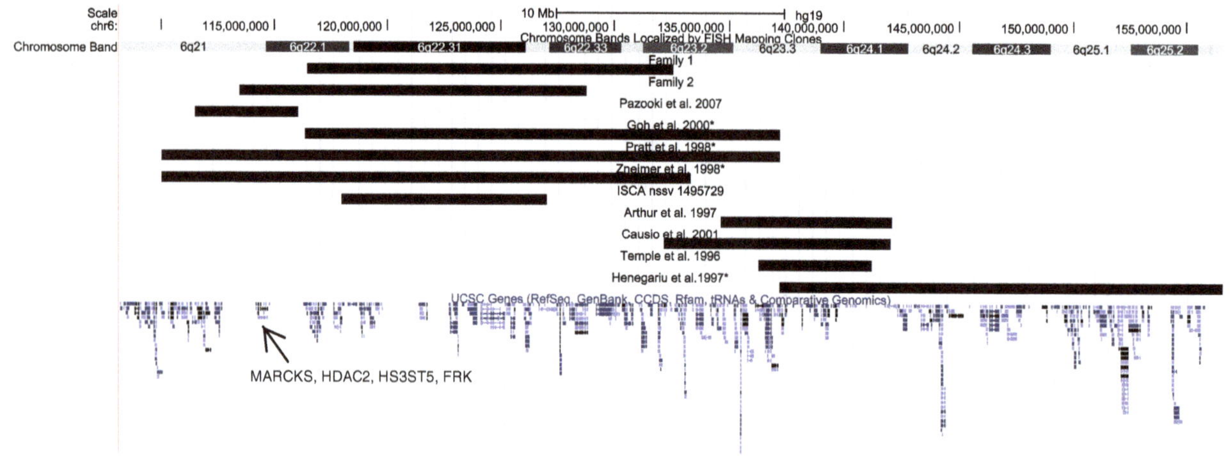


**Fig. 3** Breakpoints comparison (in GRCh37/hg19) in cases with dup 6q21q23 where molecular testing was done (minimal breakpoints based on FISH/YAC or DNA markers or given by the authors of original papers, if appropriate lifted from other genome builds)

case and patients published by Goh et al., Pratt et al. and Zneimer et al. [20, 24, 25], although the breakpoints based on karyotyping could be highly imprecise. All these patients presented with DD/mild ID and have common craniofacial features with constant hypertelorism and frequent mid-face hypoplasia with anteverted nares [20, 24, 25]. Further, the two cases reported by Pazooki et al. that only partially overlap with the duplication in family 2 also presented DD and similar dysmorphic features (hypertelorism and anteverted nares), but no congenital malformation.

### Possible candidate genes for DD/ID in 6q21q23

Although the duplicated regions are large, we conducted a gene content study to search for candidate genes that may explain the ID/learning problems in presented families. Gene lists were generated using Nexus BioDiscovery Copy Number 7.5 and the data were uploaded and analyzed with QIAGEN's Ingenuity® Pathway Analysis (IPA®, QIAGEN Redwood City, www.ingenuity.com). A list of genes and proteins related to ID was generated using the Knowledge Base of IPA. In case of the 6q duplication in family 1, we did not find any candidate gene that may explain the ID when duplicated, which may support our hypothesis that the 6q duplication seems to be benign if present alone. However, the proximal region that was duplicated in family 2, but not in family 1 seems to have an interesting gene content. It contains four OMIM genes: *MARCKS, HDAC2, HS3ST5* and *FRK*, all involved in brain function and development [27–30]. Interestingly it was shown that *MARCKS* expression is significantly elevated (45 %) in the hippocampus of mice, which exhibit impaired hippocampus-dependent learning [27] and neuron-specific over-expression of *HDAC2* decreased dendritic spine density, synapse number, synaptic plasticity and memory formation [31]. Since all four genes are involved in neural development, one could speculate that if their expression is dosage dependent, their duplication may play a role in neurological phenotypes like ID, DD and brain malformations. To our knowledge, so far, there are no cases of whole gene duplications in *MARCKS, HDAC2* and *HS3ST5* in control populations (neither in Decipher Population CNVs, Toronto Database of Genomic Variants, nor our in house controls), and there is only one family published by Pazooki et al. carrying a smaller duplication, but overlapping also with *MARCKS, HDAC2, HS3ST5* (Fig. 3) [26]. Unfortunately these data are not enough evidence to claim that duplication of *MARCKS, HDAC2, HS3ST5* causes learning problems or ID/DD. The duplication of these genes remains a variation of unknown clinical significance, however it cannot be excluded that it may contribute to learning problems when also other genes involved in neurological phenotypes are deregulated.

### The second hit hypothesis

The variability in phenotypes in patients shown in Table 1 could be explained by different chromosome breakpoints, however the duplications in the current families show variability within a family as well. This cannot be explained by different gene content, but it may be a consequence of the presence of additional anomalies in affected individuals.

The two-hit model has been introduced to explain the phenotypic variability in genetic disorders [18, 19]. The presence of the additional hit may modify phenotype, either acting in an additive manner (independently adding new features), or by participation in the same or similar biochemical pathway causing more severe phenotypes [32]. And indeed in family 1, the 6q22.1q23.2 duplication seems to be an euchromatic variant without phenotypic consequences, as only the individuals carrying the 6q duplication and the additional susceptibility CNV showed abnormal phenotypes. Family 1 shows very high penetrance of the susceptibility locus, when both chromosome aberrations are present. Although this observation can be reassuring for the fetus, we found prediction of the fetal prognosis still problematic since the father of the fetus carried a susceptibility locus for neurodevelopmental disorder, but the paternal "additional hit" remained unknown. The fetus did not inherit the paternal SL, nevertheless the paternal "additional hit" may have been inherited and may influence the intellectual development of the child.

In family 2, the interstitial 6q duplication seems to show highly variable expression in the mother and fetus. The fetus had dysmorphic features similar to reported cases in the literature and multiple congenital malformations that were not described before. The breakpoints and gene content were identical in the mother, who only had learning difficulties in childhood. There are no healthy carriers of this duplication in this family and the *de novo* occurrence of this chromosomal duplication in the mother of the fetus may be an argument for its causality for the phenotype. The "second hit" has not been identified by microarray in this family and remains unresolved. Genetic counseling for a future pregnancy remains problematic: it is doubtful whether it is reasonable to offer an invasive prenatal test, if the "additional hit" is still unknown and if no fetal ultrasound abnormalities are present. Given these limitations, the couple has opted for preimplantation diagnosis.

## Conclusions

Finding a rare euchromatic variant or a susceptibility locus is challenging in both postnatal and prenatal settings. Our study shows that the 6q22.1q23.2 duplication may represent a private variant that is benign when present alone, but that may act as the "additional/second hit" in SL carriers. We suggest that also large benign CNVs can serve as "an additional hit" and therefore our study supports the opinion of Thomas Liehr that benign variants cannot be fully neglected in genetic analysis [17]. The presented family 1 supports "the multi-hit hypothesis" showing that the penetrance of such a SL in families known to carry an "additional hit" can be much higher than predicted [33], which may explain the conflicting conclusions on the association with an abnormal phenotype in the papers on SL [34–36]. Finding the "additional hit" within the family is therefore very important for genetic counseling and the assessment of the SL penetrance within the particular family.

### Abbreviations

CNV, copy number variation; DD, developmental delay; FISH, fluorescent in situ hybridization; ID, intellectual disability; OFC, occipitofrontal circumference; SL, susceptibility locus

### Acknowledgements

We kindly thank the families for their participation in this study.

### Funding

There was no funding available for this study.

### Authors' contributions

MIS conceived the study, made substantial contributions to conception and design, analysis and interpretation of genomic data. LvZ made substantial contributions to acquisition of data, analysis and interpretation of genomic data and participated in the drafting of the manuscript. FP participated in the drafting of the manuscript and coordinated the genetic counseling of the patients. SB and IJPvH made substantial contributions to acquisition of data and carried out analysis and interpretation of data. MK and JC performed pre-test counseling, invasive testing, perinatal management and contributed to the acquisition of phenotypic data (prenatal ultrasound scans). DVO and AK carried literature search and interpretation of data. AK carried out the analysis with IPA. MIS, LvZ, SB, FP and KEMD were responsible for the final diagnoses and reports. KEMD coordinated the genetic counseling of the patients and together with MIS supervised the study. All authors revised the manuscript critically for important intellectual content, approved the final version and agreed to be accountable for all aspects of the work in ensuring that questions related to the accuracy or integrity of any part of the work are appropriately investigated and resolved.

### Competing interests

The authors declare that they have no competing interests.

### Author details

[1]Department of Clinical Genetics, Erasmus MC, Ee2475, Wytemaweg 80, 3015 CN Rotterdam, The Netherlands. [2]Department of Clinical Genetics, University Hospital, Lille, France. [3]Department of Cytogenetics, University Hospital, Lille, France. [4]Department of Obstetrics and Gynecology, subdivision Obstetrics and Prenatal Medicine, Erasmus MC, Rotterdam, The Netherlands. [5]Stichting Prenatale Screening Zuidwest Nederland, Wytemaweg 80, Na-1509, 3015GE Na-1503 Rotterdam, The Netherlands. [6]Department of Bioinformatics Erasmus MC, Rotterdam, The Netherlands.

### References

1. Dallapiccola B, Bricarelli FD, Quartino AR, Mazzilli MC, Chisci R, Gandini E. Delineation of syndromes due to partial 6q imbalances. Trisomy 6q21 leads to qter and monosomy 6q221 leads to qter in two unrelated patients. Acta Genet Med Gemellol (Roma). 1978;27:57–66.
2. Tipton RE, Berns JS, Johnson WE, Wilroy Jr RS, Summitt RL. Duplication 6q syndrome. Am J Med Genet. 1979;3(4):325–30.
3. Turleau C, de Grouchy J. Trisomy 6qter. Clin Genet. 1981;19(3):202–6.
4. Pivnick EK, Qumsiyeh MB, Tharapel AT, Summitt JB, Wilroy RS. Partial duplication of the long arm of chromosome 6: a clinically recognisable syndrome. J Med Genet. 1990;27(8):523–6.
5. Uhrich S, FitzSimmons J, Easterling TR, Mack L, Disteche CM. Duplication (6q) syndrome diagnosed in utero. Am J Med Genet. 1991;41(3):282–3.
6. Cappon SL, Duncan AM, Khalifa MM. Interstitial 6q duplication in an adult male without growth delay or severe mental retardation. Med Sci Monit. 2000;6(3):581–5.
7. Henegariu O, Heerema NA, Vance GH. Mild "duplication 6q syndrome": a case with partial trisomy (6)(q23.3q25.3). Am J Med Genet. 1997;68(4):450–4.
8. Zweier C, Trautmann U, Ekici A, Rauch A. A 15 Mb duplication of 6q24.1-q25.3 associated with typical but milder features of the duplication 6q syndrome. Eur J Med Genet. 2008;51(4):358–61.
9. Tabet AC, Aboura A, Gerard M, Pilorge M, Dupont C, Gadisseux JF, et al. Molecular characterization of a de novo 6q24.2q25.3 duplication interrupting UTRN in a patient with arthrogryposis. Am J Med Genet A. 2010;152A(7):1781–8.

10. Sheth F, Trivedi S, Andrieux J, Blouin JL, Sheth J. Pure interstitial dup(6)(q22.31q22.31) - a case report. Ital J Pediatr. 2015;41:5.
11. Carreira IM, Ferreira SI, Matoso E, Pires LM, Ferrao J, Jardim A, et al. Copy number variants prioritization after array-CGH analysis - a cohort of 1000 patients. Mol Cytogenet. 2015;8:103.
12. Kowalczyk M, Srebniak M, Tomaszewska A. Chromosome abnormalities without phenotypic consequences. J Appl Genet. 2007;48(2):157–66.
13. Barber JC. Directly transmitted unbalanced chromosome abnormalities and euchromatic variants. J Med Genet. 2005;42(8):609–29.
14. Barber JC, Joyce CA, Collinson MN, Nicholson JC, Willatt LR, Dyson HM, et al. Duplication of 8p23.1: a cytogenetic anomaly with no established clinical significance. J Med Genet. 1998;35(6):491–6.
15. Barber JC, Mahl H, Portch J, Crawfurd MD. Interstitial deletions without phenotypic effect: prenatal diagnosis of a new family and brief review. Prenat Diagn. 1991;11(6):411–6.
16. Liehr T. Benign & Pathological Chromosomal Imbalances, 1st Edition Microscopic and Submicroscopic Copy Number Variations (CNVs) in Genetics and Counseling. Academic Press; 2013.
17. Liehr T. Cytogenetically visible copy number variations (CG-CNVs) in banding and molecular cytogenetics of human; about heteromorphisms and euchromatic variants. Mol Cytogenet. 2016;9:5.
18. Girirajan S, Rosenfeld JA, Cooper GM, Antonacci F, Siswara P, Itsara A, et al. A recurrent 16p12.1 microdeletion supports a two-hit model for severe developmental delay. Nat Genet. 2010;42(3):203–9.
19. Veltman JA, Brunner HG. Understanding variable expressivity in microdeletion syndromes. Nat Genet. 2010;42(3):192–3.
20. Goh DL, Tan AS, Chen JY, Van Den Berghe JA. Dysmorphic sibs trisomic for the region 6q22.1– > 6q23.3. J Med Genet. 2000;37(11):889–92.
21. Arthur EI, Zlotogora J, Lerer I, Dagan J, Marks K, Abeliovich D. Transient neonatal diabetes mellitus in a child with invdup(6)(q22q23) of paternal origin. Eur J Hum Genet. 1997;5(6):417–9.
22. Causio F, Fischetto R, Carnevale F, Pansini A, Rocchi M. Trisomy 6q syndrome: a case with a < < de novo > > 6q23 tandem duplication. Genet Couns. 2001;12(2):145–50.
23. Temple IK, Gardner RJ, Robinson DO, Kibirige MS, Ferguson AW, Baum JD, et al. Further evidence for an imprinted gene for neonatal diabetes localised to chromosome 6q22-q23. Hum Mol Genet. 1996;5(8):1117–21.
24. Pratt VM, Roberson JR, Weiss L, Van Dyke DL. Duplication 6q21q23 in two unrelated patients. Am J Med Genet. 1998;80(2):112–4.
25. Zneimer SM, Ziel B, Bachman R. Partial trisomy of chromosome 6q: an interstitial duplication of the long arm. Am J Med Genet. 1998;80(2):133–5.
26. Pazooki M, Lebbar A, Roubergues A, Baverel F, Letessier D, Dupont JM. Pure familial 6q21q22.1 duplication in two generations. Eur J Med Genet. 2007;50(1):60–5.
27. McNamara RK, Hussain RJ, Simon EJ, Stumpo DJ, Blackshear PJ, Abel T, et al. Effect of myristoylated alanine-rich C kinase substrate (MARCKS) overexpression on hippocampus-dependent learning and hippocampal synaptic plasticity in MARCKS transgenic mice. Hippocampus. 2005;15(5):675–83.
28. Jawerka M, Colak D, Dimou L, Spiller C, Lagger S, Montgomery RL, et al. The specific role of histone deacetylase 2 in adult neurogenesis. Neuron Glia Biol. 2010;6(2):93–107.
29. Mochizuki H, Yoshida K, Gotoh M, Sugioka S, Kikuchi N, Kwon YD, et al. Characterization of a heparan sulfate 3-O-sulfotransferase-5, an enzyme synthesizing a tetrasulfated disaccharide. J Biol Chem. 2003;278(29):26780–7.
30. Chandrasekharan S, Qiu TH, Alkharouf N, Brantley K, Mitchell JB, Liu ET. Characterization of mice deficient in the Src family nonreceptor tyrosine kinase Frk/rak. Mol Cell Biol. 2002;22(14):5235–47.
31. Guan JS, Haggarty SJ, Giacometti E, Dannenberg JH, Joseph N, Gao J, et al. HDAC2 negatively regulates memory formation and synaptic plasticity. Nature. 2009;459(7243):55–60.
32. Kumar RA. Two-hit wonder: a novel genetic model to explain variable expressivity in severe pediatric phenotypes. Clin Genet. 2010;78(6):517–9.
33. Rosenfeld JA, Coe BP, Eichler EE, Cuckle H, Shaffer LG. Estimates of penetrance for recurrent pathogenic copy-number variations. Genet Med. 2013;15(6):478–81.
34. Stefansson H, Meyer-Lindenberg A, Steinberg S, Magnusdottir B, Morgen K, Arnarsdottir S, et al. CNVs conferring risk of autism or schizophrenia affect cognition in controls. Nature. 2014;505(7483):361–6.
35. Hashemi B, Bassett A, Chitayat D, Chong K, Feldman M, Flanagan J, et al. Deletion of 15q11.2(BP1-BP2) region: Further evidence for lack of phenotypic specificity in a pediatric population. Am J Med Genet A. 2015;167A(9):2098–102.
36. Vanlerberghe C, Petit F, Malan V, Vincent-Delorme C, Bouquillon S, Boute O, et al. 15q11.2 microdeletion (BP1-BP2) and developmental delay, behaviour issues, epilepsy and congenital heart disease: a series of 52 patients. Eur J Med Genet. 2015;58(3):140–7.

2

# A maternally inherited 8.05 Mb Xq21 deletion associated with Choroideremia, deafness, and mental retardation syndrome in a male patient

Siying Liang[1†], Nan Jiang[1†], Shuo Li[1†], Xiaohu Jiang[2] and Dongyi Yu[1*]

**Abstract**

**Background:** Deletions in Xq21 cause various congenital defects in males including choroideremia, deafness and mental retardation, depending on their size and gene content. Until now only a limited number of patients with Xq21 deletions has been reported.

**Case presentation:** Here we describe a 17-year-old male with choroideremia, deafness, and mental retardation syndrome. Using SNP arrays, an 8.05 Mb deletion in Xq21 was identified inherited from the apparently healthy mother. The deleted region harbors 12 OMIM genes, of which *POU3F4, CHM,* and *ZNF711* might have contributed to the patient's phenotype including hearing loss, poor vision, and intellectual disability. Moreover, the patient's mother exhibits a normal phenotype while carrying the same deletion, which is often observed in previous studies on female carriers in families with this syndrome.

**Conclusions:** Our study confirms the causative effect between the Xq21 deletion in males and choroideremia, deafness and mental retardation.

**Keywords:** Xq21, Choroideremia, Deafness, Mental retardation, SNP arrays

## Background

X-chromosome deletions can result in serious congenital defects. Males seldom exhibit these defects, as deletions on the X chromosome are essentially lethal in male embryos discarded at an early embryonic stage. Even though high-resolution SNP array analysis has been performed to identify small deletions on the X chromosome, the clinical significance of Xq21 deletions in males is still poorly understood. It has been shown that a contiguous gene Xq21 deletion, including *POU3F4, CHM* and *ZNF711* genes, could result in choroideremia, deafness, and mental retardation syndrome. This deletion produces degeneration of the choriocapillaris, the retinal pigment epithelium, and the photoreceptor of the eye, as well as inner ear abnormality with progressive mixed hearing loss and intellectual disability. In the last decades, only six cases with Xq21 deletions have been reported [1–3]. Despite the severe symptoms exhibited by male probands, most female carriers are non-symptomatic or express only a mild phenotype [2].

Here we describe the case of a 17-year-old male with mental retardation, choroideremia, hearing impairment, cochlear deformity, and facial anomalies. Analysis by SNP array, identified an 8.05 Mb contiguous gene deletion in Xq21 harboring *POU3F4, CYLC1, RPS6KA6, HDX, APOOL, SATL1, ZNF711, POF1B, CHM, DACH2, KLHL4,* and *CPXCR1* genes. The same deletion was identified in the apparently healthy mother. Our data contribute to further understanding the correlation between Xq21 deletions and the abnormal phenotypes. Furthermore, we present all the Xq21 deletion cases previously described in order to review the matter of genotype-phenotype correlations.

* Correspondence: yudongyi0532@163.com
†Equal contributors
[1]Genetic Testing Center, Qingdao Women and Children's Hospital, Qingdao University, #217, Liaoyangxi Road, Qingdao 266034, China

## Case presentation

The patient was born by spontaneous delivery after an uneventful pregnancy (birth weight 3.350 kg and occipitofrontal circumference 35.5 cm) to phenotypically normal parents. He showed global development delay since infancy. He learned to speak at 18 months old and to walk at 2.5 years old. During childhood, he showed severe learning impairment and social disabilities. However, he was able to react to verbal words and to carry out brief communications. He has a narrow forehead, slightly drooping eyelids, short palpebral fissures, and prominent ears (Fig. 1). His IQ level is below 40, according to the Wechsler Intelligence Scale test, and his general cognitive ability is also low. His vision test result was out of the normal scale, indicating poor sight. His hearing test showed moderate hearing impairment with 60 dB of hearing loss. Ophthalmoscopy showed partial degeneration of the eye choroid (Fig. 2a). High resolution CT (HRCT) imaging showed that the base turn of the cochlea was shortened, the second turn and the apical turn were merged or unclearly divided, and the modiolus was absent, which evidently supported for the inner ear malformation (Fig. 2b). The patient's mother also underwent the tests described above. However, her results were normal and there was no evidence suggesting that she might exhibit choroideremia, or hearing impairment in the future.

## Methods

Peripheral blood samples of the patient and his mother were used for genomic DNA extraction. Briefly, genomic DNA was isolated from whole blood using DNA Blood Mini Kit (Qiagen, Germany). Chromosomal microarray analysis was performed using Cytoscan 750 K chip, (Affymetrix, USA) according to manufacturer's instructions. CMA was performed with CytoScan 750 K array (Affymetrix, Santa Clara, CA, USA) according to the manufacturer's recommendations. The platform is composed of 550,000 non-polymorphic CNV probes and more than 200,000 SNP probes with an average resolution of 100 kb. The data was analyzed using chromosome analysis software ChAS (Affymetrix, USA). Primers flanking the deleted fragment, *POU3F4*and *CPXCR1*, were designed using Primer 5.0 (Premier, Canada) and were used to validate the deletion by PCR and agarose electrophoresis. Data collection were performed via searching in DECIPHER database (https://decipher.sanger.ac.uk/) and ISCA (https://www.clinicalgenome.org/) in order to identify cases of patients carrying similar deletions [4].

## Results

SNP array analysis detected an 8.05 Mb deletion in the long arm of the X chromosome at Xq21.1-21.31 (Fig. 3) in both the patient and his mother. The genomic position of this deletion according to GRCh37/hg19 was Chr X: 80,817,978-88,868,979. The deleted region harbors 12 genes, including *POU3F4, CYLC1, RPS6KA6, HDX, APOOL, SATL1, ZNF711, POF1B, CHM, DACH2, KLHL4* and *CPXCR1*(Table 1). The PCR result confirmed the SNP array data.

## Discussion

Patients with choroideremia, deafness, and mental retardation were first described by Ayazi [1]. In a kindred (XL-45), two brothers and their maternal uncle exhibited this syndrome, while the females had only characteristic retinal changes. The second kindred (XL-62) was reported by Nussbaum [2], in which two matrilineal first cousins had choroideremia, mental retardation, deafness, and short stature. Nussbaum found that affected members from both kindreds, XL-45 and XL-62, carried similar size deletions in Xq21. Following fine mapping studies revealed that the deleted region contained putative loci for choroideremia, X-linked deafness-2 (DFNX2), and non-specific X-linked mental retardation. These loci are currently known as genes *CHM* and *POU3F4* [5]. Another case was reported by Song et al. [3], in which a 3-year-old boy showed deafness and mild mental retardation, while genetic analysis confirmed the presence of a 16 Mb Xq21 deletion. In this kindred (SV-08-20), the carrier mother had only mild high-tone hearing loss. To the best of our knowledge, so far, our patient is the seventh reported case with this syndrome. Although the genetic deletion and clinical phenotype are highly typical compared to the previous reports, there are still notable distinctions. For instance, in our case the patient's mother exhibits no

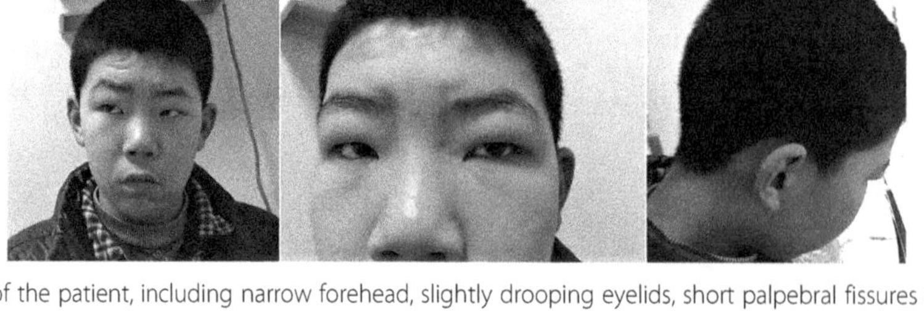

**Fig. 1** Facial dysmorphism of the patient, including narrow forehead, slightly drooping eyelids, short palpebral fissures and prominent ears

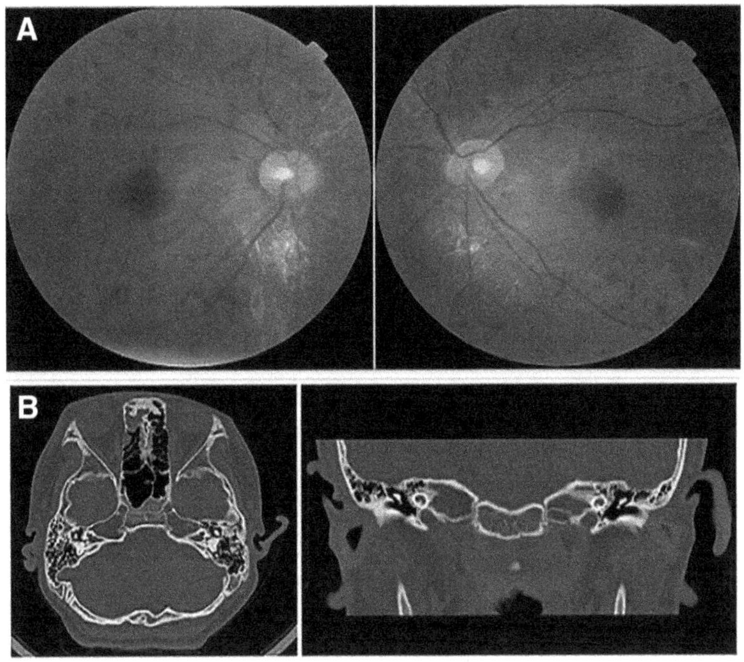


**Fig. 2** **a** Ophthalmoscopy photos of the patient showed the partial degeneration of the choroid in both eyes. **b** High-resolution CT imaging showed the cochlea deformity of the patient, including the short base turn of the cochlea, unclear division between the second turn and the apical turn of the cochlea and the absence of the modiolus

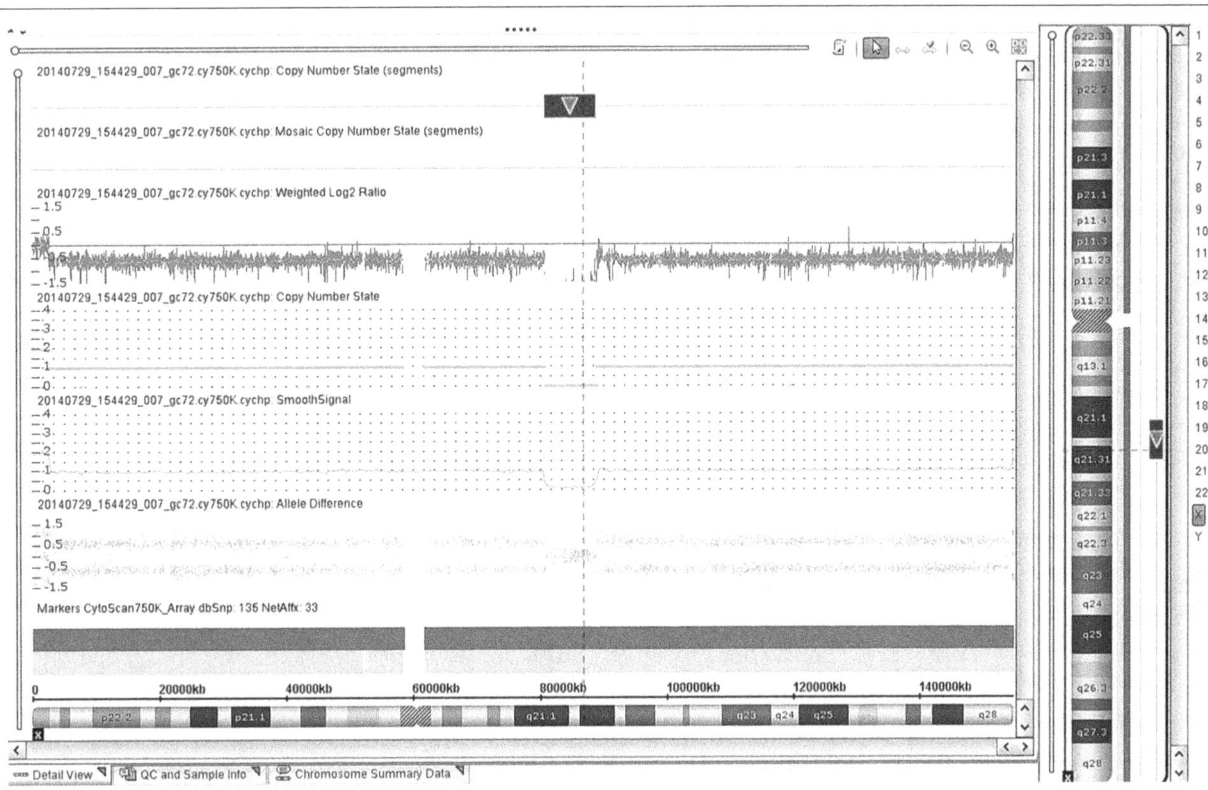


**Fig. 3** Detected by SNP arrays analysis, an 8.05 Mb deletion on the long arm of the X chromosome at Xq21 in the patient

**Table 1** OMIM genes included in the deletion, protein products and function and disease caused

| Gene | Protein | Protein function | Disease |
|---|---|---|---|
| POU3F4 | POU class 3 homeobox 4 | Inner ear development | Non-syndromic hearing loss |
| CYLC1 | Cylicin, basic protein of sperm head cytoskeleton 1 | Spermatid differentiation | None |
| RPS6KA6 | Ribosomal protein S6 kinase A6 | Activation of the mitogen-activated kinase cascade | None |
| HDX | Highly divergent homeobox | Unknown | None |
| APOOL | Apolipoprotein O like | Lipoprotein complexes circulation | None |
| SATL1 | Spermidine/spermine N1-acetyl transferase-like 1 | Unknown | None |
| ZNF711 | Zinc finger protein 711 | Similarity to protein that acts as a transcriptional activator | Mental retardation, X-linked type 97 |
| POF1B | Premature ovarian failure, 1B | Germ cell division | Premature ovarian failure |
| CHM | Rab escort protein 1 | Regulation of vesicular traffic | Choroideremia |
| DACH2 | Dachshund family transcription factor 2 | Regulation of organogenesis and myogenesis | None |
| KLHL4 | Kelch like family member 4 | Banding domain of actin | None |
| CPXCR1 | CPX chromosome region, candidate 1 | Contains a motif similar to motifs in zinc finger protein | None |

symptoms, which is consistent with most of the female carriers in XL-62 but not with those in XL-45. A detailed comparison of all the seven cases and female carriers is made in Table 2.

As deafness and choroideremia are commonly observed in all the recorded cases, *POU3F4* and *CHM* gene deletions are two basic indexes for diagnosis. *POU3F4* gene encodes POU-III class factor 4, a transcription factor that mediates epigenetic signals, which induce striatal neuron-precursor differentiation. By generating non-functional products, mutations in this gene often lead to DFNX2, which is characterized by conductive and sensorineural progressive hearing loss and pathognomonic temporal bone deformity, including dilatation of the inner auditory canal and fistulous connection between the internal dilatation auditory canal and the cochlear basal turn [6]. Accordingly, our patient showed inner ear deformity with short base turn of the cochlea, unclear division within the cochlea and the absence of the modiolus, which is a typical consequence of *POU3F4* deletion.

*CHM* gene defect is a confirmed cause of choroideremia, an X-linked disease leading to progressive vision loss. *CHM* encodes REP1, a subunit of geranylgeranyl transferase that affects the regulation of vesicular traffic. Deletions and point mutations in *CHM* generate a truncated product and result in degeneration of the choriocapillaris, retinal pigment epithelium, and eye photoreceptors [7]. Despite the strong pathogenicity in male patients, mutations in *CHM* do not have the same effect on female carriers. This might be a consequence of the non-random inactivation of the X chromosome, which has been validated by Carrel and Willard in their studies on *CHM*-inactivation escaping pattern [8].

Notably in previous reports, all male probands exhibited prominent phenotypes, including both choroideremia and

**Table 2** Detailed comparison of the phenotype, the deleted region and the genes included in the probands and female carriers in the reported kindreds

| Kindred | Phenotype of male patients | Phenotype of female carriers | Deleted region in Chr X | Refered OMIM genes | Reference |
|---|---|---|---|---|---|
| XL-45 | Choroideremia, mental retardation, deafness | Retinal changes of choroiderenia | Between DXS232 and DXS95 (fine mapping) DXS232 and DXS95 DXS232 and DXS95 | Not reported | Ayazi,1981 Nussbaum,1987 |
| XL-62 | Choroideremia, short stature, mental retardation, deafness | Mild high frequency sensorineural hearing loss (seen in only one out of four) | Between DXS72 and DXS214 (fine mapping) DXS232 and DXS95 DXS232 and DXS95 | Not reported | Nussbaum, 1987 |
| SV-08-20 | Severe bilateral hearing loss, central hypotonia, developmental delay, mild mental retardation, vesicoureteral reflux | Mild high-tone hearing loss | 16 Mb Xq21 (estimated by PCR) | *POU3F4, CHM* | Song, 2010 |
| Present case | Choroideremia, mental retardation, hearing impairments, cochlea deformity, facial anomalies | Normal | 8.05 Mb Xq21 Chr X: (80,817,978-88,868,979) | *CHM, POU3F4, ZNF711, POF1b* | - |

hearing impairment, while the female carriers of each kindred exhibited only one of the clinical characteristics and their symptoms were milder. In our case, the mother manifests no symptoms, similar to the female carriers in kindred XL-62. This diversity of female carrier's phenotypes shows that although a regressive inheritance pattern is clear, the exact influence of gene loss towards female carriers is still unpredictable.

*ZNF711* is a member of the zinc-finger gene family. It has been proved that the ZNF711 protein interacts, as a cofactor, with demethylase PHF8 in binding to target genes, thus suggesting a role for *ZNF711* in transcriptional modulation [9]. Although limited in clinical case reports, *ZNF711* gene loss is believed to be causative to non-specific X-linked mental retardation(MRX97). By exon sequencing of the X chromosome in 208 families with X-linked mental retardation, Tarpey et al. 2009. identified two truncating mutations of *ZNF711* in two families with MRX97 [10]. Clinical reports of sporadic cases also support this pathogenetic connection [11]. Recently in 11 male patients from two new found MRX97 families, Van der Welf et al. [12] identified a frameshift deletion and a missence mutation in *ZNF711* which both predict the deleterious effect and cause the disease. By expression analysis of cell culture, they also showed that these mutations induced differential expression of genes known to be expressed in the brain compared to controls, which adds evidence to *ZNF711* as a transcription factor. In our case, our patient exhibits severe intellectual disabilities and facial dysmorphism, which are coincided with the phenotype of MRX97. Considering of other pathogenetic genes (*POU3F4* and *CHM*) have no independent effect to mental retardation, *ZNF711* loss may have contributed majorly to the MRX97 phenotype of our patient.

We continued to search in the Decipher and ISCA databases for similar size deletions at Xq21.1 and identified 11 deletions with certain pathogenicity. Although most of them have concurrent phenotypes, none is exactly corresponds to the phenotypes of our patient. A notable fact is that deletions which does not contain *ZNF711* are

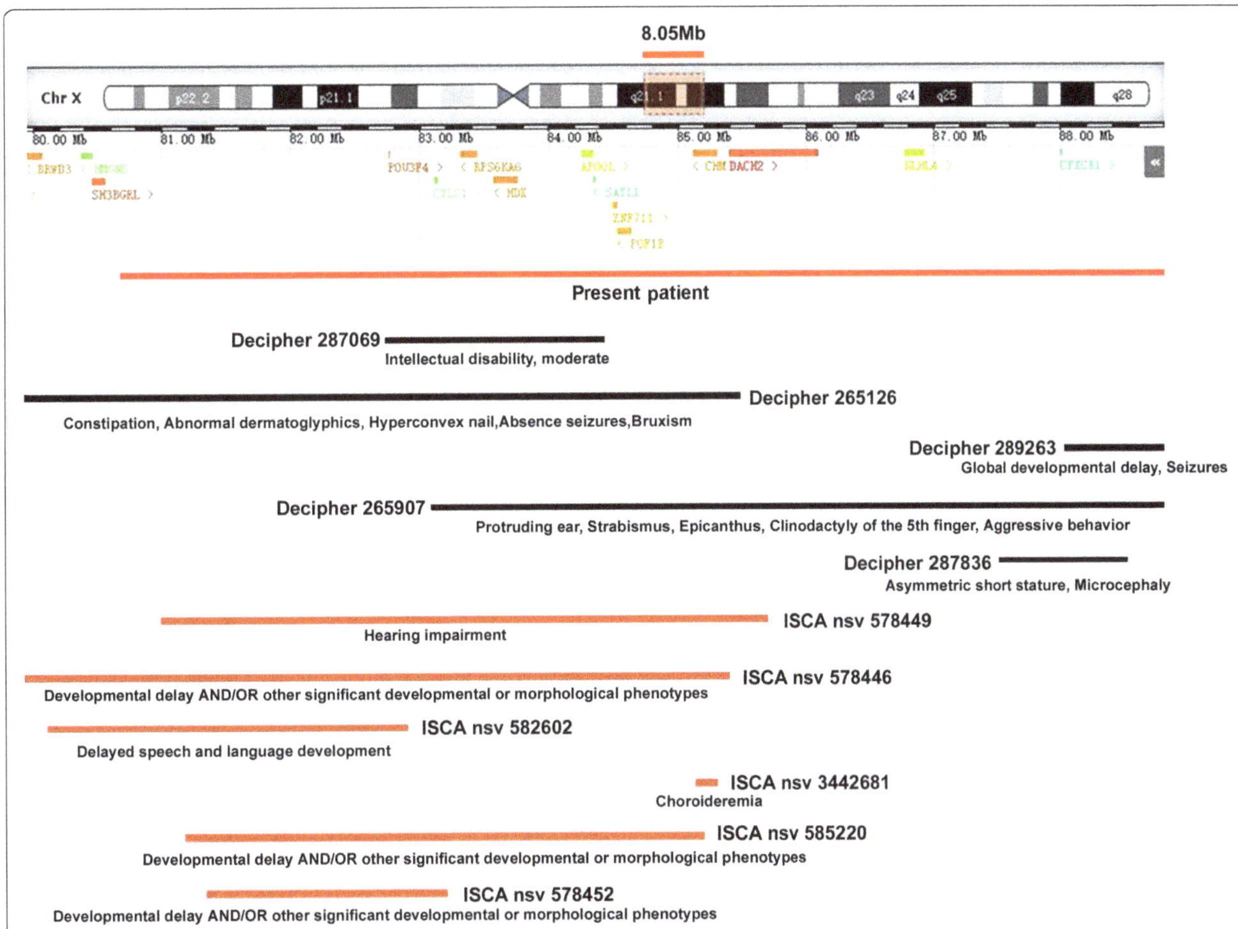


**Fig. 4** Xq21.1 deletion. The upper part of the figure illustrates the exact locations of the protein coding genes included in this region. The lower part of the figure schematically represents the Xq21.1 deleted region in our patient(in *red*) and other deletions reported in the Decipher(in *black*) and ISCA database(in *red*). The ID of each patient is reported. The clinical features of the patients are reported in parentheses below the corresponding deletion as described in Decipher (https://decipher.sanger.ac.uk/) and ISCA (https://www.clinicalgenome.org/)

often not associated with mental retardations (Decipher 289,263, 287,836, ISCA 582602, 3,442,681, and 578,452, Fig. 4) or only with moderate MD (Decipher 287,069, Fig. 4). This furtherly suggests that *ZNF711* gene loss might be an independent cause to mental retardation.

## Conclusion

In conclusion, our male patient carrying the 8.05 Mb Xq21 deletion exhibits a typical phenotype of choroideremia, deafness, and mental retardation syndrome, an association which has been demonstrated by previous cases. Meanwhile, as it is commonly observed in other female carriers, the mother of our patient, who carries the same deletion, is non-symptomatic. Additionally, comparing to previous reports our patient has a more compact deleted genome region which contains less OMIM genes. This may help to prune down the causative genes of disease phenotypes. Although our study confirms the causative effect of the Xq21 deletion in males with multiple congenital defects, more cases are needed to be studied in order to clarify the consequences of gene loss in this chromosomal region and the effects on the phenotype.

### Abbreviation

*APOOL*: Apolipoprotein O like; ChAS: Chromosome analysis suite (Affymetrix); *CHM*: Rab escort protein 1; Chr: Chromosome; CPXCR1: CPX chromosome region, candidate 1; *CYLC1*: Cylicin, basic protein of sperm head cytoskeleton 1; *DACH2*: Dachshund family transcription factor 2; DFNX2: Deafness, X-linked 2; HDX: Highly divergent homeobox; HRCT: High-resolution computed tomography; IQ: Intelligence quotient; KLHL4: Kelch like family member 4; OMIM: Online Mendelian inheritance in man; PCR: Polymerase chain reaction; *POF1B*: Premature ovarian failure, 1B; *POU3F4*: POU class 3 homeobox 4; *RPS6KA6*: Ribosomal protein S6 kinase A6; *SATL1*: Spermidine/spermine N1-acetyl transferase-like 1; SNP: Single-nucleotide polymorphism; Xq21: X chromosome long arm q band 21; *ZNF711*: Zinc finger protein 711

### Acknowledgments

We thank the patient and his family for their participation in this study.

### Funding

Not applicable.

### Authors' contributions

By carrying out molecular genetic tests, helping in the clinical examination of the patient and writing manuscript, Siying L,NJ and Shuo.L have contributed equally to this articles. XJ helped in data research for revision. DY conceived of the study and helped to draft the manuscript. All authors read and approved the final manuscript.

### Competing interests

The authors declare that they have no competing interests.

### Author details

[1]Genetic Testing Center, Qingdao Women and Children's Hospital, Qingdao University, #217, Liaoyangxi Road, Qingdao 266034, China. [2]Qingdao Women and Children's Hospital, Qingdao University, Qingdao, China.

### References

1. Ayazi S. Choroideremia, obesity, and congenital deafness. Am J Ophthalmol. 1981;92(1):63–9.
2. Nussbaum RL, Lesko JG, Lewis RA, Ledbetter SA, Ledbetter DH. Isolation of anonymous DNA sequences from within a submicroscopic X chromosomal deletion in a patient with choroideremia, deafness, and mental retardation. Proc Natl Acad Sci U S A. 1987;84(18):6521–5.
3. Song MH, Lee HK, Choi JY, Kim S, Bok J, Kim UK. Clinical evaluation of DFN3 patients with deletions in the POU3F4 locus and detection of carrier female using MLPA. Clin Genet. 2010;78(6):524–32.
4. Firth HV, Richards SM, Bevan AP, et al. DECIPHER: database of chromosomal imbalance and phenotype in humans using Ensembl resources. Am J Hum Genet. 2009;84(4):524–33.
5. Bach I, Robinson D, Thomas N, Ropers HH, Cremers FP. Physical fine mapping of genes underlying X-linked deafness and non fra (X)-X-linked mental retardation at Xq21. Hum Genet. 1992;89(6):620–4.
6. Phelps PD, Reardon W, Pembrey M, Bellman S, Luxom L. X-linked deafness, stapes gushers and a distinctive defect of the inner ear. Neuroradiology. 1991;33(4):326–30.
7. McTaggart KE, Tran M, Mah DY, Lai SW, Nesslinger NJ, MacDonald IM. Mutational analysis of patients with the diagnosis of choroideremia. Hum Mutat. 2002;20(3):189–96.
8. Carrel L, Willard HF. Heterogeneous gene expression from the inactive X chromosome: an X-linked gene that escapes X inactivation in some human cell lines but is inactivated in others. Proc Natl Acad Sci U S A. 1999;96(13):7364–9.
9. Kleine-Kohlbrecher D, Christensen J, Vandamme J, et al. A functional link between the histone demethylase PHF8 and the transcription factor ZNF711 in X-linked mental retardation. Mol Cell. 2010;38(2):165–78.
10. Tarpey PS, Smith R, Pleasance E, et al. A systematic, large-scale resequencing screen of X-chromosome coding exons in mental retardation. Nat Genet. 2009;41(5):535–43.
11. Jin Z, Yu L, Geng J, Wang J, Jin X, Huang H. A novel 47.2 Mb duplication on chromosomal bands Xq21.1-25 associated with mental retardation. Gene. 2015;567(1):98–102.
12. Van der Werf IM, Van Dijck A, Reyniers E, et al. Mutations in two large pedigrees highlight the role of ZNF711 in X-linked intellectual disability. Gene. 2017;605:92–8.

3

# Enlarged NT (≥3.5 mm) in the first trimester – not all chromosome aberrations can be detected by NIPT

Malgorzata I. Srebniak[1*], Merel C. de Wit[2], Karin E. M. Diderich[1], Lutgarde C. P. Govaerts[1], Marieke Joosten[1], Maarten F. C. M. Knapen[2,3], Marnix J. Bos[1], Gerda A. G. Looye-Bruinsma[1], Mieke Koningen[1], Attie T. J. I. Go[2], Robert Jan H. Galjaard[1] and Diane Van Opstal[1]

**Abstract**

**Background:** Since non-invasive prenatal testing (NIPT) in maternal blood became available, we evaluated which chromosome aberrations found in our cohort of fetuses with an enlarged NT in the first trimester of pregnancy (tested with SNP microarray) could be detected by NIPT as well.

**Method:** 362 fetuses were referred for cytogenetic testing due to an enlarged NT (≥3.5 mm). Chromosome aberrations were investigated using QF-PCR, karyotyping and whole genome SNP array.

**Results:** After invasive testing a chromosomal abnormality was detected in 137/362 (38 %) fetuses. 100/362 (28 %) cases concerned trisomy 21, 18 or 13, 25/362 (7 %) an aneuploidy of sex chromosomes and 3/362 (0.8 %) triploidy. In 6/362 (1.6 %) a pathogenic structural unbalanced chromosome aberration was seen and in 3/362 (0.8 %) a susceptibility locus for neurodevelopmental disorders was found. We estimated that in 2–10 % of fetuses with enlarged NT a chromosome aberration would be missed by current NIPT approaches.

**Conclusion:** Based on our cohort of fetuses with enlarged NT we may conclude that NIPT, depending on the approach, will miss chromosome aberrations in a significant percentage of pregnancies. Moreover all abnormal NIPT results require confirmatory studies with invasive testing, which will delay definitive diagnosis in ca. 30 % of patients. These figures are important for pretest counseling enabling pregnant women to make informed choices on the prenatal test. Larger cohorts of fetuses with an enlarged NT should be investigated to assess the additional diagnostic value of high resolution array testing for this indication.

**Keywords:** Array, Microdeletion, NIPT, Nuchal translucency, NT, Submicroscopic chromosomal abnormalities, Prenatal diagnosis

**Abbreviations:** CNV, Copy number variation; CRL, Crown rump length; CV, Chorionic villi; DD, Developmental delay; GMDD, Generalized mosaicism with discrepant direct results; ID, Intellectual disability; MLPA, Multiplex ligation-dependent probe amplification; NIPT, Non-invasive prenatal test; NT, Nuchal translucency; QF-PCR, Quantitative fluorescence-polymerase chain reaction; RAD, Rapid aneuploidy detection; SL, Susceptibility locus

* Correspondence: m.srebniak@erasmusmc.nl
[1]Department of Clinical Genetics, Erasmus Medical Center, Wytemaweg 80, 3015, CN, Rotterdam, The Netherlands
Full list of author information is available at the end of the article

## Background

Nuchal translucency (NT) measurement is widely used as a marker of fetal abnormalities both of chromosomal and non-chromosomal origin [1–3]. A fetal NT > 99th percentile is by definition found in about 1 % of pregnancies [4]. Enlarged NT is not only associated with aneuploidies and other chromosome abnormalities, but also with a number of genetic syndromes, as well as with structural congenital anomalies, mainly cardiac defects [3, 5, 6]. The majority of fetuses with NT ≥ 3.5 mm have a normal karyotype and the pregnancy outcome is highly dependent on the absence of anomalies on expert fetal ultrasound examination [7]. Since non-invasive prenatal testing (NIPT) in maternal blood became available, we evaluated which chromosome aberrations found in our cohort of fetuses with an enlarged NT in the first trimester of pregnancy (tested with SNP microarray) could be detected by NIPT as well. The results of this study can be used in pretest counseling, which can be helpful for making informed choice between invasive and non-invasive genetic testing.

## Methods

362 women carrying a fetus with an enlarged NT (≥3.5 mm) in the first trimester were prospectively referred for Illumina SNP genotyping array as described before [8, 9]. Fetal material was obtained through chorionic villi sampling (311 cases) or amniocentesis (51 cases) after the NT was measured as a part of the first trimester combined screening or as part of the routine first trimester crown rump length (CRL) measurement for pregnancy dating. Samples collected in our central location and 3 satellite hospitals between 1st September 2011 until 31st March 2016 that were routinely referred for SNP array testing (0.15 Mb resolution) were included in this cohort. All cytogenetic tests were done in one central laboratory. This cohort overlaps slightly with the cohort published before [10]. To create a homogenous cohort as much as possible we excluded the following cases:

- fetuses referred for hydrops foetalis,
- fetuses referred for enlarged NT with co-existing congenital anomalies evident on the CRL scan or the NT scan

All samples were tested with QF-PCR or MLPA to detect common aneuploidies (rapid aneuploidy detection - RAD). When RAD detected trisomy 21 or 13, such samples were karyotyped (GTG banding analysis) to assess the recurrence risk. Cases of triploidy or trisomy 18 were not further tested. All cases showing normal RAD results or sex-chromosomal aneuploidy were tested with Illumina SNP array (HumanCytoSNP-12 or Infinium_CytoSNP_850K with analysis resolution of ca. 0.15 Mb) as described before [8].

To answer our research question we have divided chromosome aberrations in the following groups:

1) autosomal aneuploidies
2) sex-chromosome aneuploidies that may be detected by NIPT when sex-chromosomes analysis is included in the test
3) triploidy
4) pathogenic structural unbalanced chromosome aberrations (both microscopic and submicroscopic)
5) susceptibility loci for neurodevelopmental disorders.

Further, we evaluated which aberrations would theoretically be missed by current NIPT approaches (NIPT tests were not routinely performed in this cohort). To be able to make this assessment, for the purpose of this paper, we assumed that all non-mosaic aneuploidies (both autosomal and sex-chromosomal) would be detectable by current NIPT [11] as well as structural unbalanced aberrations larger than 10 Mb [12, 13]. We report estimated percentages of abnormal cases missed by particular NIPT approaches with Agresti–Coull (adjusted Wald) 95 % confidence intervals, which have higher coverage probability than large-sample Wald intervals, in particular for small proportions [14, 15].

## Results

The distribution of chromosomal abnormalities according to NT within the study population is presented in Table 1. The diagnostic flow was shown in Fig. 1. 38 % (137/362) of the cases showed abnormal cytogenetic results, which are presented in Table 2. The most common aberration was trisomy 21 (17 % 63/362) and in total in 28 % (100/362) of the cases an autosomal aneuploidy was detected (trisomy 21, 18 or 13). In 6/362 (1.6 %) a pathogenic unbalanced structural chromosome aberration was found: 5 were microscopically visible (>10 Mb) and 1 was submicroscopic (an atypical 22q11 microdeletion) [16]. There were three cases (3/362, 0.8 %) that showed a susceptibility locus for a neurodevelopmental disorder (2 cases of 15q11 microdeletion and one case of 16p11.2 microdeletion), these aberrations are probably not related to the enlarged NT.

Table 2 also shows the estimated percentage of cases that could be missed by current NIPT approaches in each category of chromosome aberrations. Based on our estimation a chromosomal anomaly would be undetected by NIPT in about 2–10 % of patients, depending on the approach used (Table 3).

## Discussion

Nuchal fluid accumulation may be caused by several factors, therefore, diverse genetic abnormalities may be expected in such fetuses. Taking this and numerous advantages of genomic microarrays [17] into account we

**Table 1** Distribution of chromosomal abnormalities according to NT within the study population ($n = 362$)

| NT in mm | Number of cases in the cohort (%) | Number of cases with chromosome aberrations (% within the category) |
|---|---|---|
| 3.5–4.4 | 179 (49 %) | 35 (19 %) |
| 4.5–5.4 | 68 (19 %) | 32 (47 %) |
| 5.5–6.4 | 42 (11.6 %) | 30 (71 %) |
| 6.5–7.4 | 24 (6.6 %) | 14 (58.3 %) |
| 7.5–8.4 | 14 (3.9 %) | 6 (43 %) |
| ≥8.5 | 10 (2.8 %) | 6 (60 %) |
| unknown (hygroma colli, where NT measurement was not specified) | 25 (7 %) | 14 (56 %) |
| Total | 362 | 137 (38 %) |

have chosen a whole genome SNP array technique for cytogenetic investigations in cases of an enlarged NT [8, 9]. In the present study, we prospectively investigated the frequency of (sub) microscopic aberrations in this group of fetuses. Since non-invasive prenatal testing (NIPT) in maternal blood became available and the patients can face a choice between an invasive and non-invasive testing, we evaluated how high the risks of missing a pathogenic chromosome finding can be in a cohort of fetuses with enlarged NT measurement.

### Autosomal aneuploidies and triploidy

Although most of the anomalous fetuses showed trisomy 13, 18 or 21 (100/137, 73 %) and NIPT seems to be an excellent and safe test with a high positive predictive value in this selected high risk group, there are some drawbacks that have to be taken into account. One has to be aware of the risk of false-negative NIPT results for the common trisomies [18, 19]. 3.5 % of Down/Patau/Edwards syndrome cases would potentially be missed by NIPT due to generalized mosaicism with discrepant direct results (GMDD) [20]. Therefore, as shown in Table 2, at least 3 trisomic cases in the cohort presented in this paper (3.5 % out of 100 cases) would potentially be also missed if this cohort was tested with NIPT as a first-tier test. Additionally, other potential causes for false-negative NIPT results such as a low fetal DNA fraction (e.g. due to a high maternal body mass index) or technical failures, should also be taken into account [21]. The detection of triploidy is problematic as well. Although are SNP approaches are able to detect triploidy [22, 23], in our knowledge, there are no data showing that this could be achieved in assays based on whole genome shallow sequencing.

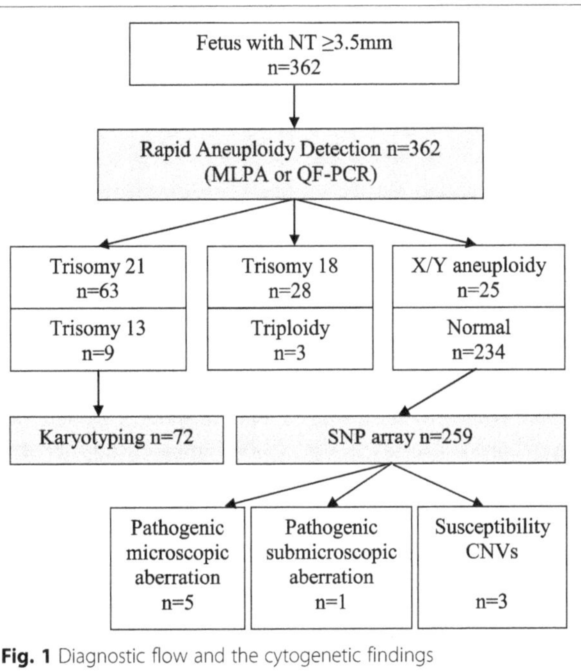


**Fig. 1** Diagnostic flow and the cytogenetic findings

### Sex-chromosome aneuploidies

The second most common group of aberrations in fetuses with an enlarged NT is monosomy X (5.5 % 20/362, Table 2). Gil and colleagues showed that cfDNA tests could detect monosomy X in about 90 % of the cases [24], so at least 2 cases of monosomy X (10 % out of 20 cases) would be missed in this cohort. An accurate non-invasive detection of fetal monosomy X remains problematic due to several reasons. First of all, chromosomal mosaicism is common in sex chromosomal aneuploidy [25]. A low percentage of abnormal cells in the cytotrophoblast and co-existence of different abnormal cell lines may mask the actual chromosome aberration (e.g. 45,X/47,XXX) and lead to false negative results. There is also a maternal factor influencing the results as normal adult females show an age-related loss of X-chromosomes [26]. This mosaicism of chromosome X influences the positive predictive value in case of a monosomy X detection [27]. Moreover, finding sufficient Y-chromosome loci that are informative for copy number quantification may be difficult [28], causing monosomy X detection to be highly dependent on the NIPT method used. These difficulties are reflected in the recent literature that showed very limited follow-up of monosomy X cases diagnosed non-invasively [21, 29]. So although some authors suggest that there are accurate methods to detect fetal sex chromosomal aneuploidy in maternal plasma [30, 31], recent clinical experience shows low positive predictive value for monosomy X. This situation can be expected since the fetal DNA in maternal plasma is derived from the cytotrophoblast of chorionic villi (CV) and cytogenetic studies in CV already showed that sex-chromosomal aneuploidy in the

**Table 2** Results of cytogenetic testing in fetuses with enlarged NT (≥3.5 mm) or hygroma colli in the first trimester in fetuses referred for cytogenetic testing

| Type of chromosome aberration | Number of fetuses $n = 362$ | Potential detection by current NIPT approaches | % of anomalies that are going to be missed due to placental mosaicism or current testing resolution (>7–10 Mb) |
|---|---|---|---|
| Autosomal aneuploidy | | Yes | 3.5 % is likely to be missed [20, 49, 50]<br>0.8 % (3/362) |
| Trisomy 21 | 63 (17 %) | | |
| Trisomy 18 | 28 (7.7 %) | | |
| Trisomy 13 | 9 (2.5 %) | | |
| Sex-chromosomal aneuploidy | | Yes (if X/Y analysis are included) | 10 % of monosomy X are likely to be missed [24]<br>0.5 % (2/362)<br>Mosaic samples are most probably missed<br>0.5 % (2/362) |
| Monosomy X[a] | 20 (5.5 %) | | |
| XXX | 2 (0.5 %) | | |
| XXY | 1 (0.3 %) | | |
| Mosaic X/XY | 2 (0.5 %) | | |
| Triploidy | 3 (0.8 %) | Yes (if SNP approach is applied) | Most of the current approaches cannot detect triploidy, and so far it is not possible to combine targeted SNP analysis with high coverage and whole genome profiling with high resolution<br>0.8 % (3/362) |
| Pathogenic unbalanced chromosome aberrations:<br>1) 46,XY,der [9] t (9;13) (q33.1;q12.11),-13 (NT 4.9 mm; 116 Mb gain at 9p24-q33))<br>2) 46,XX,del [8] (p23.1) inv dup [8] (p11.21p23.1) (NT 4.6 mm; 28 Mb gain at 8p)<br>3) 45,XX,der [4] t (4;15) (q32.1;q13.3),-15dn (hygroma colli; 34 Mb loss at 4p))<br>4) arr [hg19] 9p24.3p22.2 (46,587-18,277,618) x1 (NT 5.2 mm; 18 Mb loss at 9p)<br>5) arr [hg19] 1q32.1q44 (202,542,202-249,218,992) x3,9p24.3p24.1 (46,587-7,017,391) x1 (NT 3.6 mm, 47 Mb gain at 1q, 7 Mb loss 9p)<br>6) atypical 22q11 microdeletion of paternal origin arr [hg19] 22q11.21 (21,111,299-21,463,730) x1 pat (NT 4.3 mm, >0.5 Mb) | 6 (1.6 %) | Larger than 10 Mb Yes (if whole genome profiling with resolution of 10 Mb is applied) | 1/6 cases would be potentially missed: 0.3 % (1/362) |
| Susceptibility loci for neurodevelopmental disorders:<br>1) 15q11 microdeletion of NIPA1/NIPA2 of paternal origin arr [hg18] 15q11.2 (20,191,584-21,025,923) x1pat (NT 4.7 mm)<br>2) 15q11 microdeletion of NIPA1/NIPA2 of maternal origin arr [hg19] 15q11.2 (22,299,434-23,272,733) x1mat (NT 4.4 mm)<br>3) *de novo* 16q11.2 microdeletion arr [hg19] 16p11.2 (29,595,483-30,198,151) x1dn (hygroma colli) | 3 (0.8 %) | No | So far genome wide detection of submicroscopic aberrations is not feasible. All will be missed<br>0.8 % (3/362) |
| Total number abnormal cases | 137 (38 %) | | |

[a]One case showed also isochromosome Xp (case published before in [51])

cytotrophoblast of CV (STC-villi, short term cultured villi) is often not representative for the actual fetal karyotype [19, 32].

#### Pathogenic unbalanced structural aberrations

Although an enlarged NT was observed in fetuses with unbalanced translocations, no significant differences were seen in a study that evaluated the role of nuchal translucency (NT) in the prediction of unbalanced translocation in offspring of couples carrying balanced translocations [33]. A recent study of Christiansen and colleagues showed that the distributions for NT measurements in case of an aberration other than trisomy 21, 13 or 18 more closely resembled that of the normal population [34]. So the detection of rare unbalanced chromosome anomalies in cohorts with an enlarged NT may be co-incidental. Nevertheless karyotypically visible unbalanced chromosome aberrations are likely to be detected by whole genome profiling NIPT approaches [12, 13, 35]. Unfortunately it is difficult to assess how many may be missed due to their mitotic origin and absence in the cytotrophoblast.

The incidence of pathogenic submicroscopic chromosomal abnormalities in fetuses with an enlarged NT has been studied by only few groups [36–41] resulting in

**Table 3** Percentage of abnormal cases missed by particular NIPT approaches. Additionally as 3.5 % of trisomy 13, 18 and 21 would be missed due to placental mosaicism 3/362 (0.8 %) cases were included in all NIPT options. As susceptibility CNVs are not the primary reason for invasive testing they were not included in the number of cases with structural anomalies that would be missed by NIPT

| Type of NIPT testing | Percentage of patients in our cohort that would show false negative results with NIPT | 95 % CI for percentage LL, UL | Number of cases that would be missed in our cohort |
|---|---|---|---|
| Targeted approach for trisomy 13, 18 and 21 | 10 % (37/362) | 7.48, 13.80 | 34 + 3/362 (20x monosomy X, 5x other sex chromosomal aneuploidy, 3x triploidy, 6x structural anomalies + 3/362 (0.8 %) based on placental mosaicism) |
| Targeted approach for common aneuploidies of chromosomes 13, 18, 21, X/Y | 4 % (14/362) | 2.26, 6.44 | 11 + 3/362 (2x mosaic sex chromosomal aneuploidy, 3x triploidy, 6x structural anomalies + 3/362 (0.8 %) based on placental mosaicism) |
| Targeted approach for common aneuploidies of chromosomes 13, 18, 21, X/Y and triploidy | 3 % (11/362) | 1.64, 5.42 | 8 + 3/362 (2x mosaic sex chromosomal aneuploidy, 6x structural anomalies + 3/362 (0.8 %) based on placental mosaicism) |
| Whole genome profiling with a resolution of ca. 10 Mb | 2 % (7/362) | 0.09, 4.02 | 4 + 3/362 (3x triploidy and 1x submicroscopic anomaly will be missed + 3/362 (0.8 %) based on placental mosaicism) |

*CI* confidence interval, *LL* lower limit, *UL* upper limit

conflicting conclusions [42, 43]. These differences in frequencies of chromosomal aberrations in published cohorts were observed before [42] and it may be a consequence of both cohort selection and differences in array design. Many of previously reported cohorts were either retrospectively tested and highly selected [38, 39] or included a heterogeneous group of fetuses with and without additional ultrasound anomalies detected in both first and second trimester [36, 38, 44, 45]. Our results show that the prevalence of submicroscopic aberrations in fetuses with enlarged NT resembles the prevalence in fetuses without ultrasound anomalies. This confirms previous results published by Huang and colleagues [39]. Therefore, in our opinion larger unselected cohorts with enlarged NT should be published to assess the actual risk of a pathogenic submicroscopic unbalanced chromosome aberration when an enlarged NT is diagnosed in the first trimester.

### Susceptibility loci for neurodevelopmental disorders

We did not take the susceptibility loci for neurodevelopmental disorders into account for the calculations shown in Table 3. Susceptibility CNVs are quite often found in prenatal array testing [46], however there is no study that showed any relationship with an enlarged NT. Finding additional predisposition factors may play a role in decision making in pregnancy, however it is less likely that one would choose invasive testing with a primary aim to investigate these. Therefore we assume that missing these findings is not the most important incentive for deciding on the prenatal test. Moreover the frequency of susceptibility CNVs in this cohort (0.8 % 3/362) resembles more the frequency in fetuses without ultrasound anomalies (1.3 %) [47] than those with ultrasound anomalies (2.7 %) [10].

## Conclusions

Since most (73 %; 100/137) chromosome aberrations in cases of an enlarged NT (≥3.5 mm) in the first trimester involved trisomy 21, 18 and 13, NIPT at first sight seems to be an appropriate test. However, our study confirms the previously published data by Lichtenbelt and colleagues [48] and shows that because of current limitations of NIPT (depending on the type of analysis) in ca. 2–10 % of cases with an enlarged NT a chromosome aberration will be missed by non-invasive testing. Moreover since the risk for a chromosome aberration is high (1:3) and since aberrant NIPT requires confirmatory studies due to the origin of the cfDNA, therefore NIPT as compared to invasive testing will delay a final diagnosis in about 30 % of patients. The limitations of NIPT should be clearly addressed in the pre-test counseling: possible diagnostic delay, the risk for false negative and false positive results and the fact that false-positive cases of monosomy X in enlarged NT fetuses may cause additional anxiety.

#### Acknowledgements
We would like to thank all clinicians for referring the patients and laboratory technicians for their dedicated work to achieve rapid prenatal results. We would like to thank Marike Polak for the statistical calculations done during the manuscript preparation.

#### Funding
There was no funding available for this study.

#### Authors' contributions
MIS conceived the study, made substantial contributions to conception and

design, analysis and interpretation of genomic data and drafted the manuscript. KEMD, LCPG, MJ, MJB, GAGL, MK and DVO made substantial contributions to acquisition of data, analysis and interpretation of genomic data. MJ, ATJIG and RJHG coordinated the counseling of the patients. MCdW, KEMD, LCPG, MJ, MFCMK and ATJIG made substantial contributions to acquisition of clinical data. MCdW, MFCMK and ATJIG performed pre-test counseling, invasive testing, perinatal management and contributed to the acquisition of phenotypic data (prenatal ultrasound scans). DVO supervised the study and carried literature search. MIS and DVO were responsible for the final diagnoses and reports. All authors revised the manuscript critically for important intellectual content, approved the final version and agreed to be accountable for all aspects of the work in ensuring that questions related to the accuracy or integrity of any part of the work are appropriately investigated and resolved.

#### Competing interests
The authors declare that they have no competing interests.

#### Author details
[1]Department of Clinical Genetics, Erasmus Medical Center, Wytemaweg 80, 3015, CN, Rotterdam, The Netherlands. [2]Department of Obstetrics and Gynecology, Erasmus Medical Center, Wytemaweg 80, 3015, CN, Rotterdam, The Netherlands. [3]Foundation Prenatal Screening Southwest region of The Netherlands, Wytemaweg 80, Na-1509, 3015, CN, Rotterdam, The Netherlands.

#### References
1. Nicolaides KH, Azar G, Byrne D, Mansur C, Marks K. Fetal nuchal translucency: ultrasound screening for chromosomal defects in first trimester of pregnancy. BMJ. 1992;304(6831):867–9.
2. Snijders RJ, Noble P, Sebire N, Souka A, Nicolaides KH. UK multicentre project on assessment of risk of trisomy 21 by maternal age and fetal nuchal-translucency thickness at 10–14 weeks of gestation. Fetal medicine foundation first trimester screening group. Lancet. 1998;352(9125):343–6.
3. Souka AP, Von Kaisenberg CS, Hyett JA, Sonek JD, Nicolaides KH. Increased nuchal translucency with normal karyotype. Am J Obstet Gynecol. 2005; 192(4):1005–21.
4. Senat MV, Bussieres L, Couderc S, Roume J, Rozenberg P, Bouyer J, et al. Long-term outcome of children born after a first-trimester measurement of nuchal translucency at the 99th percentile or greater with normal karyotype: a prospective study. Am J Obstet Gynecol. 2007;196(1):53. e1-6.
5. McAuliffe FM, Hornberger LK, Winsor S, Chitayat D, Chong K, Johnson JA. Fetal cardiac defects and increased nuchal translucency thickness: a prospective study. Am J Obstet Gynecol. 2004;191(4):1486–90.
6. Burger NB, Bekker MN, de Groot CJ, Christoffels VM, Haak MC. Why increased nuchal translucency is associated with congenital heart disease: a systematic review on genetic mechanisms. Prenat Diagn. 2015;35(6):517–28.
7. Bilardo CM, Muller MA, Pajkrt E, Clur SA, van Zalen MM, Bijlsma EK. Increased nuchal translucency thickness and normal karyotype: time for parental reassurance. Ultrasound Obstet Gynecol. 2007;30(1):11–8.
8. Srebniak MI, Boter M, Oudesluijs GO, Cohen-Overbeek T, Govaerts LC, Diderich KE, et al. Genomic SNP array as a gold standard for prenatal diagnosis of foetal ultrasound abnormalities. Mol Cytogenet. 2012;5(1):14.
9. Srebniak M, Boter M, Oudesluijs G, Joosten M, Govaerts L, Van Opstal D, et al. Application of SNP array for rapid prenatal diagnosis: implementation, genetic counselling and diagnostic flow. Eur J Hum Genet. 2011; 19(12):1230–7.
10. Srebniak MI, Diderich KE, Joosten M, Govaerts LC, Knijnenburg J, de Vries FA, et al. Prenatal SNP array testing in 1000 fetuses with ultrasound anomalies: causative, unexpected and susceptibility CNVs. Eur J Hum Genet. 2016; 24(5):645–51.
11. Boon EM, Faas BH. Benefits and limitations of whole genome versus targeted approaches for noninvasive prenatal testing for fetal aneuploidies. Prenat Diagn. 2013;33(6):563–8.
12. Straver R, Sistermans EA, Holstege H, Visser A, Oudejans CB, Reinders MJ. WISECONDOR: detection of fetal aberrations from shallow sequencing maternal plasma based on a within-sample comparison scheme. Nucleic Acids Res. 2014;42(5):e31.
13. Zhao C, Tynan J, Ehrich M, Hannum G, McCullough R, Saldivar JS, et al. Detection of fetal subchromosomal abnormalities by sequencing circulating cell-free DNA from maternal plasma. Clin Chem. 2015;61(4):608–16.
14. Agresti A, Coull BA. Approximate is better than "exact" for interval estimation of binomial proportions. Am Stat. 1998;52(2):119–26.
15. Brown LD, Cai TT, DasGupta A, Agresti A, Coull BA, Casella G, et al. Interval estimation for a binomial proportion - comment - rejoinder. Stat Sci. 2001; 16(2):101–33.
16. Verhagen JM, Diderich KE, Oudesluijs G, Mancini GM, Eggink AJ, Verkleij-Hagoort AC, et al. Phenotypic variability of atypical 22q11.2 deletions not including TBX1. Am J Med Genet A. 2012;158A(10):2412–20.
17. Srebniak MI, Van Opstal D, Joosten M, Diderich KE, de Vries FA, Riedijk S, et al. Whole-genome array as a first-line cytogenetic test in prenatal diagnosis. Ultrasound Obstet Gynecol. 2015;45(4):363–72.
18. Sepulveda W. Discordant results between fetal cell-free DNA in maternal plasma and chorionic villus sampling in a first-trimester fetus with increased nuchal translucency and megacystis. Ultrasound Obstet Gynecol. 2014; 44(3):369.
19. van den Berg C, Van Opstal D, Polak-Knook J, Galjaard RJ. (Potential) false-negative diagnoses in chorionic villi and a review of the literature. Prenat Diagn. 2006;26(5):401–8.
20. Van Opstal D, Srebniak MI, Polak J, de Vries F, Govaerts LC, Joosten M, et al. False negative NIPT results: risk figures for chromosomes 13, 18 and 21 based on chorionic villi results in 5967 cases and literature review. PLoS One. 2016;11(1):e0146794.
21. Dar P, Curnow KJ, Gross SJ, Hall MP, Stosic M, Demko Z, et al. Clinical experience and follow-up with large scale single-nucleotide polymorphism-based noninvasive prenatal aneuploidy testing. Am J Obstet Gynecol. 2014; 211(5):527. e1- e17.
22. Nicolaides KH, Syngelaki A, Gil M, Atanasova V, Markova D. Validation of targeted sequencing of single-nucleotide polymorphisms for non-invasive prenatal detection of aneuploidy of chromosomes 13, 18, 21, X, and Y. Prenat Diagn. 2013;33(6):575–9.
23. Ryan A, Hunkapiller N, Banjevic M, Vankayalapati N, Fong N, Jinnett KN, et al. Validation of an Enhanced Version of a Single-Nucleotide Polymorphism-Based Noninvasive Prenatal Test for Detection of Fetal Aneuploidies. Fetal Diagn Ther. 2016. [Epub ahead of print]
24. Gil MM, Quezada MS, Revello R, Akolekar R, Nicolaides KH. Analysis of cell-free DNA in maternal blood in screening for fetal aneuploidies: updated meta-analysis. Ultrasound Obstet Gynecol. 2015;45(3):249–66.
25. Forabosco A, Percesepe A, Santucci S. Incidence of non-age-dependent chromosomal abnormalities: a population-based study on 88965 amniocenteses. Eur J Hum Genet. 2009;17(7):897–903.
26. Russell LM, Strike P, Browne CE, Jacobs PA. X chromosome loss and ageing. Cytogenet Genome Res. 2007;116(3):181–5.
27. Wang Y, Chen Y, Tian F, Zhang J, Song Z, Wu Y, et al. Maternal mosaicism is a significant contributor to discordant sex chromosomal aneuploidies associated with noninvasive prenatal testing. Clin Chem. 2014;60(1):251–9.
28. Benn P, Cuckle H, Pergament E. Non-invasive prenatal testing for aneuploidy: current status and future prospects. Ultrasound Obstet Gynecol. 2013;42(1):15–33.
29. Futch T, Spinosa J, Bhatt S, de Feo E, Rava RP, Sehnert AJ. Initial clinical laboratory experience in noninvasive prenatal testing for fetal aneuploidy from maternal plasma DNA samples. Prenat Diagn. 2013;33(6):569–74.
30. Samango-Sprouse C, Banjevic M, Ryan A, Sigurjonsson S, Zimmermann B, Hill M, et al. SNP-based non-invasive prenatal testing detects sex chromosome aneuploidies with high accuracy. Prenat Diagn. 2013;33(7): 643–9.
31. Yu SC, Chan KC, Zheng YW, Jiang P, Liao GJ, Sun H, et al. Size-based molecular diagnostics using plasma DNA for noninvasive prenatal testing. Proc Natl Acad Sci U S A. 2014;111(23):8583–8.
32. Van Opstal D, Srebniak MI. Cytogenetic confirmation of a positive NIPT result: evidence-based choice between chorionic villus sampling and amniocentesis depending on chromosome aberration. Expert Rev Mol Diagn. 2016;16(5):513–20.
33. Arigita M, Grande M, Mula R, Borobio V, Sanchez A, Soler A, et al. Nuchal translucency thickness in the prediction of unbalanced translocations. Prenat Diagn. 2014;34(10):982–5.

34. Christiansen M, Ekelund CK, Petersen OB, Hyett J, Eastwood N, Ball S, et al. Nuchal translucency distributions for different chromosomal anomalies in a large unselected population cohort. Prenat Diagn. 2016;36(1):49–55.
35. Bayindir B, Dehaspe L, Brison N, Brady P, Ardui S, Kammoun M, et al. Noninvasive prenatal testing using a novel analysis pipeline to screen for all autosomal fetal aneuploidies improves pregnancy management. Eur J Hum Genet. 2015;23:1286–93.
36. Schou KV, Kirchhoff M, Nygaard U, Jorgensen C, Sundberg K. Increased nuchal translucency with normal karyotype: a follow-up study of 100 cases supplemented with CGH and MLPA analyses. Ultrasound Obstet Gynecol. 2009;34(6):618–22.
37. Pan M, Han J, Zhen L, Yang X, Li R, Liao C, et al. Prenatal diagnosis of fetuses with increased nuchal translucency using an approach based on quantitative fluorescent polymerase chain reaction and genomic microarray. Eur J Obstet Gynecol Reprod Biol. 2015;197:164–7.
38. Leung TY, Vogel I, Lau TK, Chong W, Hyett JA, Petersen OB, et al. Identification of submicroscopic chromosomal aberrations in fetuses with increased nuchal translucency and apparently normal karyotype. Ultrasound Obstet Gynecol. 2011;38(3):314–9.
39. Huang J, Poon LC, Akolekar R, Choy KW, Leung TY, Nicolaides KH. Is high fetal nuchal translucency associated with submicroscopic chromosomal abnormalities on array CGH? Ultrasound Obstet Gynecol. 2014;43(6):620–4.
40. Scott F, Murphy K, Carey L, Greville W, Mansfield N, Barahona P, et al. Prenatal diagnosis using combined quantitative fluorescent polymerase chain reaction and array comparative genomic hybridization analysis as a first-line test: results from over 1000 consecutive cases. Ultrasound Obstet Gynecol. 2013;41(5):500–7.
41. Lund IC, Christensen R, Petersen OB, Vogel I, Vestergaard EM. Chromosomal microarray in fetuses with increased nuchal translucency. Ultrasound Obstet Gynecol. 2015;45(1):95–100.
42. de Wit MC, Srebniak MI, Govaerts LC, Van Opstal D, Galjaard RJ, Go AT. Additional value of prenatal genomic array testing in fetuses with isolated structural ultrasound abnormalities and a normal karyotype: a systematic review of the literature. Ultrasound Obstet Gynecol. 2014;43(2):139–46.
43. Grande M, Jansen FA, Blumenfeld YJ, Fisher A, Odibo AO, Haak MC, et al. Genomic microarray in fetuses with increased nuchal translucency and normal karyotype: a systematic review and meta-analysis. Ultrasound Obstet Gynecol. 2015;46(6):650–8.
44. Rooryck C, Toutain J, Cailley D, Bouron J, Horovitz J, Lacombe D, et al. Prenatal diagnosis using array-CGH: a French experience. Eur J Med Genet. 2013;56(7):341–5.
45. Yang X, Li R, Fu F, Zhang Y, Li D, Liao C. Submicroscopic chromosomal abnormalities in Fetuses with Increased Nuchal Translucency and Normal Karyotype. J Matern Fetal Neonatal Med. 2016;19:1–5.
46. Wapner RJ, Martin CL, Levy B, Ballif BC, Eng CM, Zachary JM, et al. Chromosomal microarray versus karyotyping for prenatal diagnosis. N Engl J Med. 2012;367(23):2175–84.
47. Van Opstal D, de Vries F, Govaerts L, Boter M, Lont D, van Veen S, et al. Benefits and burdens of using a SNP array in pregnancies at increased risk for the common aneuploidies. Hum Mutat. 2015;36(3):319–26.
48. Lichtenbelt KD, Diemel BD, Koster MP, Manten GT, Siljee J, Schuring-Blom GH, et al. Detection of fetal chromosomal anomalies: does nuchal translucency measurement have added value in the era of non-invasive prenatal testing? Prenat Diagn. 2015;35(7):663–8.
49. Grati FR, Malvestiti F, Ferreira JC, Bajaj K, Gaetani E, Agrati C, et al. Fetoplacental mosaicism: potential implications for false-positive and false-negative noninvasive prenatal screening results. Genet Med. 2014; 16(8):620–4.
50. Taylor-Phillips S, Freeman K, Geppert J, Agbebiyi A, Uthman OA, Madan J, et al. Accuracy of non-invasive prenatal testing using cell-free DNA for detection of Down, Edwards and Patau syndromes: a systematic review and meta-analysis. BMJ Open. 2016;6(1):e010002.
51. Srebniak MI, Bos MJ, de Vries FA, Heydanus R, Wessels MW, Van Opstal D. SNP array detects chromosome aberrations that we thought do not exist: the first case of an isochromosome Xp (i(X)(p10)). Prenat Diagn. 2014; 34(8):806–8.

# 4

# *MIR137* is the key gene mediator of the syndromic obesity phenotype of patients with 1p21.3 microdeletions

Arianna Tucci, Claudia Ciaccio, Giulietta Scuvera, Susanna Esposito and Donatella Milani*

**Abstract**

**Background:** Deletions in the long arm of chromosome 1 have been described in patients with a phenotype consisting primarily of obesity, intellectual disability and autism-spectrum disorder. The minimal region of overlap comprises two genes: *DPYD* and *MIR137*.

**Case presentation:** We describe a 10-year-old boy with syndromic obesity who carries a novel 1p21.3 deletion overlapping the critical region with the *MIR137* gene only.

**Conclusions:** This study suggests that *MIR137* is the mediator of the obesity phenotype of patients carrying 1p21.3 microdeletions.

**Keywords:** Obesity, Array-CGH, Genetics, *MIR137*, 1p21.3, Intellectual disability, Autism spectrum disorder

## Background

Obesity is a complex disease that results from the interactions of a variety of hereditary and environmental factors. Heritability for obesity is high (typically 0.4 to 0.7) [1], comparable to that of other complex, polygenic diseases such as autism [2]. In most individuals, the genetic basis for obesity is complex and likely to involve the interaction of multiple genes and gene-by-environment interactions. However, there are rare examples of monogenic causes for obesity that provide insights to pathways that may account for more common causes of obesity and indicate targets for therapeutic intervention. These disorders include obesity syndromes such as Prader Willi syndrome and Bardet–Biedl syndrome and microdeletion/duplication syndromes such as 1p36 and 17p11.2, in which affected patients are usually identified by additional phenotypes, such as intellectual disability (ID), dysmorphic features or other developmental abnormalities. Gaining insight into genetic causes through the study of obesity-related disorders has provided a more comprehensive picture of the mechanisms that control food intake and energy balance related to the development of obesity (e.g., *SIM1*).

Deletions in chromosome 1p21.3 have been reported in a total of 12 individuals presenting with a variable combination of ID, autism spectrum disorders (ASD) and obesity [3–6]. The shortest region of overlap (SRO) has been restricted to two genes: dihydropyrimidine dehydrogenase (*DPYD*) and microRNA 137 (*MIR137*). The *DPYD* encodes for the rate-limiting enzyme in the catabolism of the pyrimidine bases, and mutations in this gene cause DPYD deficiency (OMIM #274270), an autosomal recessive disease of variable severity typically characterized by the presence of childhood onset neurological problems, such as developmental delay and convulsions. *MIR137* encodes for miR-137, a microRNA (miRNA) molecule involved in the post-transcriptional regulation of genes [7].

In this study, we report an additional case carrying a 1p21.3 microdeletion that presented with ID, ASD, obesity and additional clinical features. We propose the *MIR137* gene as the mediator of the obesity phenotype that presents in patients carrying chromosome 1p21.3 microdeletions.

* Correspondence: donatella.milani@policlinico.mi.it
Pediatric Highly Intensive Care Unit, Department of Pathophysiology and Transplantation, Università degli Studi di Milano, Fondazione IRCCS Ca' Granda Ospedale Maggiore Policlinico, Via Commenda 9, 20122 Milano, Italy

## Case presentation

The proband is a ten-year-old male and the first-born child of healthy non-consanguineous parents. The family history was unremarkable for neurological disorders, behavioral problems, and congenital anomalies.

He was born at 39 weeks of gestation via elective caesarian section. His birth weight was 2800 g (10-25th centile) and his length, occipital frontal circumference and APGAR scores were not reported but were said to be normal. At birth, no medical problems were recorded. Postnatally, his growth was normal; global psychomotor delay was noted: the boy took his first steps at the age of 20 months and said his first words at the age of 36 months. In infancy, he had several episodes of febrile convulsions, which spontaneously resolved at the age of 3 years. During a routine heart examination, a heart murmur was noticed, which prompted further tests. An echocardiogram showed a bicuspid aortic valve, with mild stenosis of the aortic root.

At the age of 9, he attended the fifth year of primary school due to speech disorder and anxiety. Neuropsychiatric assessment revealed anxiety, normal non verbal cognitive function, specific language impairment and fine motor skills disturbances, requiring weekly psychomotricity sessions. His growth parameters were as follows: weight was 39.3 kg (75th centile), height 147.2 cm (97th centile), body mass index (BMI) was 18.13 kg/m$^2$. At the age of 10, the boy weighted 48 kg (>97th centile), height was 154 cm (>97th centile), head circumference was 58 cm (>97th centile) and BMI was 20.6. Pubic hair appearance, growth spurt and weight gain were noted. The boy was hospitalized, and further tests were performed, confirming precocious puberty of central origin: a radiograph of the hand and wrist, which showed advanced bone age (bone age of 13 years, biological age 9 years and 5 months); renal echography, adrenal glands and tests, which were normal, and the LHRH test, which showed an LH response. The boy started agonist LHRH therapy. Brain magnetic resonance imaging (MRI) showed increased cerebrospinal fluid (CSF) spaces posteriorly to the cerebellum and a moderate focal increase of CSF in the anterior temporal horns and in the lamina of the quadrigeminal cistern. The pituitary gland was normal.

Chromosome analysis by array-CGH (a-CGH) revealed a 5.2-Mb deletion on chromosome 1p21.3p21.1 (chromosome 1:98,456,293-103,682,084 – hg19). a-CGH was performed using a Cytochip ISCA 180 K Oligo platform (BlueGnome Ltd.). a-CGH analysis of the parents revealed the de novo origin of the deletion.

## Conclusions

Deletions at 1p21.3 have been recognized as a cause of childhood obesity syndrome. Twelve patients carrying 1p21.3 deletions have been described in the literature to date [3–6], presenting with mild to moderate ID (100 %), obesity or a tendency to obesity, with a weight 3 or more standard deviations above the mean (92 %), ASD (92 %) and mild dysmorphic features (67 %) (Fig. 1 and Table 1). The minimal overlapping region was restricted to a chromosomal segment of 1.22 Mb, which includes the *DPYD* and *MIR137* genes. *DPYD* was proposed as the gene contributing to the phenotype [3, 5], based on the assumption that its haploinsufficiency would contribute to the development of a neuropsychiatric phenotype, which also leads to obesity. However, the case herein presented and the patient recently reported by Pinto et al. [6] carried a deletion overlapping in the critical region only at the *MIR137*, which suggests that this is the gene underlying the phenotype of patients carrying deletions at 1p21.3.

miRNAs are noncoding 21–23 nucleotide small RNAs that are highly conserved and involved in several biological processes, such as cell proliferation, apoptosis, cell differentiation and morphogenesis [8]. They regulate posttranscriptional processes via sequence-specific interactions with the untranslated regions (UTRs) of cognate messenger RNA targets [7, 9]. Each individual miRNA can regulate many mRNAs, and conversely, each mRNA can be targeted by a number of miRNAs. The involvement of miR-137 in obesity, ID and ASD could be explained at two different levels. First, miR-137 regulates a multitude of genes in the central nervous system (CNS) [10]. Specifically, miR-137 has been shown to be involved in

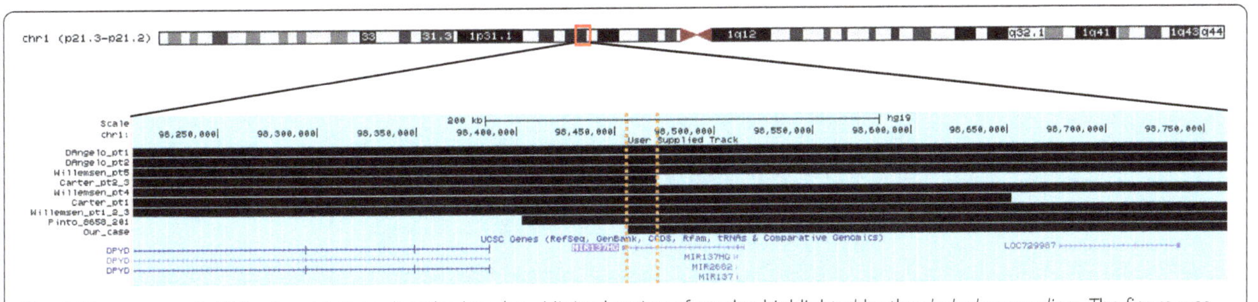


**Fig. 1** Chromosome 1p21.3 microdeletions described to date. Minimal region of overlap highlighted by the *dashed orange lines*. The figure was drawn according to the UCSC Genome Browser on Human Feb. 2009 (GRCh37/hg19) assembly

**Table 1** Clinical features of patients carrying overlapping 1p21.3 deletions

| | Carter pt 1 | Carter pt 2, pt 3 | Willemsen pt 1, pt2, pt 3 | Willemsen pt 4 | Willemsen pt 5 | D'Angelo pt 1 | D'Angelo pt 2 | Pinto pt 8658_201 | Our case |
|---|---|---|---|---|---|---|---|---|---|
| Chromosome Position on chr 1 (hg19) | 97,559,579–98,652,079 | 96,969,562–98,471,225 | 97,727,412–99,477,412 | 97,547,412–98,957,412 | 96,497,412–98,947,412 | 93,919,217–99,846,176 | 95,696,444–107,755,879 | 98,403,034–101,151,364 | 98,456,293–103,682,084 |
| Age | 13 years 9 months | 7 years, 5 years | 42 years, 38 years, NA | 33 years | 18 years | 15 years | 8 years 8 months | NA | 10 years |
| Gender | M | M, F | M, M, F | M | F | F | F | F | |
| Intellectual disability | Severe language delay | Severe language delay | Borderline, Mild-moderate | Mild | Moderate | Language delay | Severe language delay | Severe language delay | Mild |
| Autism spectrum disorder | + | + | + | + | + | NA | + | + | + |
| Weight | NA | > > $97^{th}$ centile 50th centile, | $90^{th}$, >$98^{th}$ centile | $98^{th}$ centile | >$98^{th}$ centile | >$95^{th}$ centile | >$95^{th}$ centile | Overweight | Overweight |
| Dysmorphic features | NA | + | + | + | + | + | - | NA | - |
| Ocular problems | NA | NA | Myopia, astigmatism | Myopia, astigmatism | / | Myopia | / | NA | Hypermetropy |
| Precocious puberty | NA | NA | - | - | - | - | + | NA | + |
| Others | / | Small joint hypermobility, macrocephaly | / | / | / | / | / | High pain intolerance | Bicuspic aortic valve |

modulating neurogenesis, with a dose-dependent effect [11]. Moreover, the miR137 targets Ezh2, a H3-K27 methyltransferase involved in the regulation of neuroprogenitor cell maintenance and differentiation [12]. Notably, mutations in the *EZH2* gene cause Weaver syndrome, another syndromic overgrowth disorder characterized by ID, dysmorphic features and obesity [13]. Although the role of neuronal noncoding RNAs in the energy control of the body is not fully understood, recently, the hypothalamic miR-103 has been shown to protect against hyperphagic obesity in mice [14]. Therefore, the role of miR-137 in the control of food intake or energy accumulation and expenditure in the CNS can be speculated.

At a peripheral level, recent studies have shown that miRNAs are dysregulated in obese adipose tissue [15]. Furthermore, during adipogenesis, miRNAs regulate fat cell development by accelerating or inhibiting adipocyte differentiation. In addition, miRNAs may regulate the commitment to the adipogenic lineage in multipotent stem cells and therefore govern the numbers of fat cells [16].

Ninety-two percent of the cases carrying 1p21.3 deletion present with ASD. miR-137 is a brain expressed miRNA [17, 18] that regulates several protein coding genes that are important for brain function, and involved in the pathogenesis of neuropsychiatric disorders including schizophrenia [17, 19]. Functional studies indicate that miR-137 is involved in controlling neuronal differentiation and maturation [20, 21] as well as synapse development [22], all of which have been implicated on the pathogenesis of autism [20, 23]. Of note, lymphoblastoid cell lines from patients carrying 1p21.3 deletion involving the miR-137 gene have reduced levels of miR-137 [4]. miR-137 is highly expressed in the hippocampus, occipital cortex, and frontal cortex in human post-mortem tissue, as well as in the synaptosomal fractions in mouse brain preparations, providing further evidence that miR-137 plays a role in synapse formation during brain development [4].

Several studies have implicated miRNA in autism. A number of miRNAs have shown differing expression levels in samples from autistic individuals compared to matched controls [24, 25], suggesting that dysregulation of miRNAs could be related to autism. Furthermore, miR-137 has been recently implicated in ASD via a genome-wide meta-analysis that considered single nucleotide polymorphism data across five psychiatric disorders (ASD, attention deficit-hyperactivity disorder, bipolar disorder, major depressive disorder, and schizophrenia), and found an association between mir-137 and both schizophrenia and ASD [26].

Lastly, Devanna and Vernes provided support for miR-137 as an autism candidate by showing that the RORa gene, a novel autism candidate gene, is regulated directly by miR-137 through targeting its 3 UTR in a site-specific manner [27].

It is therefore likely that the core clinical features of obesity and ASD in patients carrying 1p21.3 deletion are both mediated by miR-137.

The case herein described presents with clinical features not previously described in the 1p21.3 microdeletion syndrome, such as precocious puberty and bicuspid aortic valve, with mild stenosis of the aortic root. The boy carries a 1p21.3 deletion, which extends 5 Mb proximally to the SRO and includes a number of genes. *PALMD* and *S1PR1* encode for proteins that are expressed during normal embryonic heart development and morphogenesis. Specifically, PALMD has been associated with aortic root size [28], while S1PR1 has an important role in the regulation of sprouting angiogenesis and vascular maturation. It inhibits sprouting angiogenesis to prevent excessive sprouting during blood vessel development [29]. With regard to precocious puberty, we found two DECIPHER patients that carried deletions partially overlapping with our case and precocious puberty: case 260349, which presented with precocious puberty and specific learning disability and carrying a deletion at chr1:97,000,749–99,813,665; case 254871 presented with ASD, ID, precocious puberty and spotty hyperpigmentation, carrying the deletion at chr1:97019762–102447536. The SRO among these microdeletions includes the SNX7, PLPPR4 and PLPPR5 genes. Both PLPPR4 and PLPPR5 encode for a lipid phosphate phosphatase enzyme specifically expressed in neurons and located in the membranes of outgrowing axons, important for axonal outgrowth during development and regenerative sprouting [30, 31].

In summary, with this study, we present a case carrying a novel 1p31.3 microdeletion, and we propose that the miRNA miR137 is the mediator of the obesity, ASD and ID phenotype. Further studies are warranted to elucidate the molecular mechanisms by which miR-137 mediates the phenotype, both in the CNS and the adipose tissue.

### Abbreviations

ASD: Autism-spectrum disorders; BMI: Body mass index; CNS: Central nervous system; CSF: Cerebrospinal fluid; ID: Intellectual disability; MRI: Magnetic resonance imaging; SRO: Shortest region of overlap; UTRs: Untraslated regions

### Acknowledgements

We thank the patient and his parents for their kind cooperation.

### Funding

Not applicable.

### Authors' contributions

AT performed the paediatric evaluation of the patient, wrote the manuscript and analysed the SNP array result; CC and GS analysed the SNP array result and e and critically read the manuscript; SE revised the manuscript critically;

DM initiated the study, performed the paediatric evaluation of the patient, made substantial contribution to study design and revised the manuscript critically. All authors read and approved the final manuscript.

### Competing interests

The authors declare that they have no competing interests.

### References


1. Maes HH, Neale MC, Eaves LJ. Genetic and environmental factors in relative body weight and human adiposity. Behav Genet. 1997;27(4):325–51.
2. Santangelo SL, Tsatsanis K. What is known about autism: genes, brain, and behavior. Am J Pharmacogenomics Genomics. 2005;5(2):71–92.
3. D'Angelo CS, Moller Dos Santos MF, Alonso LG, Koiffmann CP. Two new cases of 1p21.3 deletions and an unbalanced translocation t(8;12) among individuals with syndromic obesity. Mol Syndromol. 2015;6(2):63–70.
4. Willemsen MH, Vallès A, Kirkels LAMH, Mastebroek M, Olde Loohuis N, Kos A, Wissink-Lindhout WM, de Brouwer APM, Nillesen WM, Pfundt R, Holder-Espinasse M, Vallée L, Andrieux J, Coppens-Hofman MC, Rensen H, Hamel BCJ, van Bokhoven H, Aschrafi A, Kleefstra T. Chromosome 1p21.3 microdeletions comprising DPYD and MIR137 are associated with intellectual disability. J Med Genet. 2011;48(12):810–8.
5. Carter MT, Nikkel SM, Fernandez BA, Marshall CR, Noor A, Lionel AC, Prasad A, Pinto D, Joseph-George AM, Noakes C, Fairbrother-Davies C, Roberts W, Vincent J, Weksberg R, Scherer SW. Hemizygous deletions on chromosome 1p21.3 involving the DPYD gene in individuals with autism spectrum disorder. Clin Genet. 2011;80(5):435–43.
6. Pinto D, Delaby E, Merico D, Barbosa M, Merikangas A, Klei L, Thiruvahindrapuram B, Xu X, Ziman R, Wang Z, Vorstman JAS, Thompson A, Regan R, Pilorge M, Pellecchia G, Pagnamenta AT, Oliveira B, Marshall CR, Magalhaes TR, Lowe JK, Howe JL, Griswold AJ, Gilbert J, Duketis E, Dombroski BA, De Jonge MV, Cuccaro M, Crawford EL, Correia CT, Conroy J, Conceição IC, Chiocchetti AG, Casey JP, Cai G, Cabrol C, Bolshakova N, Bacchelli E, Anney R, Gallinger S, Cotterchio M, Casey G, Zwaigenbaum L, Wittemeyer K, Wing K, Wallace S, van Engeland H, Tryfon A, Thomson S, Soorya L, Rogé B, Roberts W, Poustka F, Mouga S, Minshew N, McInnes LA, McGrew SG, Lord C, Leboyer M, Le Couteur AS, Kolevzon A, Jiménez González P, Jacob S, Holt R, Guter S, Green J, Green A, Gillberg C, Fernandez BA, Duque F, Delorme R, Dawson G, Chaste P, Café C, Brennan S, Bourgeron T, Bolton PF, Bölte S, Bernier R, Baird G, Bailey AJ, Anagnostou E, Almeida J, Wijsman EM, Vieland VJ, Vicente AM, Schellenberg GD, Pericak-Vance M, Paterson AD, Parr JR, Oliveira G, Nurnberger JI, Monaco AP, Maestrini E, Klauck SM, Hakonarson H, Haines JL, Geschwind DH, Freitag CM, Folstein SE, Ennis S, Coon H, Battaglia A, Szatmari P, Sutcliffe JS, Hallmayer J, Gill M, Cook EH, Buxbaum JD, Devlin B, Gallagher L, Betancur C, Scherer SW. Convergence of genes and cellular pathways dysregulated in autism spectrum disorders. Am J Hum Genet. 2014;94(5):677–94.
7. Bartel DP. MicroRNAs: target recognition and regulatory functions. Cell. 2009;136(2):215–33.
8. Ambros V. The functions of animal microRNAs. Nature. 2004;431(7006):350–5.
9. Plasterk RHA. Micro RNAs in animal development. Cell. 2006;124(5):877–81.
10. Guella I, Sequeira A, Rollins B, Morgan L, Torri F, van Erp TGM, Myers RM, Barchas JD, Schatzberg AF, Watson SJ, Akil H, Bunney WE, Potkin SG, Macciardi F, Vawter MP. Analysis of miR-137 expression and rs1625579 in dorsolateral prefrontal cortex. J Psychiatr Res. 2013;47(9):1215–21.
11. Szulwach KE, Li X, Smrt RD, Li Y, Luo Y, Lin L, Santistevan NJ, Li W, Zhao X, Jin P. Cross talk between microRNA and epigenetic regulation in adult neurogenesis. J Cell Biol. 2010;189(1):127–41.
12. Sher F, Rössler R, Brouwer N, Balasubramaniyan V, Boddeke E, Copray S. Differentiation of neural stem cells into oligodendrocytes: involvement of the polycomb group protein Ezh2. Stem Cells Dayt Ohio. 2008;26(11):2875–83.
13. Tatton-Brown K, Hanks S, Ruark E, Zachariou A, Duarte SDV, Ramsay E, Snape K, Murray A, Perdeaux ER, Seal S, Loveday C, Banka S, Clericuzio C, Flinter F, Magee A, McConnell V, Patton M, Raith W, Rankin J, Splitt M, Strenger V, Taylor C, Wheeler P, Temple KI, Cole T, Douglas J, Rahman N, Childhood Overgrowth Collaboration. Germline mutations in the oncogene EZH2 cause Weaver syndrome and increased human height. Oncotarget. 2011;2(12):1127–33.
14. Vinnikov IA, Hajdukiewicz K, Reymann J, Beneke J, Czajkowski R, Roth LC, Novak M, Roller A, Dörner N, Starkuviene V, Theis FJ, Erfle H, Schütz G, Grinevich V, Konopka W. Hypothalamic miR-103 protects from hyperphagic obesity in mice. J Neurosci Off J Soc Neurosci. 2014;34(32):10659–74.
15. Xie H, Sun L, Lodish HF. Targeting microRNAs in obesity. Expert Opin Ther Targets. 2009;13(10):1227–38.
16. McGregor RA, Choi MS. microRNAs in the regulation of adipogenesis and obesity. Curr Mol Med. 2011;11(4):304–16.
17. Forero DA, vanderVen K, Callaerts P, Del-Favero J. miRNA genes and the brain: implications for psychiatric disorders. Hum Mutat. 2010;31(11):1195–204.
18. Liang Y, Ridzon D, Wong L, Chen C. Characterization of microRNA expression profiles in normal human tissues. BMC Genomics. 2007;8:166.
19. Wright C, Calhoun VD, Ehrlich S, Wang L, Turner JA, Perrone-Bizzozero NI. Meta gene set enrichment analyses link miR-137-regulated pathways with schizophrenia risk. Front Genet. 2015;6:147.
20. Mariani J, Coppola G, Zhang P, Abyzov A, Provini L, Tomasini L, Amenduni M, Szekely A, Palejev D, Wilson M, Gerstein M, Grigorenko EL, Chawarska K, Pelphrey KA, Howe JR, Vaccarino FM. FOXG1-dependent dysregulation of GABA/Glutamate neuron differentiation in autism spectrum disorders. Cell. 2015;162(2):375–90.
21. Smrt RD, Szulwach KE, Pfeiffer RL, Li X, Guo W, Pathania M, Teng ZQ, Luo Y, Peng J, Bordey A, Jin P, Zhao X. MicroRNA miR-137 regulates neuronal maturation by targeting ubiquitin ligase mind bomb-1. Stem Cells. 2010; 28(6):1060–70.
22. Collins AL, Kim Y, Bloom RJ, Kelada SN, Sethupathy P, Sullivan PF. Transcriptional targets of the schizophrenia risk gene MIR137. Transl Psychiatry. 2014;4:e404.
23. Penzes P, Cahill ME, Jones KA, VanLeeuwen JE, Woolfrey KM. Dendritic spine pathology in neuropsychiatric disorders. Nat Neurosci. 2011;14(3):285–93.
24. Sarachana T, Zhou R, Chen G, Manji HK, Hu VW. Investigation of posttranscriptional gene regulatory networks associated with autism spectrum disorders by microRNA expression profiling of lymphoblastoid cell lines. Genome Med. 2010;2(4):23.
25. Abu-Elneel K, et al. Heterogeneous dysregulation of microRNAs across the autism spectrum. Neurogenetics. 2008;9(3):153–61.
26. Cross-Disorder Group of the Psychiatric Genomics Consortium. Identification of risk loci with shared effects on five major psychiatric disorders: a genome-wide analysis. Lancet. 2013;381(9875):1371–9.
27. Devanna P, Vernes SC. A direct molecular link between the autism candidate gene RORa and the schizophrenia candidate MIR137. Sci Rep. 2014;4:3994.
28. Vasan RS, Glazer NL, Felix JF, Lieb W, Wild PS, Felix SB, Watzinger N, Larson MG, Smith NL, Dehghan A, Grosshennig A, Schillert A, Teumer A, Schmidt R, Kathiresan S, Lumley T, Aulchenko YS, König IR, Zeller T, Homuth G, Struchalin M, Aragam J, Bis JC, Rivadeneira F, Erdmann J, Schnabel RB, Dörr M, Zweiker R, Lind L, Rodeheffer RJ, Greiser KH, Levy D, Haritunians T, Deckers JW, Stritzke J, Lackner KJ, Völker U, Ingelsson E, Kullo I, Haerting J, O'Donnell CJ, Heckbert SR, Stricker BH, Ziegler A, Reffelmann T, Redfield MM, Werdan K, Mitchell GF, Rice K, Arnett DK, Hofman A, Gottdiener JS, Uitterlinden AG, Meitinger T, Blettner M, Friedrich N, Wang TJ, Psaty BM, van Duijn CM, Wichmann HE, Munzel TF, Kroemer HK, Benjamin EJ, Rotter JI, Witteman JC, Schunkert H, Schmidt H, Völzke H, Blankenberg S. Genetic variants associated with cardiac structure and function: a meta-analysis and replication of genome-wide association data. JAMA. 2009;302(2):168–78.
29. Mendelson K, Zygmunt T, Torres-Vázquez J, Evans T, Hla T. Sphingosine 1-phosphate receptor signaling regulates proper embryonic vascular patterning. J Biol Chem. 2013;288(4):2143–56.
30. Sciorra VA, Morris AJ. Roles for lipid phosphate phosphatases in regulation of cellular signaling. Biochim Biophys Acta. 2002;1582(1–3):45–51.
31. Broggini T, Nitsch R, Savaskan NE. Plasticity-related gene 5 (PRG5) induces filopodia and neurite growth and impedes lysophosphatidic acid- and nogo-A-mediated axonal retraction. Mol Biol Cell. 2010;21(4):521–37.

5

# Effect of SP600125 on the mitotic spindle in HeLa Cells, leading to mitotic arrest, endoreduplication and apoptosis

Donia Mili*, Kaouthar Abid, Imed Rjiba and Abderraouf Kenani

**Abstract**

**Background:** The JNK inhibitor SP600125 strongly inhibits cell proliferation in many human cancer cells by blocking mitosis progression and inducing cell death. Despite, all this study, the mechanism by which SP600125 inhibits mitosis-related effects in human cervical cells (HeLa cells) remains unclear. In this study, we investigated the effects of SP600125 on the cell viability, cell cycle, and on the spindle assembly during mitosis in HeLa cells.

**Methods:** To explore this approach, we used a viability test, an immunofluorescence microscopy to detect Histone phosphorylation and mitotic spindle aberrations. Apoptosis was characterised using Western Blotting.

**Results:** Treatment of HeLa cells with varying concentrations of SP600125 induces significant G2/M cell cycle arrest with elevated phosphorylation of histone H3 within 48 h, and endoreduplication after 48 h. SP600125 also induces significant abnormal mitotic spindle. High concentrations of SP600125 (20 μM) induce disturbing microtubule assembly in vitro. Additionally, SP600125- induced delayed apoptosis and cell death was accompanied by significant poly ADP-ribose polymerase (PARP) cleavage and caspase-3 activation in the late phase (at 72 h).

**Conclusion:** Our results confirmed that SP600125 induce mitosis arrest in G2/M, endoreduplication, mitotic spindle aberrations and apoptosis.

**Keywords:** SP600125, HeLa cells, Mitotic spindle, Apoptosis

## Background

Faithful transmission of genetic information during mitosis is ensured by the spindle assembly checkpoints [1]. Cell cycle progression to the G1, S, and G2/M phases is controlled by those cell cycle checkpoints that ensure the correct order and transition timing of the mitotic spindle [2]. After G2/M arrest, a significant subpopulation of pRb-negative cells demonstrated an excessive amount of 4 N DNA, known as endoreduplication [3]. Many agents are known for their effect of endoreduplication: agents that interfere with spindle assembly (eg. Microtubule polylerisation inhibitors eg., colchicines), the enzyme poisons (eg: amsacrine, and Adriamycin), catalytic inhibitors (eg: merbarone, aclarubicin) and physical agents that damage DNA, such as X-rays. Some of these microtubule-interfering agents, such as nocodazole and paclitaxel, induce significant endoreduplication due to the sister chromatid miss-segregation [4].

SP600125 is an anthrapyrazolone inhibitor of JNK that competes with ATP to inhibit the phosphorylation of c-Jun. Although JNK appears to be involved in cell proliferation, there is no evidence linking JNK activation to specific phases of the cell cycle. In fact, in Jurkat cells, JNK activity increased in G2/M checkpoint and was demonstrated to be responsible for apoptotic Bcl-2 phosphorylation [5]. Recent studies have focused on the effects of JNK in the promotion of cell death, and it has been reported that the JNK-antisense oligonucleotide inhibits tumour growth and induces regression in a high number of cases [6, 7].

Some research indicates that JNK activity is essential to maintain proliferation and diploidy in cancer cells. However, the induction mechanisms of G2/M arrest,

* Correspondence: doniamili@gmail.com
UR 12ES08 "Signalisation Cellulaire et Pathologies" Faculté de Médecine Monastir, Université de Monastir, Monastir, Tunisie

endoreduplication, and apoptosis due to SP600125 still unclear [8].

In this study, we investigated the relationships between polyploid giant cells and apoptosis in human cervical cells treated with SP600125. We tried to explore the effects of SP600125 in G2/M phase arrest, endoreduplication, and delayed apoptosis via disorganization of the mitotic spindle assembly.

## Methods

### Reagents

The specific JNK inhibitor SP600125 was purchased from Sigma (S5567). The inhibitor was reconstituted in DMSO to make a 10 mM stock solution, and DMSO (0.1%) was used as a control vehicle. MTT, Hoechst 33258. (861405 Sigma Aldrich), were purchased from Sigma (St. Louis, MO). Triton and FBS were purchased from GIBCO (Gaithersburg, MD). An enhanced chemiluminescence (ECL) kit was purchased from Amersham (Arlington Heights, IL). Rabbit Anti-Histone H3 (phospho S10) antibody (ab47297). Primary antibodies were detected using an anti-mouse and anti-rabbit secondary antibodies conjugated with Alexa Fluorescent.

### Cell lines and cell culture

HeLa human carcinoma epithelial cell lines were obtained from the American type culture collection (ATCC. CCL-2). Cells were grown in DMEM supplemented with 10% heat-inactivated FBS and 1% penicillin- streptomycin (GIBCO) in 5% CO2 at 37 °C. Cells were seeded at $5 \times 10^4$ cells/ml and treated with SP600125 at the indicated times. Cell growth was determined using MTT assays.

### Immunofluorescence analysis

For immunofluorescence analysis, Firstly, we brought the cells, already cultured and transfected on a glass coverslip in a 24-well plate. The cells were washed three times with phosphate-buffered saline (PBS) and then fixed with PBS containing 4% paraformaldehyde at room temperature for 30 min. The fixed cells were washed with PBS containing 0.1% Triton X-100 and then blocked with 1 mg/ml NaBH4 in PBS. After been blocked, the cells were incubated for 1 h with the primary antibodies, mouse monoclonal anti-α-tubulin (F2168 clone DM1A purified immunoglobulin, monoclonal anti-α-tubulin-FITC antibody produced in mouse, Sigma Aldrich).

The cells were then washed three times with PBS containing 0.1% Triton X-100 and incubated with a secondary antibody, Alexa-fluor 488 anti- Mouse antibody (62197 Sigma Aldrich) and Alaxa-fluor 568 anti-rabbit Antibody (SAB1102713 Sigma Aldrich) for 20 min, at room temperature and away from light.

For DNA staining, cells were incubated with 5 μg/ml Hoechst 33342 for 5 min prior to fixation. Glass coverslip was mounted on a glass slide with the Fluor save (Calbiochem 34 5789) and examined under a fluorescence microscope.

### Statistical analysis

All data from cell counts, MTT assays, PARP and caspase-3 activity experiments were derived from at least three independent experiments. Images were visualized with a Zeiss Axiovert 200 M inverted microscope. Images were captured using CoolSnap HQ (Photometrics) black and white camera driven by the Metamorph software (Universal Imaging) then downloaded into Photoshop. Image J (1.49 V) was used to quantify the Western blots. Statistical analyses were conducted using Sigma Plot software, and values are presented as mean ± SD. Significant differences between groups were determined using an unpaired Student's t-test. A value of $^*P < 0.05$ was accepted as an indication of statistical significance.

## Results

### SP600125 induces a dose-dependent inhibition in cell viability and expansion of cell size in human HeLa cells

Recent studies have shown that SP600125, a pharmacological inhibitor of JNK, causes cell viability inhibition in certain cell types, including breast cancer [8], multiple myeloma [9], and B-lymphoma [10]. To verify this effect on cervical cells, HeLa cell line was treated with varying concentrations of SP600125 for 24 h, 48 h and 72 h. Cell viability and morphological changes were assessed using MTT assays and microscopy (Fig. 1).

As shown in Fig. 1(a, a', a") significant inhibition of cell viability in a dose/time-dependent manner was observed in HeLa cell line. DMSO (0.1%), used as a vehicle control, did not affect cell viability or morphology.

In other hand, when cells were examined under phase contrast microscopy, after 48H of incubation cells treated with 20 μM SP600125 presented with swelling, condensed nucleus and modest apoptotic shrinkage at 48 h, compared to control cells (Fig. 1b). To confirm that SP600125 inhibited JNK activity, we realised a Western blot analysis using p-c-Jun antibodies in HeLa cells extract after their incubation with SP600125 during 48H. As shown in Fig. 1c, treatment with 20 μM SP600125 almost completely supressed c-Jun phosphorylation after 48 h. These results indicate that SP600125 causes antiproliferative effects with an apoptotic cell morphology in cervical cells through inhibition of JNK activity.

### SP600125 treatment induces persistence of histone H3 phosphorylation in HeLa cells during mitosis

Some research has shown that Serine 10 ($Ser^{10}$) phosphorylation of histone H3 has emerged as a sensitive

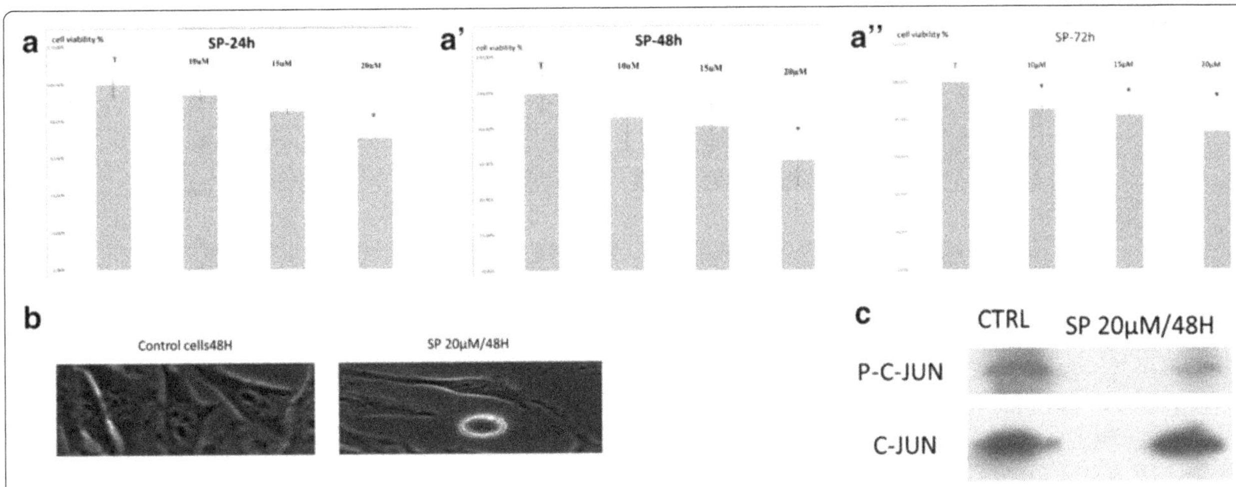


**Fig. 1** **a** HeLa cells were plated at 5 × 104 cells/ml and incubated for 24 h. Cells were treated with the indicated concentrations of SP600125 and the cell viability was measured using a metabolic-dye-based MTT assay. Each point represents the mean ± SD of three independent experiments. Significance was determined using Student's test (*$P < 0.05$ vs. vehicle control). **a'** HeLa cells were plated at 5 × 104 cells/ml and incubated for 48 h. Cells were treated with the indicated concentrations of SP600125 and the cell viability was measured using a metabolic-dye-based MTT assay. Each point represents the mean ± SD of three independent experiments. Significance was determined using Student's test (*$P < 0.05$ vs. vehicle control). **a''**: HeLa cells were plated at 5 × 104 cells/ml and incubated for 72 h. Cells were treated with the indicated concentrations of SP600125 and the cell viability was measured using a metabolic-dye-based MTT assay. Each point represents the mean ± SD of three independent experiments. Significance was determined using Student's test (*$P < 0.05$ vs. vehicle control). **b** Cells were incubated with the indicated concentrations of SP600125. After a 48 h-incubation, cells were sampled and examined under light microscopy. Magnification × 200. **c** After HeLa cells were treated with SP600125 for the indicated time, expression of c-Jun and phosphorylated c-Jun was detected using Western blot analysis

marker for mitotic cells [11]. In mammalian cells, site-specific phosphorylation of H3 at Ser$^{10}$ has been shown to initiate bulk phosphorylation during prophase, become maximal during metaphase, diminish during anaphase and is lost during telophase. Drugs that induce the phosphorylation of H3 also initiate premature chromosomal condensation in cell lines. Also, drug-induced dephosphorylation of H3 were correlated with chromosome relaxation [12].

In this study, we tried to use this approach by using antibodies highly selective to the amino-terminus of H3 in a phosphorylated Ser$^{10}$ form. As shown in Fig. 2a, Ser$^{10}$ phosphorylation of histone H3 was retained in HeLa cells at 48 h. SP600125 time-specifically induced G2/M phase arrest at 48 h with histone H3 phosphorylation on Ser$^{10}$ as a G2/M arrest marker, and then induced endoreduplication at 48 h (Fig. 2b). Finaly HeLa cells presented significant signs of apoptosis and endoreduplication.

### SP600125 induces the formation of aberrant mitotic spindle

Microtubules (MTs) play an important role in cell replication and division, maintenance of cell shape, and cellular movement. Microtubules are composed of α-, β-tubulin, and microtubule-associated proteins (MAPs). They are in an unstable steady state of a highly dynamic process of polymerization and depolymerization, and disrupting the dynamics of microtubules leads to endoreduplication.

In order to examine the MTs assembly in SP600125-mediated endoreduplication, we reasoned that the mitotic spindle itself might be a target of SP600125 effect. To respond to this question, we examined whether mitotic cells treated with 20 μM SP600125 displayed many changes in tubulin polymerization. Treatment with SP600125 increased the abnormal structure and promoted an increased intensity of α-tubulin staining, measured by indirect immunofluorescence (Fig. 3). Immunofluorescence analysis does not clearly provide a quantitative measure of tubulin polymerization in the cell but it shows the formation of aberrant structures: mini spindle with shifted chromosomes, mini spindle and spindle with reduced density of microtubules, multipolar spindle as shown in Fig. 3 [13].

### SP600125 induces apoptosis in HeLa cells after endoreduplication and aneuploidy

To assess whether delayed apoptosis contributed to the viability inhibition effects of SP600125, we investigated the effects of SP600125 on apoptosis.

Apoptosis is controlled by a complex interplay between many proteins. Bcl-2, a 26-kDa integral membrane oncoprotein, was the first anti-apoptosis gene product discovered. Several research has demonstrated that overexpression of Bcl-2 protein protects cells from apoptosis in some cell lines [12]; although a recent

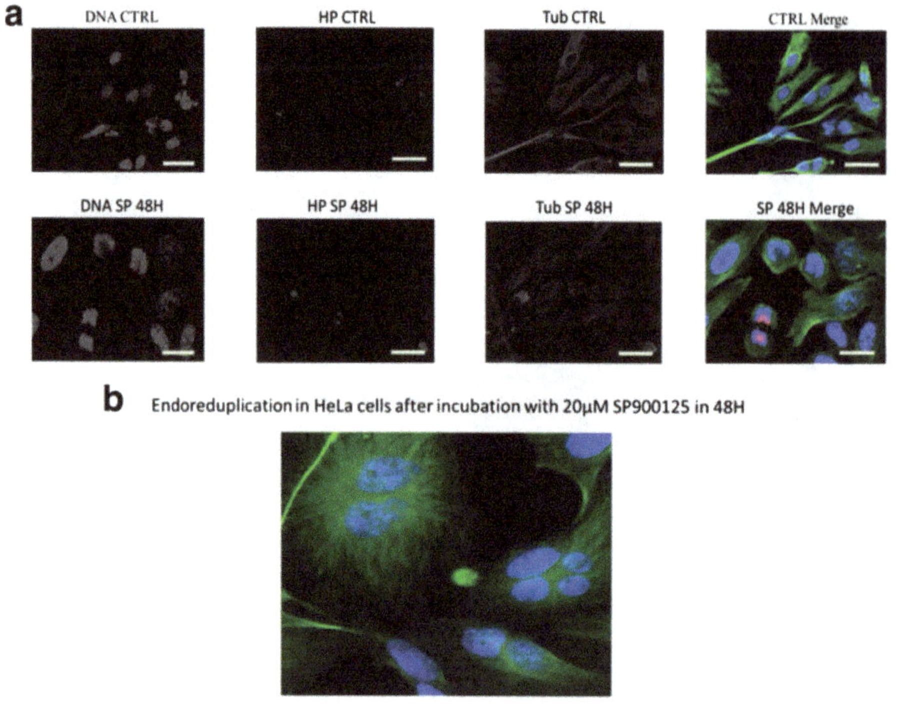


**Fig. 2** **a** Histone 3 Phosphorylation was analyzed using immunofluorescent staining in HeLa cells treated with 20 μM SP600125 for the indicated times. Cells were fixed, permeabilized, and stained. Tubulin tagged with IgG anti-tubulin, H3 phosphorylated was stained with Rabbit Anti-Histone H3 (phospho S10) antibody (ab47297). Primary antibodies was detected using an anti-mouse and anti- rabbit secondary antibodies conjugated with Alexa Fluorescent (*Green* for tubulin and *Red* for H3P). Cells were analyzed using fluorescence microscopy (×400). Hoechst 33258 was used for nuclear staining. **b** Endoreduplication detected using Immunofluorescence in HeLa cells treated with 20 μM SP600125 for 48H. Tubulin tagged with IgG anti-tubulin. Primary antibody was detected using an anti- mouse secondary antibody conjugated with Alexa Fluorescent (*Green* for tubulin)

report indicates that the level of this oncoprotein is not always correlated with an increased ability of the cell to resist death-promoting stimuli [14]. Recently, some research, reported that treatment with either okadaic acid, a potent inhibitor of phosphatase, or the antitubulin agent paclitaxel induced in Bcl-2 protein phosphorylation and induction of programmed cell death in lymphoid cells. Suggesting that Bcl-2 phosphorylation may change its antiapoptotic function. Whereas anticancer drugs damaging DNA do not [12].

In this study, in HeLa cells, SP600125 (20 μM) induced an increase in the multinuclear giant cell population (>4 N DNA) (Fig. 4b) and the caspase-3 activation (Fig. 4a) in a time-dependent manner. Western blot analysis also demonstrated that SP600125 caused PARP cleavage and Bcl-2 downregulation (Fig. 4c), suggesting that the inhibitory effects of SP600125 on cervical cell viability are dependent on apoptosis.

## Discussion

SP600125 has been implicated in G2/M arrest and apoptosis, but its precise role remains unknown [15]. The present study provides the mechanism to explain the induction of G2/M arrest, endoreduplication, and delayed apoptosis caused by SP600125 in cervical cells.

As shown in Fig. 2a, we have demonstrated that SP600125 (I- arrests G2/M phases with phosphorylation of histone H3 at 24 h; (II- suggesting that SP600125 induces endoreduplication; (III- promotes spindle aberrations, a critical process in cell division; and (IV- induces delayed apoptosis in HeLa cells. Therefore, SP600125 has a strong anticancer effect against cervical cells in a dose- and time-dependent manner by disturbing tubulin polymerization and disrupting the organization of the microtubule mitotic cytoskeleton.

The G2/M checkpoint is especially important in protecting normal cells from tumour formation driven by the accumulation of mutations [16]. Therefore, elimination of the checkpoint increases the sensitivity of human tumour cell lines to anticancer agents. Some studies have reported that the G2/M arrest induced by SP600125 may be due to inhibition of cyclin B/Cdk1 kinase activity through an increase in p21 levels [17, 18]. Increased JNK activity is important for the dissociation of p21 and JNK, following which cells enter into the S phases [8].

Using biochemical and immunofluorescence methods, we have shown that SP60015 significantly increases tubulin disorders. Microtubules are crucial cellular and structural components that induce cellular development, division, and movement [19]. Therefore, microtubule-

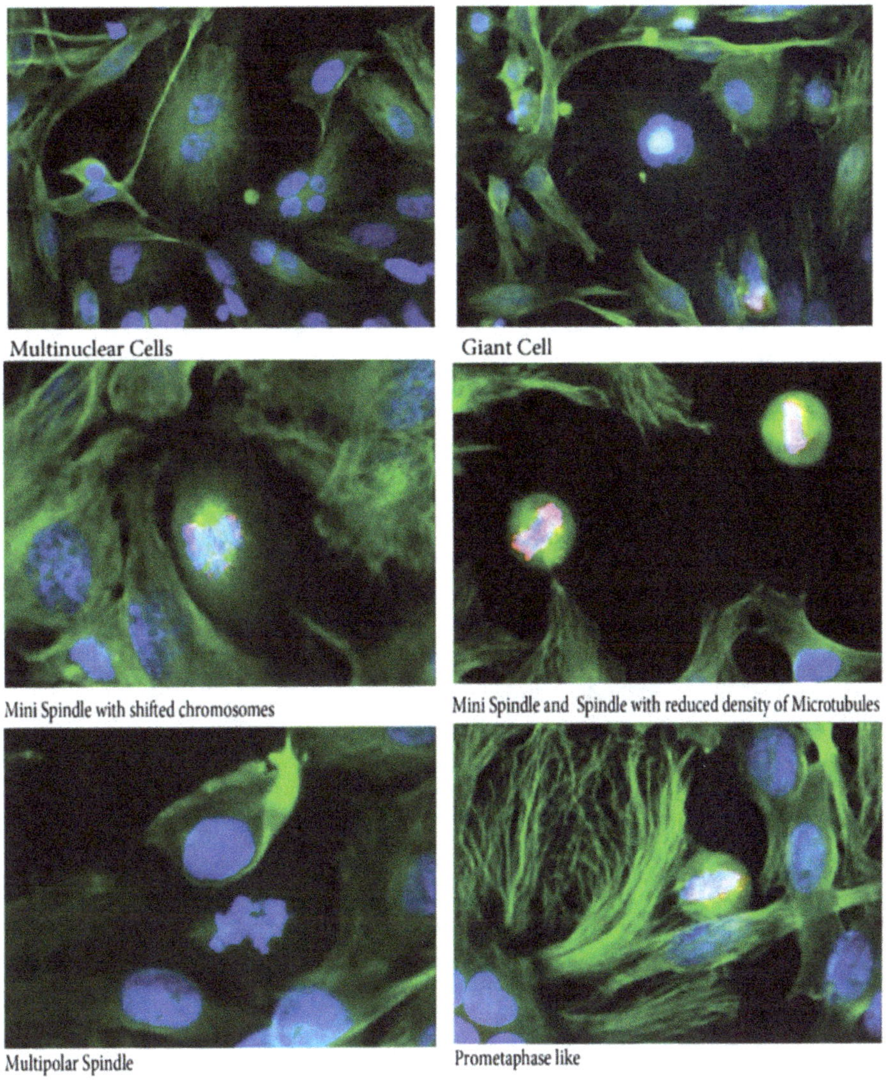


**Fig. 3** Immunofluorescence analysis shows clearly the formation of aberrant mitotic spindle structure. Spindle perturbation in HeLa cells after SP600125, Tubulin tagged with IgG anti-tubulin (*green* fluorescence), and DNA labelled with Hoechst

disrupting agents provide a novel approach to cancer chemoprevention and/or cancer therapy.

Recently, certain cancer chemotherapy agents have been found to exert their anticancer activities by disrupting the dynamics of microtubule assembly, thus perturbing the formation and function of the mitotic spindle apparatus and arresting cells in mitosis [20, 21]. This action of SP600125 is similar to that of paclitaxel, which binds to tubulin and increases tubulin polymerization, causing cells to arrest in the G2/M phase thereby blocking cell cycle progression [13]. Our results strongly support the idea that SP600125 inhibits cell proliferation by inhibiting mitosis through disturbing tubulin polymerization.

Tumour cells often evade apoptosis by overexpressing anti-apoptotic proteins, such as Bcl-2, which give them a survival advantage [22]. Recently, contrasting results have been reported. In fact, decreased or phosphorylated Bcl-2 is implicated in the resistance of human ovarian cancer cells to tubulin polymerizing agents, such as paclitaxel [23, 24]. Other reports have shown that Bcl-2 phosphorylation is a common event in mitosis [14].

Our results have shown that the level of endogenous Bcl-2 expression does not affect SP600125-induced endoreduplication up to 24 h (Fig. 4c).

## Conclusion

In conclusion, our findings indicate a role for both targeting (tubulin polymerization) and signalling (Bcl-2) in human cervical cells for SP600125. Increased p-histone H3 protein expressions were found to be responsible for SP600125-induced G2/M arrest at 48 h and high

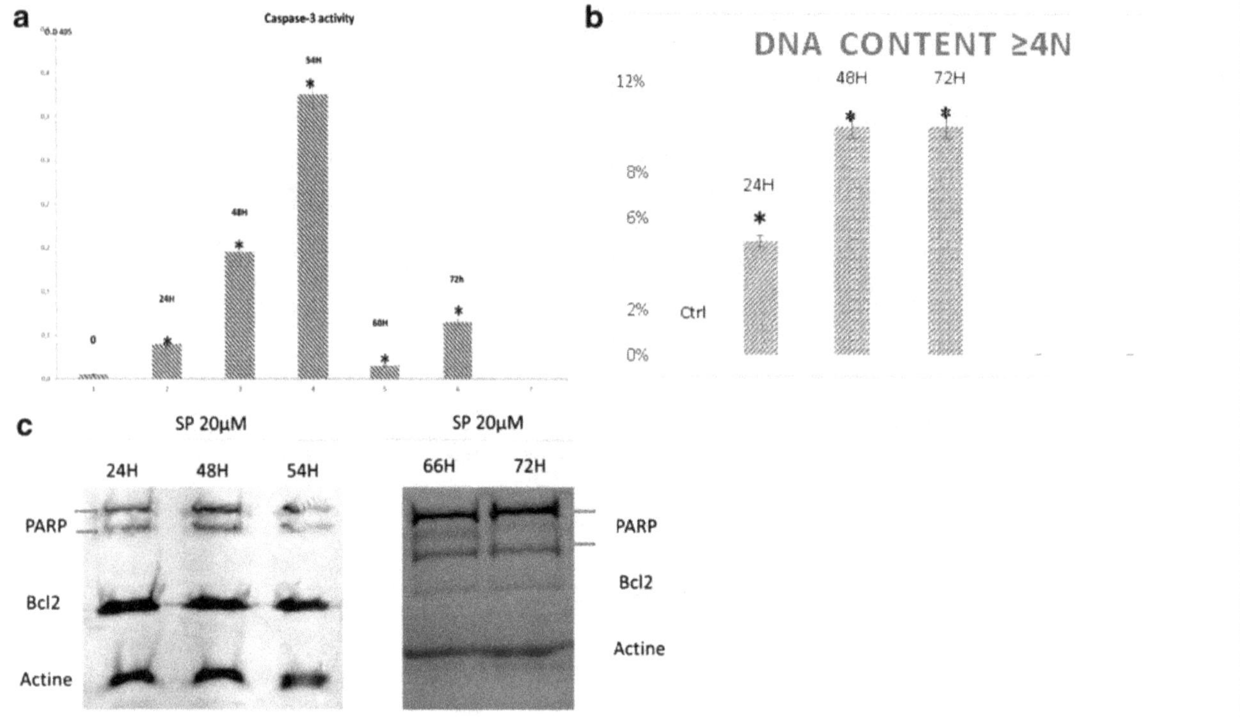


**Fig. 4** **a** SP 20 µM, after 48 h of treatment with SP600125, the caspase-3 activity was assayed using a caspase assay kit, following the manufacturer's protocol. **b** Quantification of Multinucleated cells observed because of the SP600125 incubation (20 µM). Time dependent experience. The average value ± SD from three independent experiments is also shown. Asterisks indicate significant differences (* $p < 0.05$) calculated by the Duncan's t-test. **c** Equal amounts of cell lysate (60 µg) were resolved using SDS-PAGE, transferred to nitrocellulose, and probed with specific antibodies (anti-PARP and anti-Bcl-2). Actin was used as an internal loading control

SP600125-induced endoreduplication at 48 h. SP600125-induced delayed apoptosis was related to Bcl-2 expression, which was closely related to endoreduplication. Further studies are necessary to clarify the exact mechanisms that are induced by SP600125 involved in specific stages of cell apoptosis.

### Abbreviations
ATP: Adenosine triphosphate; DNA: Deoxyribonucleic acid; H3: Histone 3; JNK: Jun kinase; MAPs: Microtubules associated proteins; MTs: Microtubules; PARP: Poly ADP-ribose polymerase (PARP); Ser: Serine

### Acknowledgements
We gratefully acknowledge the financial support of the University of Monastir and the scientific support of the INSERM.

### Funding
The study was part of a project funded by Unité 836 INSERM, eq7, Grenoble France and l'Unité de recherche UR 12ES08 "Signalisation Cellulaire et Pathologies" in the faculty of Medecine Monastir, Tunisia. The research team declares that the copyrights are reserved to this two teams and that all views, scientific findings, conclusions, and recommendations mentioned in the study represent the sole opinion of the research team.

### Authors' contribution
INSERM U836 conceived of the study and participated in its design. Donia Mili and Kaouthar Abid carried all the techniques used in this research and helped to draft the manuscript. Imed Rjiba and Abderraouf Kenani interpreted the molecular and the statistical results, and corrected the manuscript. All authors read and approved the final manuscript.

### Competing interest
The authors declare that they have no conflicts of interest with the contents of this article.

### References
1. Zhou J, Yao J, Joshi HC. Attachment and tension in the spindle assembly checkpoint. J Cell Sci. 2002;115:3547–55.
2. Elledge SJ. Cell Cycle Checkpoints: Preventing an Identity Crisis. SCIENCE. 1996;274:1664-72.
3. Niculescu III AB, Chen X, Smeets M, Hengst L, Prives C, Reed SI. Effects of p21Cip1/Waf1 at Both the G1/S and the G2/M Cell Cycle Transitions: pRb Is a Critical Determinant in Blocking DNA Replication and in Preventing Endoreduplication. Mol Cell Biol. 1997;18(1):629–43.
4. Jordan MA, Toso RJ, Thrower D, Wilson L. Mechanism of mitotic block and inhibition of cell proliferation by taxol at low concentrations. Cell Biol. 1993;90:9552–6.
5. Du L, Lyle CS, Obey TB, Gaarde WA, Muir JA, Bennett BL, Chambers TC. Inhibition of Cell Proliferation and Cell Cycle Progression by Specific Inhibition of Basal JNK Activity EVIDENCE THAT MITOTIC Bcl-2 PHOSPHORYLATION IS JNK-INDEPENDENT. The Journal Of Biological Chemistry. 2004;279(19):11957–66.
6. Shin M, Yan C, Boyd D. An inhibitor of c-jun aminoterminal kinase (SP600125) represses c-Jun activation, DNA-binding and PMA-inducible 92-kDa type IV collagenase expression. Biochim Biophys Acta. 2002;1589:311–6.
7. Bennett BL, Sasaki DT, Murray BW, O'Leary EC, Sakata ST, Xu W, Leisten JC, Motiwala A, Pierce S, Satoh Y, Bhagwat SS, Manning AM, Anderson DW. SP600125, an anthrapyrazolone inhibitor of Jun N-terminal kinase. Cell Biol. 2001;98(24):13681–6.

8. Mingo-Sion AM, Marietta PM, Koller E, Wolf DM, Van Den Berg CL. Inhibition of JNK reduces G2/M transit independent of p53, leading to endoreduplication, decreased proliferation, and apoptosis in breast cancer cells. Oncogene. 2004;23:596–604.
9. Hideshima T, Hayashi T, Chauhan D, Akiyama M, Richardson P, Anderson K, Anderson K. Biologic sequelae of c-Jun NH2-terminal kinase (JNK) activation in multiple myeloma cell lines. Oncogene. 2003;22:8797–801.
10. Sarah M. Jacobs-Helber STS. Jun N-terminal kinase promotes proliferation of immature erythroid cells and erythropoietin-dependent cell lines. Blood. 2004;104(3):696-703.
11. Hendzel MJ, Wei Y, Mancini MA, Van Hooser A, Ranalli T, Brinkley BR, Bazett-Jones DP, Bazett-Jones DP, Allis CD. Mitosis-specific phosphorylation of histone H3 initiates primarily within pericentromeric heterochromatin during G2 and Spreads in an ordered fashion coincident with mitotic chromosome condensation. Chromosoma. 1997;106:348–60.
12. Haldar S, Basu A, Croce CM. Bcl2 is the guardian of microtubule integrity. Cancer Res. 1997;57:229–23.
13. Demidenko ZN, Kalurupalle S, Hanko C, Lim CU, Broude E, Blagosklonny MV. Mechanism of G1-like arrest by low concentrations of paclitaxel: next cell cycle p53-dependent arrest with sub G1 DNA content mediated by prolonged mitosis. Oncogene. 2008;27:4402–10.
14. Bassik MC, Scorrano L, Oakes SA, Pozzan T, Korsmeyer SJ. Phosphorylation of BCL-2 regulates ER Ca2þ homeostasis and apoptosis. EMBO J. 2004;23:1207–16.
15. Jacobs-Helber SM, Sawyer ST. Jun N-terminal kinase promotes proliferation of immature erythroid cells and erythropoietin-dependent cell lines. Blood. 2004;104(3):696–703.
16. Da'i M, Jenie UA, Supardjan AM, Kawaichi M, Meiyanto E. T47D cells arrested at G2M and Hyperploidy Formation Induced by a Curcumin's Analogue PGV-1. Indonesian Journal of Biotechnology. 2007;12(2):1005–12.
17. Choi YH, Lee WH, Park KY, Zhang L. p53-independent Induction of p21 (WAF1/CIP1), Reduction of Cyclin B1 and G2/M Arrest by the Isoflavone Genistein in Human Prostate Carcinoma Cells. Jpn J Cancer Res. 2000;91:164–73.
18. Taylor WR, Stark GR. Regulation of the G2/M transition by p53. Oncogene. 2001;20:1803–15.
19. Huang S, Shu L, Dilling MB, Easton J, Harwood FC, Ichijo H, Houghton PJ. Sustained Activation of the JNK Cascade and Rapamycin-Induced Apoptosis Are Suppressed by p53/p21Cip1. Mol Cell. 2003;11:1491–501.
20. Gascoigne KE, Taylor SS. How do anti-mitotic drugs kill cancer cells? J Cell Sci. 2009;122:2579–85.
21. Jordan MA, Wilson L. Microtubules as a target for anticancer drugs. Nat Rev Cancer. 2004;4:253–65.
22. Warr MR, Shore GC. Small-molecule Bcl-2 antagonists as targeted therapy in oncology. Curr Oncol. 2008;15(6):256–61.
23. Petrangolini G, Cassinelli G, Pratesi G, Tortoreto M, Favini E, Supino R, Lanzi C, Belluco S, Zunino F. Antitumour and antiangiogenic effects of IDN 5390, a novel C-seco taxane, in a paclitaxel-resistant human ovarian tumour xenograft. Br J Cancer. 2004;90:1464–8.
24. Ferlini C, Raspaqlio G, Mozzetti S, Distefano M, Filippetti F, Martinelli E, Ferrandina G, Gallo D, Ranelletti FO, Scambia G. Bcl-2 Down-Regulation Is a Novel Mechanism of Paclitaxel Resistance. Mol Pharmacol. 2003;64:51–8.

6

# A *de* novo duplication of chromosome 9q34.13-qter in a fetus with Tetralogy of Fallot Syndrome

Jing Liu, Hao Hu, Na Ma, Zhengjun Jia, Yuchun Zhou, Jiancheng Hu and Hua Wang*

**Abstract**

**Background:** Partial duplications of the distal 9q have been rarely reported in literatures. The key features included characteristic facial appearance, long fingers and toes, slight psychomotor retardation, heart murmur et al. But rare severe congenital heart defects (CHD) such as TOF were reported to be associated with 9qter duplications.

**Case presentation:** A 23-year-old woman was referred for genetic counseling and prenatal diagnosis at $25^{3/7}$ weeks of gestation due to her male fetus, diagnosed as Tetralogy of Fallot Syndrome (TOF) by prenatal ultrasound. SNP (Single nucleotide polymorphism) array revealed that the male fetus had a *de* novo 5.47 Mb duplication at 9q34.13-qter. Meanwhile, non-invasive prenatal testing (NIPT) using low coverage whole genome massively parallel sequencing of circulating cell-free fetal DNA (cffDNA) showed consistent results. Multiplex ligation-dependent probe amplification (MLPA) also confirmed the duplication at 9qter.

**Conclusion:** In this paper, we present an Asian fetus with TOF caused by a *de* novo 5.47 Mb duplication at 9q34.13-qter. Duplication of 9q34.13-qter should be considered as an etiological diagnosis in the case of TOF. Our prenatal diagnostic findings provide important information for genetic counseling on the male fetus and future pregnancies in this family. Chromosomal microarray analysis (CMA) remains the first-tier clinical diagnostic test for prenatal fetus with suspicious syndromes. We also highlight the high potential application of NIPT in the screening of sub-chromosomal rearrangement.

**Keywords:** TOF, 9qter duplication, SNP array, Non-invasive prenatal testing, Prenatal diagnosis

## Background

Partial duplications of the long arm of chromosome 9 have been rarely reported in literatures. Turleau et al. first reported this new syndrome in 1975 [1]. The duplications of the distal 9q are even rare, since Alldedice et al first demonstrated the relationship between 9q34 duplications and phenotypic abnormalities [2]. The key features included slight psychomotor retardation, characteristic facial appearance, fingers and toes, heart murmur et al. But rare severe congenital heart defects (CHD) such as TOF were reported to be associated with these duplications. Amarillo et al. first reported the disrupted *RXRA* and complex microduplication of 9q (9q+) in a patient with TOF, suggesting that *RXRA* at 9q34.2 may be a critical locus in 9q + -associated CHD [3]. Here we present a male fetus with TOF who was found to have a *de* novo 5.47 Mb duplication at 9q34.13-qter detected by SNP array, which was confirmed by NIPT based on low coverage whole genome massively parallel sequencing and MLPA. A literature review was performed to refine correlation of CHD and 9q34 duplications. Our prenatal diagnostic findings provide important information for genetic counseling on the male fetus and future pregnancies in this family, and highlight the predictive values of NIPT in the screening of sub-chromosomal rearrangement.

## Case presentation

A gravida 2, para 1 woman came to our clinical genetics center for genetic counseling at $25^{3/7}$ weeks of gestation. This is her second pregnancy. A first round prenatal ultrasound revealed that the male fetus (II:2) (Fig. 1a) had multiple defects: ventricular septal defect (VSD) and

* Correspondence: wanghua213@aliyun.com
Prenatal Diagnosis Center of Province Hunan, The Maternal and Child Health Care Hospital of Hunan province, Changsha, Hunan 410008, People's Republic of China

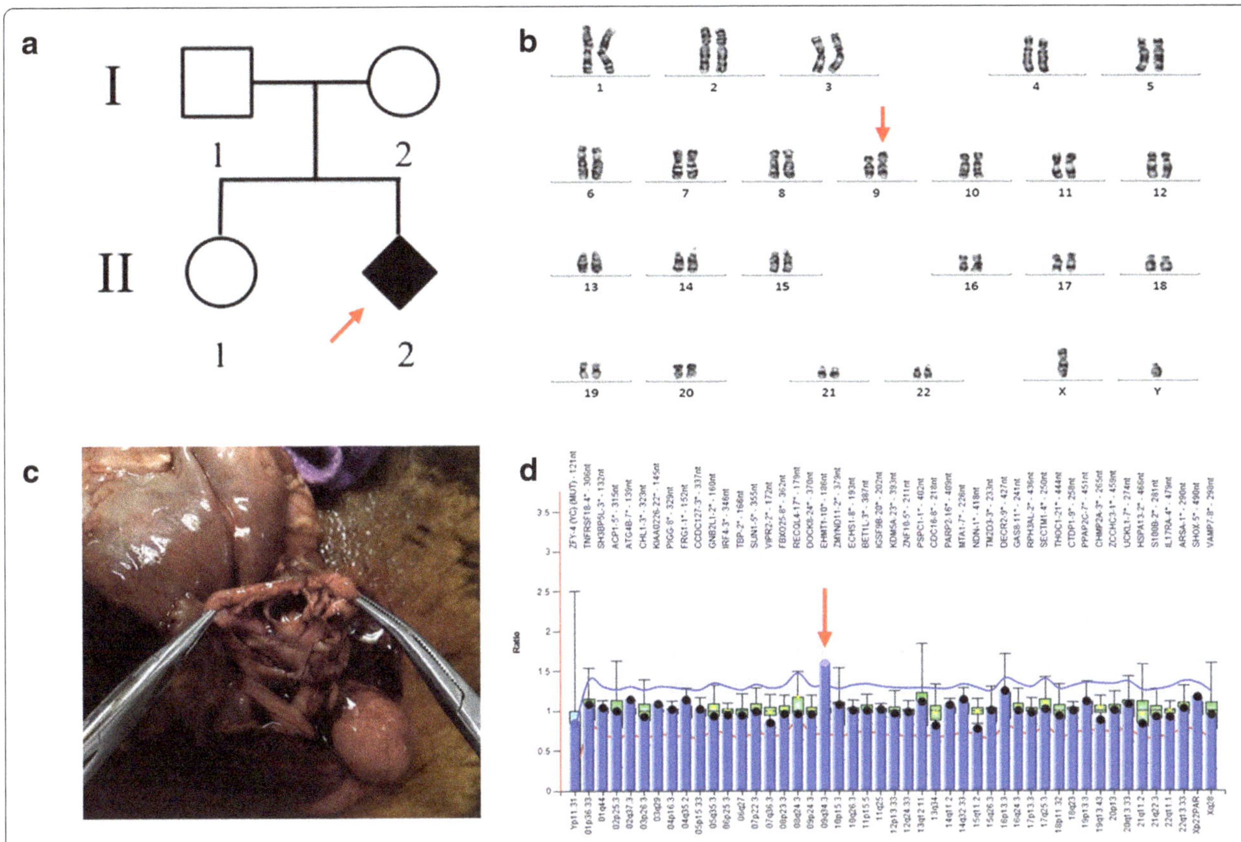


**Fig. 1 a** The pedigree of this family. The red arrow indicates the proband; **b** G-banded karyotype of the affected fetus shows a inv(9)(p11q13) which was inherited from his mother; **c** Anatomical features of heart: VSD; **d** MLPA result reveals that the peak height ratio of patient at 9q34.3 is 1.5, which means a duplication at this region

pulmonary stenosis. Biparietal diameter was 6.76 cm (50 ~ 95$^{th}$ centile) and abdominal circumference (AC) was 23.0 cm (~95$^{th}$ centile). A second round prenatal ultrasound was performed at 31 weeks of gestation, which indicated TOF.

The mother (I:2) was 23 years old and her husband (I:1) was 27 years old. Both of them were healthy non-consanguineous Chinese. Their first child (II:1) was a 2.5 years old girl, born at term by vaginal delivery after an uneventful pregnancy. Her birth weight was 3.4 kg (50 ~ 97$^{th}$ centile). No significant history of anoxia was recorded at birth. When she was 1 year old, her parents found that her pupils of each eye were not in the same size. After a series of examinations, she was diagnosed as optic nerve hypoplasia, but no genetics testing was followed up.

Amino fluid and blood samples were obtained from the fetus and the family separately after receiving informed consent. According to the genetics diagnosis and ultrasound results, this pregnancy was subsequently terminated at 32 weeks, followed by an autopsy. The male fetus' weight was 2052 g, height was 44.5 cm, head circumference was 30.6 cm, bust circumference was 26 cm, and AC was 25 cm(~5$^{th}$ centile). Facial abnormalities:a round face with small jaw, normal eye distance (19 mm), flat nasal bridge, high-arched palate. Anatomical features of heart: VSD (Fig. 1c) and displacement of the aorta to the right side over the right ventricle (about 1/2). The right outflow tract (pulmonary) was 0.7 cm, the left outflow tract (aorta) was 1.2 cm, the thickness of right ventricle was 0.5 cm, left was 1.03 cm, bicuspid valve was 1.8 cm and tricuspid valve was 2.1 cm.

## Materials and methods

After culturing amino fluid cells and peripheral blood lymphocytes obtained from the fetus and the other three family members separately, routine chromosome G-banded (320–400 bands) karyotyping analyses were performed on metaphase cells according to standard protocols.

SNP array analysis: Genomic DNA was extracted from the amino fluid cells and peripheral blood lymphocytes by using DNA Extraction Kit (Tissue and cells) and QIAamp DNA Blood Mini Kit (QIAGEN, Hilden, Germany) separately. SNP array was performed using Affymetrix CytoScan®750 K Array (Affymetrix Inc, CA,

USA), according to the manufacturer's protocol. Array results were analyzed using Chromosome Analysis Suite (ChAS; version 2.1). All genomic coordinates were taken from the February 2009 (hg19) human reference sequence (NCBI Build 37). Genes and Online Mendelian Inheritance in Man (OMIM) references were from RefSeq and OMIM entries, respectively.

The maternal peripheral blood was collected into Cell-Free DNA BCT (Streck, Inc., Omaha, NE, USA) prior to amniocentesis and centrifuged according to the protocol. The plasma was shipped to Berry Genomics in Beijing for DNA extraction and downstream low coverage whole genome massively parallel sequencing for detection of fetal sub-chromosomal anomalies.

The SALSA MLPA P070 kit was performed to determine the DNA copy number of a single DNA sequence in each of 41 human subtelomeric regions. MLPA analysis was performed following the manufacturer's instructions. The products were examined by ABI 3500dx genetic analyzer (Thermo Fisher, USA). Quantitative data were analyzed using the software of Coffalyser V8.0 (https://www.mlpa.com).

## Results

G-banded analysis of this family showed that the fetus inherited an inverted chromosome from his mother: 46, XY, inv(9)(p11q13), mat (Fig. 1b). The other two showed normal karyotypes. The SNP array result of the fetus was: arr[hg19] 9q34.13q34.3(135,550,093–141,018,648) × 3, 16p11.2(32,564,735–33,814,547) × 1 (Fig. 2a). The proximal duplication boundary was mapped within a 2.8-kb region between (nt. 135547269-135550093) at 9q34.13. The elder sister had a similar deletion at 16p11.2 as the fetus. No other pathogenic CNVs or variants of uncertain significance were identified in the parents. NIPT found a 5.6 Mb duplication in the fetus at 9q34 (Fig. 2b). MLPA analysis confirmed the duplication at 9q34.3 (Fig. 1d).

## Discussion

TOF occurs in three of every 10,000 live births. It is the most common cause of cyanotic cardiac disease in patients beyond the neonatal age, and accounts for up to one-tenth of all congenital cardiac lesions [4]. According to previous study, about 10 % of CHD in children with multiple congenital defects and/or intellectual disability

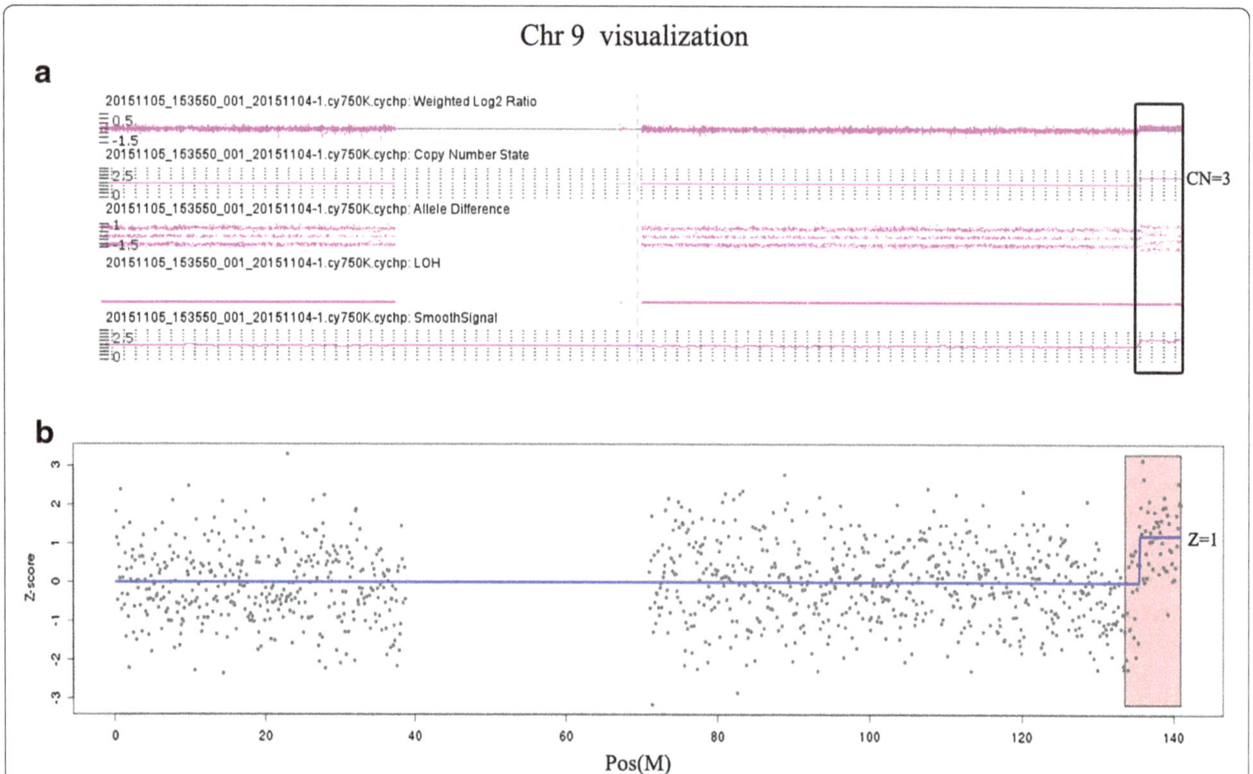


**Fig. 2** The ideograph of chromosome 9 in our patient with 9q34.13-34.3 gain. **a** CMA (Affymetrix ChAS Browser) detects a copy number gain at 9qter. The black frame region shows: 9q34.13q34.3(135,550,093-141,018,648) x3; weighted $\log_2$ ratio (WLR) is 0.5; copy number state (CN) is 3; allele differences (AD) (1.5, 0.5, −0.5, −1.5); smooth signal (SS) is 3; **b** NIPT via low coverage whole genome massively parallel sequencing of cffDNA in maternal plasma. Z score of the red bar region is 1, which means a copy number gain of this region

are caused by trisomies 21, 18 and 13 [5]. However, none of these aberrations can be attributed to a single CHD phenotype and they are associated with different CHD at variable frequencies. With the development of CMA, aberrations smaller than 5 Mb can be detected and much more submicroscopic copy number variations were found to be associated with TOF, such as 22q11.2 deletion/duplication, 1q21.1 duplication, 1q32.2 deletion, 13q13.1–13.2 deletion et al. [6–8]. Genes disrupted by and within these CNVs thus represent excellent candidate genes for CHD/TOF.

In this case, the male fetus with TOF was found to have a *de* novo 5.47 Mb duplication at distal 9q34 and a 1.25 Mb deletion at 16p11.2. There was no OMIM gene within the deletion of 16p11.2. According to the database of genomic variants (DGV; http://dgv.tcag.ca), this deletion was thought to be a benign variant. 9qter duplications have been reported to be pathological for many times since 1975 [1, 2]. Until now, there were almost 50 cases reported in DECIPHER (Database of Chromosomal Imbalance and Phenotype in Human using Ensembl Resources), which overlapped with the 9qter region we have found. A 3.0–3.4 Mb region (9q34.11-34.13) was proposed to be critical for the presentation of several phenotypes associated with 9q34 duplications [9, 10]. The key features included characteristic facial appearance, long fingers and toes, slight psychomotor retardation, heart murmur et al.

We have compared the previously reported 9q34 duplications with similar sizes or within the region we detected. Besides other symptoms, congenital heart defects were not common among the 9q34 duplications (less than 1/3 of all the previous patients). Including our case, there were only three patients with 9qter duplications showing TOF. The other two reports were described in DECIPHER #284022 and by Amarillo [4]. Amarillo also conducted a literature review to refine the correlation of CHD and partial trisomy 9q, suggesting 9q34.2 region to be the critical locus for 9q + -associated CHD and *RXRA* to be a possible candidate gene for CHD. Another patient (DECIPHER #301594) with duplication of 9q34.13-34.2 (inherited from his unaffected father) loci that involves disruption of *RXRA* showed abnormality of the ventricular septum. This also provided an evidence to support *RXRA* to be a possible candidate gene for CHD. In our case, the 5.47 Mb interval contains 92 OMIM genes, including *RXRA*. However, the proximal breakpoint maps to the intron 1 of *GTF3C4* (*604892) at 9q34.13, which was first reported by Hsieh [11]. Until now, there is no evidence indicating its relationship with heart development.

According to previous reports, even the same duplications of 9q34 in the same family have different phenotypes [9], so phenotypic variabilities among patients with cardiac structural defects may be attributed to incomplete penetrance or epigenetic events. Additional expression studies are needed to determine the role of these genes and the region in the development of CHD.

The existence of cffDNA in maternal circulation [12] and the recent advent of massive parallel sequencing technologies [13] have enabled NIPT. Peters et al. first showed proof of concept that a fetal with a 4.2-Mb deletion on chromosome 12 between bands 12p11.22 and 12p12.1 can be identified by means of noninvasive analysis of DNA in maternal plasma [14]. Liang et al. also proved the feasibility of low-coverage massive parallel CNV sequencing for the diagnosis of chromosome disease syndromes [15]. Helgeson et al. developed a novel algorithm to identify fetal microdeletion events in maternal plasma. They tested 175,393 samples, and 55 subchromosomal deletions were reported. Their results demonstrated high positive predictive values for noninvasive testing of rare sub-chromosomal deletions [16]. In this case, we also applied the NIPT to detect the fetal sub-chromosomal arrangements, and we got a positive result. This work also proved that NIPT might be expanded into the detection of sub-chromosomal copy number variations.

## Conclusion

In this study, duplication of 9q34.13-qter should be considered as the etiology for this TOF. The results provide valuable information for genetic counselors to achieve molecular diagnosis of prenatal anomalies and make more accurate predictions about the clinical outcomes. CMA remains the first-tier clinical diagnostic test for prenatal fetus with suspicious syndromes. We also highlight the high potential application of NIPT in the screening of sub-chromosomal rearrangement.

### Abbreviations

AC, abdominal circumference; cffDNA, cell-free fetal DNA; CHD, congenital heart defects; CNV, copy number variation; MLPA, multiplex ligation-dependent probe amplification; NIPT, non-invasive prenatal testing; OMIM, Online Mendelian Inheritance in Man; SNP, single nucleotide polymorphism; TOF, Trilogy of Fallot Syndrome; VSD, ventricular septal defect

### Acknowledgments

We thank this family for their contribution. We also thank laboratory staffs at Department of Prenatal diagnosis center-The Maternal and Child Health Care Hospital of Hunan Province. This study is funded by the Program of Health and Family Planning Commission of Hunan Province (B2015-102). The funding is used in the design of the study and collection.
This study was supported by grant from Health and Family Planning Commission of Hunan Province (B2015-102).

### Authors' contributions

JL and NM played a role in the molecular genetic experiments and drafted the manuscript. HH and ZJJ had major roles in the design of the study and analysis of clinical data. YCZ and JCH participated in karyotypes analysis. HW participated in the design and coordination of the study. All authors read and approved the final manuscript.

**Competing interests**
The authors declare that they have no competing interests.

**References**

1. Turleau C, De Grouchy J, Chavin-Colin F, et al. Partial trisomy 9q: a new syndrome [J]. Humangenetik. 1975;29(3):233–41.
2. Allderdice PW, Eales B, Onyett H, et al. Duplication 9q34 syndrome [J]. Am J Hum Genet. 1983;35(5):1005.
3. Amarillo IE, O'Connor S, Lee CK, et al. De novo 9q gain in an infant with tetralogy of Fallot with absent pulmonary valve: Patient report and review of congenital heart disease in 9q duplication syndrome [J]. Am J Med Genet A. 2015;167(12):2966–74.
4. Perry LW, Neill CA, Ferencz C. EUROCAT Working Party on [J]. Congenital Heart Disease: Perspective in Pediatric Cardiology. Epidemiol Congenit Heart Dis Baltimore-Washington Infant Stud. 1981;89:33–62.
5. Hartman RJ, Rasmussen SA, Botto LD, et al. The contribution of chromosomal abnormalities to congenital heart defects: a population-based study [J]. Pediatr Cardiol. 2011;32(8):1147–57.
6. Greenway SC, Pereira AC, Lin JC, et al. De novo copy number variants identify new genes and loci in isolated sporadic tetralogy of Fallot [J]. Nat Genet. 2009;41(8):931–5.
7. Mercer-Rosa L, Paridon SM, Fogel MA, et al. 22q11.2 deletion status and disease burden in children and adolescents with tetralogy of Fallot [J]. Circ Cardiovasc Genet. 2015;8:74. CIRCGENETICS. 114.000819.
8. Costain G, Silversides CK, Marshall CR, et al. 13q13.1–q13.2 deletion in tetralogy of Fallot: Clinical report and a literature review [J]. Int J Cardiol. 2011;146(2):134–9.
9. Mizuno S, Fukushi D, Kimura R, et al. Clinical and genomic characterization of siblings with a distal duplication of chromosome 9q (9q34.1-qter) [J]. Am J Med Genet A. 2011;155(9):2274–80.
10. Mundhofir FEP, Smeets D, Nillesen W, et al. Monosomy 9pter and trisomy 9q34.11qter in two sisters due to a maternal pericentric inversion [J]. Gene. 2012;511(2):451–4.
11. Hsieh YJ, Kundu TK, Wang Z, et al. The TFIIIC90 subunit of TFIIIC interacts with multiple components of the RNA polymerase III machinery and contains a histone-specific acetyltransferase activity [J]. Mol Cell Biol. 1999;19(11):7697–704.
12. Lo YMD, Corbetta N, Chamberlain PF, et al. Presence of fetal DNA in maternal plasma and serum [J]. Lancet. 1997;350(9076):485–7.
13. Mardis ER. A decade's perspective on DNA sequencing technology [J]. Nature. 2011;470(7333):198–203.
14. Peters D, Chu T, Yatsenko SA, et al. Noninvasive prenatal diagnosis of a fetal microdeletion syndrome [J]. N Engl J Med. 2011;365(19):1847–8.
15. Liang D, Peng Y, Lv W, et al. Copy number variation sequencing for comprehensive diagnosis of chromosome disease syndromes [J]. J Mol Diagn. 2014;16(5):519–26.
16. Helgeson J, Wardrop J, Boomer T, et al. Clinical outcome of subchromosomal events detected by whole-genome noninvasive prenatal testing [J]. Prenat Diagn. 2015;35(10):999–1004.

# Chromosome 12q13.13q13.13 microduplication and microdeletion

Jie Hu[1,2*], Zhishuo Ou[1], Elena Infante[3], Sally J. Kochmar[1], Suneeta Madan-Khetarpal[3], Lori Hoffner[4], Shafagh Parsazad[1] and Urvashi Surti[1,2,4]

**Abstract**

**Background:** Duplications or deletions in the 12q13.13 region are rare. Only scattered cases with duplications and/or deletions in this region have been reported in the literature or in online databases. Owing to the limited number of patients with genomic alteration within this region and lack of systematic analysis of these patients, the common clinical manifestation of these patients has remained elusive.

**Case presentation:** Here we report an 802 kb duplication in the 12q13.13q13.13 region in a 14 year-old male who presented with dysmorphic features, developmental delay (DD), mild intellectual disability (ID) and mild deformity of digits. Comparing the phenotype of our patient with those of reported patients, we find that patients with the 12q13.13 duplication or the deletion share similar phenotypes, including dysmorphic facies, abnormal nails, intellectual disability, and deformity of digits or limbs. However, patients with the deletion appear to have more severe deformity of digits or limbs.

**Conclusions:** Deletion and duplication of the 12q13.13 region may represent novel contiguous gene alteration syndromes. All seven reported 12q13.13 deletions and three of four duplications are de novo and vary in size. Therefore, these genomic alterations are not due to non-allelic homologous recombination.

**Keywords:** 12q13.13 Microdeletion/Microduplication, Array *CGH*, *HOXC*, *SPT7*, *SP1*

## Background

There are only a handful of patients with a copy number variation (CNV) in the 12q13.13 or 12q13.13q13.2 region reported in the literature. Due to the variable sizes and number of genes involved in these CNVs, the common clinical features of these patients have not been identified. In the present study, we report one patient with a small 12q13.13q13.13 duplication and review genomic alterations and clinical features of additional four patients with a duplication and seven patients with a deletion, all of which are reported in the literature or in the DECIPHER (Database of genomic variation and phenotype in humans using ensembl resources) and dbVar (genomic structural variation) databases. The common clinical features are detailed. The duplication and deletion of the 12q13.13q13.2 region may represent novel microdeletion and duplication syndromes.

* Correspondence: jhu@upmc.edu
[1]Center for Clinical Genetics and Genomics, Pittsburgh Cytogenetics Laboratory, Magee-Womens Hospital of UPMC, Pittsburgh, PA 15213, USA
[2]Department of Obstetrics, Gynecology & Reproductive Sciences, University of Pittsburgh School of Medicine, Pittsburgh, PA 15213, USA
Full list of author information is available at the end of the article

## Case presentation

Our patient is a 14 year 8-month-old male with dysmorphic features and a history of developmental delay, learning difficulties and disruptive behaviors. He was born at 35 weeks gestation to a 21-year-old gravida 1, para 0 mother. The mother denied any use of medications. Fetal ultrasounds were normal. His birth weight was 2637 g. He had mild jaundice at birth and remained in the hospital for 5 days due to breathing difficulties. He sat at 1 year of age, walked between 13 or 14 months of age, and did not speak any words until 3 and a half years of age. He had some regression of learning according to the family. At the age of 8 years he was evaluated by the Child Development Unit and diagnosed with Attention Deficit/Hyperactivity Disorder (ADHD). Genetic evaluation was performed on this patient at the age of 14 years and 8 months. At the time of the genetic evaluation, his weight was 47.2 kg (20th %ile), height was 162 cm (22nd %ile), and head circumference was 53.2 cm (30th %ile). He had dolichocephaly with prominent occiput and a long and narrow face. His eyebrows were quite heavy with medial flare. His scalp hair was somewhat sparse and fine textured. He had telecanthus, with outer canthal distance (OCD) 9.6 cm (95th %ile) and inner canthal distance (ICD) 3.9 cm (>97th %ile). The cartilage of his ears was very soft and with Darwinian tubercle bilaterally. He had esotropia, narrow and short philtrum, bifid uvula, high palate, very broad nose in the middle as well as on the tip, and receding anterior hairline with widow's peak. His genitalia was barely at the beginning of Tanner II. He also had hyperconvexed nails, collapse of arches of his feet, slight scoliosis, and quite large-looking elbows with prominent carrying angles. His skin was dry with eczema on the dorsum and numerous moles, especially under his left eye. At the time of evaluation, he was in the eighth grade but was in special education classes working at a second grade level. The representative photos of this patient are shown in Fig. 1.

The mother of the patient is 36 years old with learning disabilities. As a child, she had developmental delay and had speech therapy, occupational therapy and physical therapy. She finished high school and is attending school to become "a nurse". The maternal grandmother also had developmental delays, special education, mental health concerns, and required speech therapy. The patient's father is in his 40's. He had delays and had learning disabilities. The patient's 7-year-old and 5-year-old maternal half-sisters had no concerns reported.

## Methods

Microarray analysis was performed on purified DNA extracted from peripheral blood samples using Agilent's SurePrint G3 CGH + SNP microarray (4x180K ISCA design) platform. The array analysis followed the standard manufacturer protocols. Parental analysis was not performed because of unavailability of the samples.

## Results

The whole genome CGH + SNP microarray analysis detected a gain in copy number in the 12q13.13 region (chr12:53,304,719–54,018,772, hg19) of the long arm of chromosome 12, encompassing at least 802 kb and containing 21 OMIM genes (*KRT18, EIF4B, LOC283335, TENC1, SPRYD3, IGFBP6, SOAT2, CSAD, ZNF740, ITGB7, RARG, MFSD5, ESPL1, PFDN5, C12orf10, AAAS, SP7, SP1, AMHR2, PRR13, PCBP2, MAP3K12, TARBP, NPFF, ATF7*). The array findings are shown in the top panel of Fig. 2.

## Discussion

### Clinical features of patients with 12q13.13 duplication

Our patient had an 802 kb interstitial duplication in the 12q13.13q13.13 region. He presented with mild ID, ADHD, language difficulty and dysmorphic features including dolichocephaly, prominent occiput, bifid uvula, high arched palate, long and narrow face, high arched heavy eyebrows with medial flare, hypertelorism, esotropia, broad nose bridge and tip, short philtrum, and receding anterior

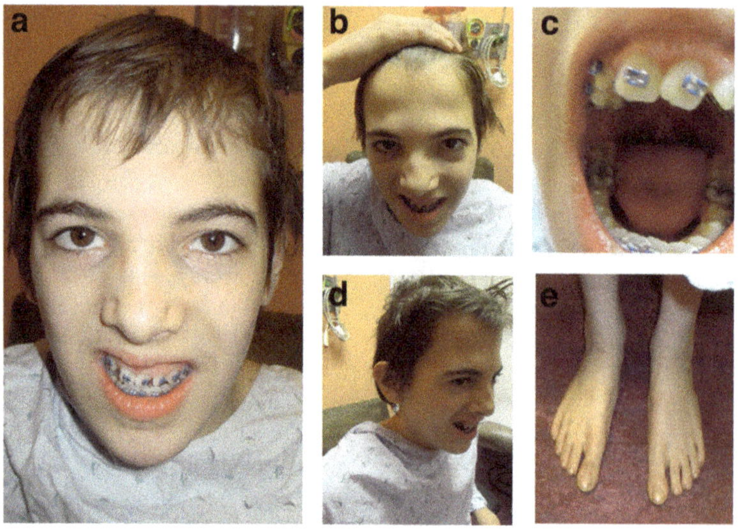


**Fig. 1** Patient at age 14 years and 8 months of age. **a** and **b**: facial features of the patient including long and narrow face, high arched heavy eyebrows with medial flare, hypertelorism, moles under left eye, broad nasal bridge and tip, short philtrum; **c**: bifid uvula and abnormal tooth; **d**: a side view of the patient showing the low-set ear; **e**: abnormal toenails

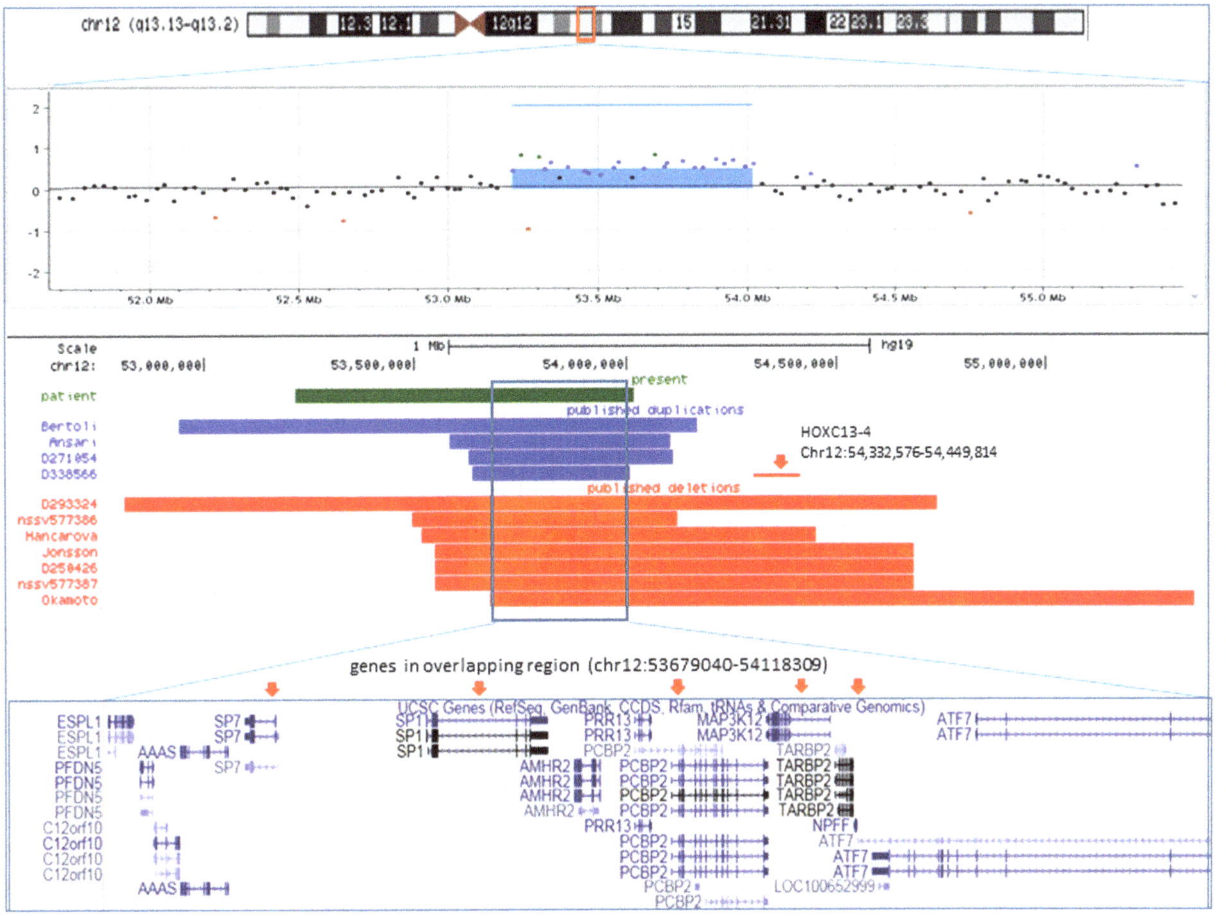


**Fig. 2** Chromosome 12q13.13 or 12q13.13q13.2 duplications and deletions found in our patient and previously reported patients. The *top panel* shows the ideogram of chromosome 12 with the 12q13.13q13.2 region marked in a *small red box*. The *scatter plot* of the Agilent array-CGH data shows an 802 kb microduplication of 12q13.13 in our patient. The schematic representation in the *middle panel* shows a comparison of the duplications and deletions involving the 12q13.13 or 12q13.13q13.2 region in the 11 reported patients and our patient. The *green bar* represents the duplication detected in our patient; the *blue bar bars* represent duplications identified in previously reported patients; the *red bars* represent deletions identified in previously reported patients. The common region shared by the deletions and the duplications is shown in a *box*. The UCSC genes in the overlapping region are shown in the *bottom panel*. The *red arrows* point to the candidate genes

hairline. He also had coned-shaped epiphyses of distal phalanges of the 2nd-5th digits, hyperconvex nails, stubby thumbs and collapse of arches of both feet.

Four patients with a similar duplication in this region were reported in the literature ([1, 2], DECIPHER 271054; DECIPHER 338566). The genome coordinates and size of the duplications, as well as phenotypes of all four reported patients and our patient are summarized in Table 1. The position of the duplications found in these patients are illustrated in the middle panel of Fig. 2. All five patients with duplication of the 12q13.3 region had ID, DD or language difficulties and dysmorphic facial features. The first patient, with a 1.2 Mb duplication in the 12q13.13q13.2 region, was reported by Bertoli et al. [2]. The duplication interval in this patient completely covers the region of duplication in our patient. Our patient and the first reported patient share some facial features including craniofacial anomalies, trigonocephaly or dolichocephaly, cleft palate or high arched plate and bifid uvula, narrow face and heavy eyebrows. In addition, mild hand and foot anomalies were also seen in our patient and the first reported patient. Some similarities with Wolf–Hirschhorn syndrome were described in Bertoli's patient, such as high nasal bridge, shallow orbits, and hypertelorism, but these were not seen in our patient. It is noted that a patient with a larger duplication (5 Mb) of this region was also reported to have Wolf-Hirschhorn syndrome-like phenotype [3]. Therefore, the variable phenotypes between our patient and the first reported patient are likely due to the size of the duplication and the genes that are involved. The second previously reported patient with a 520 kb duplication in the 12q13.13 region, was reported to have a Cornelia de Lange (CdLS)-like phenotype [1]. The third and the fourth patients reported in the

**Table 1** Laboratory findings and clinical features of 5 patients with 12q13.13 duplication

| Features | Present | Bertoli [2] | Ansari [1] | DECIPHER 271054 | DECIPHER 338566 |
|---|---|---|---|---|---|
| Age/Gender | 14/M | 6/F | NA/F | 14/M | 9/F |
| Size | 802 Kb | 1.2 Mb | 520 Kb | 484 Kb | 370 Kb |
| Chromosome regions | 12q13.13 | 12q13.13q13.2 | 12q13.13 | 12q13.13 | 12q13.13 |
| Genomic coordinates | | | | | |
| (hg18)[a] | | 51,227,241–52,353,011 | | | |
| (hg19) | 53,217,136–54,018,772 | 52,940,974–54,166,744 | 53,582,733–54,102,733 | 53,627,092–54,111,152 | 53,637,649–54,007,964 |
| # of genes | 27 | 57 | 18 | 16 | 17 |
| *HOXC* cluster | None | None | None | None | None |
| *SP1, SP7, NPFF, MAP3K12, PCBP* | Yes | Yes | Yes | Yes | Yes |
| Inheritance | Unknown | De novo | Unknown | De novo | De novo |
| Developmental Anomalies | ID, ADHD, language difficulty | ID, language difficulty | DD, ID | ID | ID |
| Craniofacial anomalies | Dolichocephaly, prominent occiput, bifid uvula, high arched palate. | Microcephaly, trigonocephaly cleft palate | | | |
| Dysmorphic facial features | Long and narrow face, high arched heavy eyebrows with medial flare, hypertelorism, esotropia, broad nasal bridge and tip, short philtrum, receding anterior hairlines, auricular tubercle | Long face, high arched eyebrows, prominent glabella, hypertelorism, prominent eye, lagoph-thalmos, shallow orbits, epicanthal folds, hypoplastic nasal alae, high nasal bridge, low-set ears, thin upper lip | CdLS-like phenotype | Abnormal face (no details described) | |
| Hand and foot anomalies | hyperconvex nails, stub thumbs, collapse of arches of feet | Small hands and feet, 2nd toe clinodactyly | | | |
| Skeletal anomalies | Mild scoliosis, coned-shaped epiphyses of distal phalanges of 2nd-5th digits | | | | |
| Other | Dry skin, eczema on dorsum | Ataxia walk, corneal sclerosis, progeroid hands | | | |

*ADHD* attention deficit hyperactivity disorder, *CdLS* Cornelia de Lange Syndrome, *DD* developmental delay, *ID* intellectual disability;
[a]hg18 nucleotide coordinates in published patients are converted into hg19 nucleotide coordinates

DECIPHER database (patients: 271,054 and 338,566) were described to have intellectual disability. In addition, the patient (271054) also had abnormal facies. No other details of the clinical features were reported in those three patients. However, it is well known that the typical facial features for CdLS patients include arched eyebrows and synophrys, some with upper limb anomalies, and small, widely spaced teeth, which are similar features observed in patients with deletion/duplication of chromosome 12q13.13 [4].

It is interesting to note that deletions of this region were also reported in seven patients ([5–7], DECIPHER patients: 293,324 and 250,426; dbVar: nssv577386 and nssv577387). A comparison of the location and size of the deletions and duplications are illustrated in the middle panel of Fig. 2. The reported laboratory findings and clinical features of those patients with deletion of the 12q13.13 region are summarized in Table 2. It appears that patients with either a deletion or a duplication of this region share some common phenotypic abnormalities, including intellectual disability, similar facial dysmorphism (long face, high palate/cleft palate) and mild limb anomalies (clinodactyly of toes and stub thumbs). However, compared to the patients with a duplication of this region, patients with a deletion of this region had more severe limb deformities including camptodactyly or flexion contracture of hand, which were reported in five of the seven patients. Club foot or valgus position of the feet was reported in one patient each (DECIPHER patient: 293,324, [6]). Moreover, heart defects which were seen in some of patients with deletion of the 12q13.13 region were not observed in patients with duplication of the same region. Other skeletal abnormalities, such as scoliosis and cone-shaped epiphyses of distal phalanges, reported in four of the seven patients with a 12q13.13 deletion ([5–7],

**Table 2** Laboratory findings and clinical features of 7 patients with 12q13.13 deletion

| Features | Okamoto 2011 [5] | Jonsson 2012 [6] | Hancarova 2013 [7] | DECHIPHER 293234 | DECHIPHER 250426 | dbVar: nssv577386 | dbVar: nssv577387 |
|---|---|---|---|---|---|---|---|
| Age/Gender | 14/M | 6/F | 5/M | Unknown | Unknown | Unknown | Unknown |
| Size | 1.7 Mb | 1.13 Mb | 0.9 Mb | 1.93 Mb | 1.13 Mb | 624.86 Kb | 988.42Kb |
| Chr. location | 12q13.13q13.2 | 12q13.13 | 12q13.13 | 12q13.13 | 12q13.13 | 12q13.13 | 12q13.13 |
| Genomic coordinates | | | | | | | |
| (hg18)[a] | 51,965,307–53,642,659 | 51,834,791–52,971,391 | 51,801,299–52,737,892 | | | | |
| (hg19) | 53,679,040–55,356,392 | 53,548,524–54,685,124 | 53,515,032–54,451,625 | 52,810,526–54,739,060 | 53,548,524–54,685,124 | 53,493,442–54,118,309 | 53,617,808–54,616,234 |
| # of genes | 61 | 33 | 21 | 81 | 42 | 34 | 44 |
| *HOXC* cluster | 9 of 9 | 9 of 9 | 9 of 9 | 9 of 9 | 9 of 9 | 0 of 9 | 9 of 9 |
| *SP1, SP7, NPFF, MAP3K12, PCBP2* | Yes | Yes | Yes | Yes | Yes | Yes | Yes |
| Inheritance | De novo | De novo | De novo | De novo | De novo | De novo | De novo |
| Developmental anomalies | ID, language difficulty | Global DD, ADHD | Mild ID | ID | ID | DD | DD |
| Growth impairment | Short stature | | Short stature, failure to thrive | | | | |
| Dysmorphic facial features | Long face, broad nose, prominent ears, low-set ears, downslanting PF, strabismus, high palate | Bilateral epicanthal folds, depressed nasal bridge, slightly bulbous and anteverted nose, short philtrum | Microcephaly, long and narrow face, hypotelorism, enophthalmos, wide nasal root, long philtrum, low-set ears, fine hair | High palate, micrognathia, epicanthal folds | Anteverted nares, depressed nasal bridge, epicanthus, short philtrum | Other significant developmental or morphological phenotypes | Malar flattening |
| Hand and foot anomalies | PIP joint flexion, camptodactyly involving 3rd and 4th fingers, inflexible DIP joints of index fingers, adducted thumbs, dislocated radial heads | Flection contracture involving digits, hands, and elbows, ulnar deviation of both hands, valgus position of both ankles, short nails | Flection contracture involving 4th and 5th fingers (right hand), ulnar deviation of both hands, hyperlaxity of joints, hypoplastic abnormal nails | Distal flection contracture, small nail, talipes equinovarus | Short nail, ulnar deviation of the hand, flexion contracture | | |
| Skeletal anomalies | Severe kyphosis, mild scoliosis | Short metacarpal and proximal phalangeal bones | Conical shaped distal phalanges, extremely long thorax, short lower limbs | | Short phalanx of finger | | Distal arthrogryposis |
| Other | Heart defect, bilateral inguinal hernias, hypodontia, persistent teeth | Umbilical hernia, pectus excavatum, subluxation at MCPIII, | Congenital heart defect, cryptorchidism, hyperelastic skin, abnormal palmar and plantar creases | Single transverse palmar crease | Umbilical hernia, pectus excavatum recurrent infections | | |

***ADHD*** **attention deficit hyperactivity disorder,** ***chr*** **chromosome,** ***DD*** **developmental delay,** ***DIP*** **distal interphalangeal,** ***ID*** **intellectual disability,** ***MCP*** **Metacarpophalangeal,** ***PF*** **palpebral fissure,** ***PIP*** **proximal interphalangeal**

**[a]hg18 nucleotide coordinates in previously reported patients are converted into hg19 nucleotide coordinates**

DECIPHER patient: 250,426), were also seen in our patient who had a duplication in this region.

### Candidate genes within the common deletion and duplication interval

There are at least 16 genes within the common overlapping region. A few of these genes are expressed in the central nervous system and/or likely to be dosage sensitive, or reported to be associated with disease by animal studies. These genes could be candidate genes for patients with deletion or duplication in this region.

The transcription factor gene (*SP1*) is most likely to be dosage sensitive (haploinsufficiency score: 0.81%) [DECIPHER]. The protein encoded by the *SP1* gene is a zinc finger transcription factor that binds to GC-rich motifs of many promoters and is then involved in a variety of cellular processes such as cell growth, apoptosis, differentiation and immune responses, DNA damage response, and chromatin remodeling (provided by RefSeq, Nov 2014). The *SP7* gene (haploinsufficiency score: 14.4%) encodes a bone specific transcription factor (osterix) which regulates osteogenesis and bone formation during embryonic development [8]. Niger et al. [9] reported that the activity of osterix (Osx/Sp7) is influenced by *Sp1*. The $sp7^{-/-}$ mutation in zebra fish causes a generalized delay in osteoblast maturation, while heterozygous zebra fishes ($sp7^{+/}-$) are not appreciably different from wild type siblings, however; they exhibit an increase in the variance of craniofacial shape [10]. Dolichocephaly and trigonocephaly are seen in our patient and the first reported patient with a duplication in the 12q13.13 region. Moreover, 'long' or 'long and narrow' facies are a common feature in patients with a deletion or duplication in the 12q13.13 region. It is known that a homozygous single base pair deletion (c.1052delA) in the *SP7* gene resulted in a child with osteogenesis imperfecta born to heterozygous carrier parents who were phenotypically normal [11]. However, the clinical features of the patients with heterozygous contiguous gene deletion/duplication involving both the *SP1* and *SP7* genes have not been investigated. Our study indicates that patients with either a deletion or a duplication of the 12q13.13 region, involving the *SP1* and *SP7* genes, share some common clinical features with those patients who have the homozygous *SP7* mutation, such as short stature, high-arched palate, mild bone deformities, mild scoliosis, and delayed motor milestones. Whether concurrent dosage changes of the *SP1* and *SP7* genes cause some of the abnormal features in these patients is unclear at present.

The *HOXC* genes are not within the common duplication interval. However, six of seven reported patients with the 12q13.13 deletion involve the *HOXC* gene cluster, which are thought to be the candidate genes for the development of skeletal anomalies and limb deformities [5–7]. Mutations or deletions involving other *HOX* genes have been well documented in developmental disorders in both humans and mice, particularly limb anomalies [12]. Our earlier study found that patients with deletion of the 3′ portion (distal) of the *HOXC* cluster including *HOXC11, HOXC10, HOXC9, HOXC8, HOXC6, HOXC5* and *HOXC4* showed no skeletal anomalies or obvious digit anomalies [13]. A recent study of multiple members from multiple generations in four families showed that the small deletions in the upstream noncoding region, with or without deletion of *HOXC13 and HOXC12,* segregated with limb deformities [14], which indicates that a putative regulatory element within that region might be deleted in those patients. Variable expressivity including club foot, vertical talus, hammertoes and syndactyly was reported in those patients. Therefore, it is possible that a deletion of the 5'of *HOXC* gene cluster may contribute to a relatively more severe phenotype in patients with the 12q13.13 deletion.

Developmental delay and intellectual disability were found in all patients with a 12q13.13 or 12q13.13q13.2 deletion/duplication. The common region for the copy number alterations in this region contains a few genes expressed in the central nervous system (*NPFF, SP1, and MAP3K12*). In addition to the *Sp1* gene the heterogeneous nuclear riboprotein E2 (*PCBP2*) gene is also predicted to be dosage sensitive with a haploinsufficiency score of 4.18% [DECHIPHER]. Although the precise phenotype-genotype correlation for these genes cannot be established, the dosage changes of these genes may contribute to the neurodevelopmental anomalies in these patients. Although parental studies were unavailable for our patient, 10 of the 11 reported deletions or duplications were found to be de novo which supports the likely pathogenic nature of these CNVs.

## Conclusions

We report one more patient with a chromosome 12q13.13 q13.13 duplication. The phenotype of this patient shows great similarity with the previously reported patients who have either a duplication or a deletion in this region, including a long face, high nasal bridge, high arched eyebrows, cleft palate, skeletal anomalies, limb deformity, language difficulty and intellectual disability. However, patients with deletion of this region have more severe skeletal anomalies, limb deformities and heart defects. Additional cases are needed to confirm these syndromes.

#### Abbreviations

*aCGH*: Array comparative genomic hybridization; ADHD: Attention deficit hyperactivity disorder; CdLS: Cornelia de Lange Syndrome; Chr: Chromosome; CNV: Copy number variation; *DD*: Developmental delay; DECIPHER: Database of genomic variation and phenotype in humans using ensembl resources; DIP: Distal interphalangeal; ICD: Inner canthal distance; ID: Intellectual disability; Kb: Kilobases; Mb: Megabases; MCP: Metacarpophalangeal; OCD: Outer canthal distance; OMIM: Online Mendelian Inheritance in Man; PF: Palpebral fissure; PIP: Proximal interphalangeal

**Acknowledgements**
We acknowledge the patient and his family participating in this study. We also thank the staff at the Pittsburgh Cytogenetics Laboratory, Magee-Womens Hospital of UPMC for their technical support. All of the authors declared that they have no competing interests.
This study makes use of data generated by the DECIPHER community. A full list of centers who contributed to the generation of the data is available from http://decipher.sanger.ac.uk.

**Funding**
Not applicable.

**Authors' contributions**
JH carried out the microarray analysis, medical chart review and data analysis. She also drafted and finalized the manuscript. EI and SM collected the medical history and helped in the review of the patient's medical chart and participated in discussion of the clinical and laboratory findings. ZO and SP carried out the literature search and formatting of the manuscript and participated in discussion of the clinical and laboratory findings. SK, LH and US discussed the results and carried out the critical reading and editing of the manuscript. All the authors have read and approved the final manuscript.

**Competing interests**
The authors declare that they have no competing interests.

**Author details**
[1]Center for Clinical Genetics and Genomics, Pittsburgh Cytogenetics Laboratory, Magee-Womens Hospital of UPMC, Pittsburgh, PA 15213, USA. [2]Department of Obstetrics, Gynecology & Reproductive Sciences, University of Pittsburgh School of Medicine, Pittsburgh, PA 15213, USA. [3]Department of Genetics, Children's Hospital of Pittsburgh of UPMC, Pittsburgh, PA 15224, USA. [4]Department of Pathology, University of Pittsburgh School of Medicine, Pittsburgh, PA 15213, USA.

**References**
1. Ansari M, Poke G, Ferry Q, Williamson K, Aldridge R, Meynert AM, et al. Genetic heterogeneity in Cornelia de Lange syndrome (CdLS) and CdLS-like phenotypes withobserved and predicted levels of mosaicism. J Med Genet. 2014;51:659–68.
2. Bertoli M, Alesi V, Gullotta F, Zampatti S, Abate MR, Palmieri C, et al. Another patient with 12q13 microduplication. Am J Med Genet A. 2013;161A:2004–8.
3. Dallapiccola B, Bernardini L, Novelli A, Mingarelli R. Phenocopy of Wolf-Hirschhorn syndrome in a patient with duplication 12q13.3q14.1. Am J Med Genet A. 2009;149A:546–8.
4. Deardorff MA, Noon SE, Krantz ID, editors. Cornelia de Lange Syndrome. Seattle: University Of Washington; 2005. p. 1993–2016.
5. Okamoto N, Tamura D, Nishimura G, Shimojima K, Yamamoto T. Submicroscopic deletion of 12q13 including HOXC gene cluster with skeletal anomalies and global developmental delay. Am J Med Genet A. 2011;155A:2997–3001.
6. Jonsson DI, Ludvigsson P, Aradhya S, Sigurdardottir S, Steinarsdottir M, Hauksdottir H. A de novo 1.13 Mb microdeletion in 12q13.13 associated with congenital distal arthrogryposis, intellectual disability and mild dysmorphism. Eur J Med Genet. 2012;55:437–40.
7. Hancarova M, Simandlova M, Drabova J, Petrak B, Koudova M, Havlovicova M, et al. Chromosome 12q13.13 deletions involving the HOXC gene cluster: phenotype and candidate genes. Eur J Med Genet. 2013;56:171–3.
8. Nakashima K, Zhou X, Kunkel G, Zhang Z, Deng JM, Behringer RR. The novel zinc finger-containing transcription factor osterix is required for osteoblast differentiation and bone formation. Cell. 2002;108:17–29.
9. Niger C, Lima F, Yoo DJ, Gupta RR, Buo AM, Hebert C, et al. The transcriptional activity of osterix requires the recruitment of Sp1 to the osteocalcin proximal promoter. Bone. 2011;49:683–92.
10. Kague E, Roy P, Asselin G, Hu G, Simonet J, Stanley A. Osterix/Sp7 limits cranial bone initiation sites and is required for formation of sutures. Dev Biol. 2016;413:160–72.
11. Lapunzina P, Aglan M, Temtamy S, Caparros-Martin JA, Valencia M, Leton R. Identification of a frameshift mutation in osterix in a patient with recessive osteogenesis imperfecta. Am J Hum Genet. 2010;87:110–4.
12. Goodman FR. Limb malformation and the human HOX genes. Am J Med Genet. 2002;112:256–65.
13. Peterson JF, Hartman J, Ghaloul-Gonzalez L, Surti U, Hu J. Absence of skeletal anomalies in siblings with a maternally inherited 12q13.13-q13.2 microdeletion partially involving the HOXC gene cluster. Am J Med Genet A. 2014;164A:810–4.
14. Alvarado DM, McCall K, Hecht JT, Dobbs MB, Gurnett CA. Deletions of 5' HOXC genes are associated with lower extremity malformations, including clubfoot and vertical talus. J Med Genet. 2016;4:1–6.

# 8

# Molecular characterization of a rare analphoid supernumerary marker chromosome derived from 7q35 → qter

Bárbara Marques[1], Cristina Ferreira[1*], Filomena Brito[1], Sónia Pedro[1], Cristina Alves[1], Teresa Lourenço[2], Marta Amorim[2] and Hildeberto Correia[1]

**Abstract**

**Background:** Analphoid supernumerary marker chromosomes (aSMC) constitute one of the smallest groups of SMC, and are characterized by a centromeric constriction but no detectable alpha-satellite DNA. These marker chromosomes cannot be properly identified by conventional banding techniques alone, and molecular cytogenetic methods are necessary for a detailed characterization. Analphoid SMC derived from chromosome 7 are extremely rare, with only five cases reported so far.

**Case presentation:** In this work we report an aSMC involving the terminal long arm of chromosome 7 in a 10-year-old boy with multiple dysmorphic features and severe development delay. Cytogenetic analysis revealed a mosaic karyotype with the presence of an extra SMC, *de novo*, in 20% of lymphocytes and 73% of fibroblast cells. Next, we performed FISH analysis with multiple DNA probes and cCGH analysis. This identified the origin of the SMC as an analphoid marker resulting of invdup rearrangement of 7q35-qter region.
Affimetrix CytoScan HD array analysis redefined the aSMC as a 15.42 Mb gain at 7q35-q36.3 (minimum tetraplicated region-chr7: 143,594,973-159,119,707; GRCh37/hg19) of maternal origin that encloses 67 OMIM genes, 16 of which associated to disease. Uniparental disomy of chromosome 7 (UPD 7) has been excluded.

**Conclusions:** We report the first patient with an aSMC(7) derived from the terminal 7q region who has been molecularly and clinically full characterized. The use of SNParray in the characterization of SMC reveals to be a powerful tool, giving information not only about copy number variation but also about loss-of-heterozygosity and parental origin. We conclude that an integrated genome-wide copy number variation analysis, if possible associated to FISH and gene expression studies, could facilitate in the future the difficult task of establishing accurate genotype-phenotype correlations and help to improve genetic counselling.

**Keywords:** Chromosome 7, Analphoid supernumerary marker chromosome, Neocentromere, Partial 7q tetrasomy, 7q duplication

* Correspondence: cristina.ferreira@insa.min-saude.pt
[1]Unidade de Citogenética, Departamento de Genética Humana, Instituto Nacional de Saúde Doutor Ricardo Jorge, I.P, Avenida Padre Cruz, 1649-016 Lisboa, Portugal
Full list of author information is available at the end of the article

## Background

Analphoid supernumerary marker chromosomes (aSMC) constitute one of the smallest groups of SMC, and are characterized by a centromeric constriction but no detectable alpha-satellite DNA [1]. These marker chromosomes cannot be clearly identified by conventional banding techniques alone, with molecular cytogenetic methods being necessary for their detailed characterization.

So far 141 aSMC have been reported encompassing 20 of the 22 autossomes and both sexual chromosomes, with 41% of these being acrocentric derivatives (from chromosomes 15 and 13) [2]. The most common aSMC are supernumerary inverted duplications (invdup) of the distal arm of a chromosome. The first aSMC derived from chromosome 7 was reported using multicolour-FISH in a patient with learning and developmental delay as well dysmorphic features [3]. Cases subsequently reported include an inverted-duplication-shaped aSMC derived from the long arm terminal region, and a derivative chromosome 7 with an interstitial deletion of the short and long arms segments showing a neocentromere in the p14 region. None of these reports included the patients' clinical description [4, 5]. Recently, Kumar et al. reported a child with dysmorphic features and developmental delay, who presented a complex chromosome rearrangement involving chromosome 7 and resulting of a class II/McClintock mechanism [6]. Louvrier et al. [7] reported a mosaic neocentric ring involving the region 7q22.1q31.1, in a child with a severe global retardation and dysmorphic features. In this case, the aSMC characterization, using arrayCGH, and the clinical description are very detailed establishing a clear genotype-phenotype correlation. In our study we used different methods in order to fully characterize an aSMC involving the terminal long arm of chromosome 7 in a patient presenting several dysmorphic features, unstable assisted broad-based walk and severe developmental delay without language acquisition. To our knowledge this is the first case reported of an aSMC(7) with an entire molecular characterization and clinical description involving the region 7q35-qter. With this study we hope to contribute for a better genotype-phenotype correlation and improved genetic counselling.

This case was submitted to the sSMC database (http://ssmc-tl.com/chromosome-7.html#N), No. 07-N-q35/1-1.

## Case presentation

The patient was a newborn male, the first child of a healthy and non-consanguineous couple, born at 28 weeks of gestation with normal somatometric parameters (weight 1167 g corresponding to P50). In the neonatal period the patient showed respiratory distress syndrome and feeding difficulties, and was diagnosed with bronchopulmonary dysplasia probably due to prematurity.

On physical examination, open and wide anterior fontanelle, bilateral eyelid edema, low-set ears, short nose with wide and depressed root, open tented, and fingers and toes nail hypoplasia were described.

The patient also showed bilateral hip dysplasia, cryptorchidism and a bilateral inguinal hernia that has already been corrected. Furthermore, the child was submitted, at 4 months of age to a colectomy for necrotizing enterocolitis, 1 month later to a tracheotomy, and at 18 months of age to a percutaneous endoscopic gastrostomy.

The patient is currently 10 years old and has severe developmental delay without language acquisition, presenting with bruxism and auto-aggressive behaviour (which started at the age of 8). The child has an unstable, assisted broad-based walk. He still depends on enteral feeding, has a tracheostomy tube for breathing and suffers from recurrent respiratory infections. The physical exam reveals an accentuation of the dysmorphic features with frontal bossing, low-set ears, straight eyebrows with synophrys and hypertelorism. There are also supernumerary teeth, divergent strabismus and anterior chamber asymmetric optic malformation (Fig. 1). Renal and cardiac malformations were excluded by ultrasound.

## Material and methods

### Cytogenetics

Cytogenetic analyses were performed on conventional giemsa-trypsin-leishman (GTL) banded metaphase chromosomes obtained from phytohemagglutinin-stimulated peripheral blood lymphocytes, from the patient and his parents, as well as skin fibroblasts from the patient by standard techniques. A karyotype was established according to the International System for Human Cytogenetic Nomenclature [8].

### Fluorescent *in situ* hybridization (FISH)

FISH analysis was performed on chromosome spreads prepared from lymphocyte and skin fibroblast cultures. FISH probes included alpha-satellite probes for all chromosomes (home made), ELN and D7S427 probes (Oncor, Gaithersburg, MD), whole chromosome painting probe (WCP) for chromosomes 2, 3, 7, 9, 10, 11,16, 17, 19 and 20 (Cambio, Cambridge, UK), subtelomeric 7q probe (TelVysion, Abbott Molecular, Abbott Park, IL, USA) and the bacterial artificial chromosome (BAC) clone RP11-298A10 (kindly supplied by Wellcome Trust Sanger Institute, Cambridge, UK). Extraction of alpha-satellite DNA for FISH probes, labelling and FISH analysis were performed following standard protocols. Extraction of BAC DNA for FISH probe, labelling and FISH analysis were performed as described earlier [9, 10].

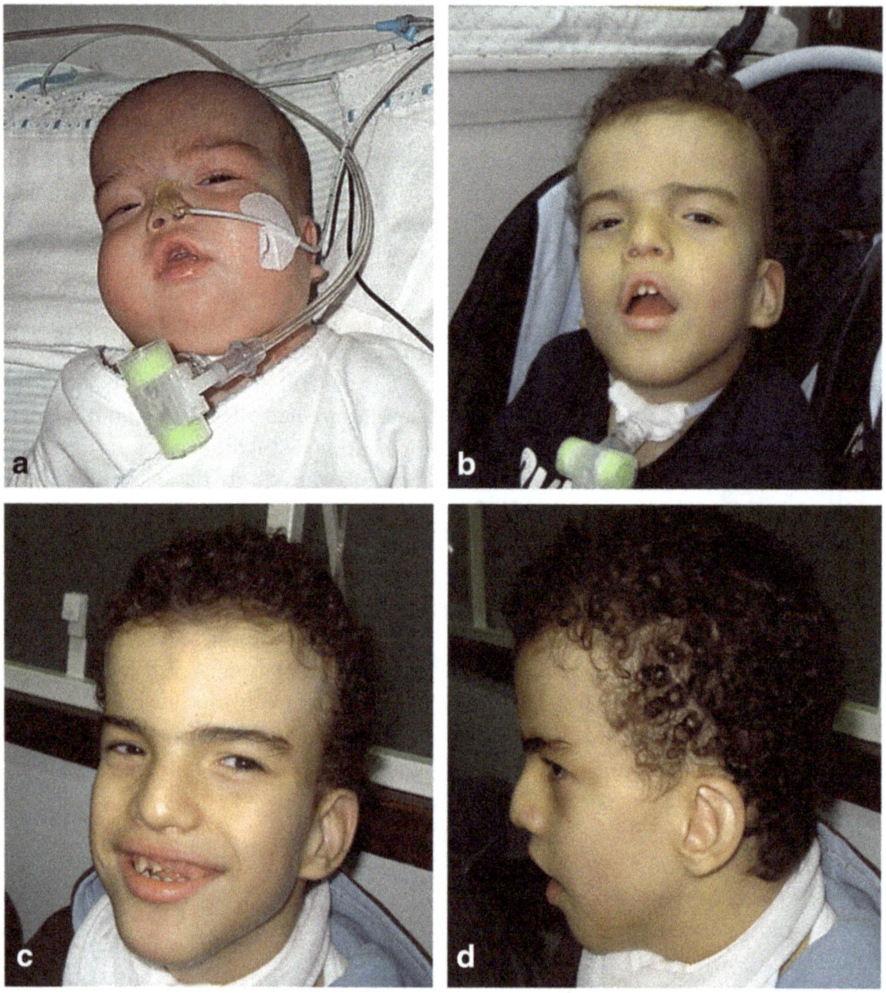

**Fig. 1** Clinical facial features of the patient at different ages. **a** At 5th months: facial edema, short nose with wide and depressed root; **b** At 4-year-old: turricephaly, curly hair, straight eyebrows with synophrys, opened tented mouth; **c** and **d** At 10-year-old: accentuation of the dysmorphic features with hypertelorism, underdeveloped crus helix, full lips and dental crowding

**Chromosomal comparative genomic hybridization (cCGH)**
Metaphase spreads were prepared from phytohemagglutinin-stimulated lymphocytes from healthy individuals, according to standard procedures. Genomic DNA was extracted from the patient's peripheral blood sample using the Wizard® genomic DNA purification Kit from Promega (Promega Corporation, WI, USA). cCGH analysis was performed according to standard procedures. The data was analyzed using ISIS-CGH software (MetaSystems, Altleisheim, Germany) with average ratio profiles of 1,25 e 0,75 and standard deviation limits.

**SNParray**
Array analysis was performed in genomic DNA extracted from peripheral blood of the patient and his parents using Affymetrix CytoScan HD® array (Affymetrix, California, USA) according to the manufacturer's recommendations (Affymetrix manual protocol Affymetrix® Cytogenetics Copy Number Assay P / N 703038 Rev. 3). CytoScan HD array contains 740,304 polymorphic (SNP, single nucleotide polymorphism) and 1,953,249 non-polymorphic (copy number probes) markers with an average intragenic marker spacing of 880 bps and intergenic marker spacing of 1737 bps. The raw data were processed using Genotyping Console v4.0 and Chromosome Analysis Suite 3.0.0.42 with NetAffx na33.1 (UCSC GRCh37/hg19) and the output data were interpreted with the UCSC Genome Browser (https://genome.ucsc.edu/; GRCh37/hg19 assembly), DECIPHER (https://decipher.sanger.ac.uk/) and ClinGen (http://www.clinicalgenome.org). The functions of the genes, which were located within the region of the genomic imbalance, were retrieved from the GeneCards (http://www.genecards.org) and OMIM (http://www.ncbi.nlm.nih.gov/omim) databases. The trio analysis to exclude uniparental disomy of chromosome 7 (UPD 7) was done using the CytoScanHD_Array

Mendelian Error Check tool and the parental origin of the aSMC was determined using MyPODFinder v.1.0.

## Results

Cytogenetic analysis revealed a mosaic karyotype with the presence of a SMC, *de novo*, in 20% of lymphocytes and 73% of skin fibroblast cells (Fig. 2a).

FISH analysis with alpha-satellite probes for all chromosomes indicated that the SMC was an analphoid marker (Fig. 2b), while the presence of euchromatic material was revealed with whole chromosome painting probe for chromosome 7 (Fig. 2c). cCGH analysis indicated that the euchromatic material had origin in the 7q35-qter region (data not shown). Hybridization with RP11-298A10 and subtelomeric 7q probes, allowed establishing that the aSMC results of an invdup rearrangement of 7q35-qter region (Fig. 2d).

Affimetrix CytoScan HD array analysis redefines the aSMC to a region of about 15.42 Mb enclosing 67 OMIM genes, 16 of which are associated to disease (Fig. 3). Trio analysis of the patient and his parents excluded the presence of UPD 7 and indicated a maternal origin of the aSMC.

Based on these results, the karyotype was established as:

mos 47,XY,+mar dn[73]/46,XY[27].ish invdup(7)(qter → q35::q35 → neo → qter)(wcp7+,D7Z1-,RP11-298A10++,TelVysion7q++).arr[GRCh37] 7q35q36.3(143218954x2,143594973_159119707x4).

## Discussion

When an SMC is discovered in a current cytogenetic analysis, its identification can be a challenging task if using FISH only. The best approach to study an SMC with euchromatic material is to use DNA microarray to determine its origin, involved region and size, followed by FISH for its characterisation. In our case, the SMC identification and characterization was made by FISH and cCGH. Afterwards, SNParray was done to mapping at submicroscopic level the genomic imbalance, to exclude the presence of UPD and to determine the parental origin. This allowed the characterization of an aSMC,

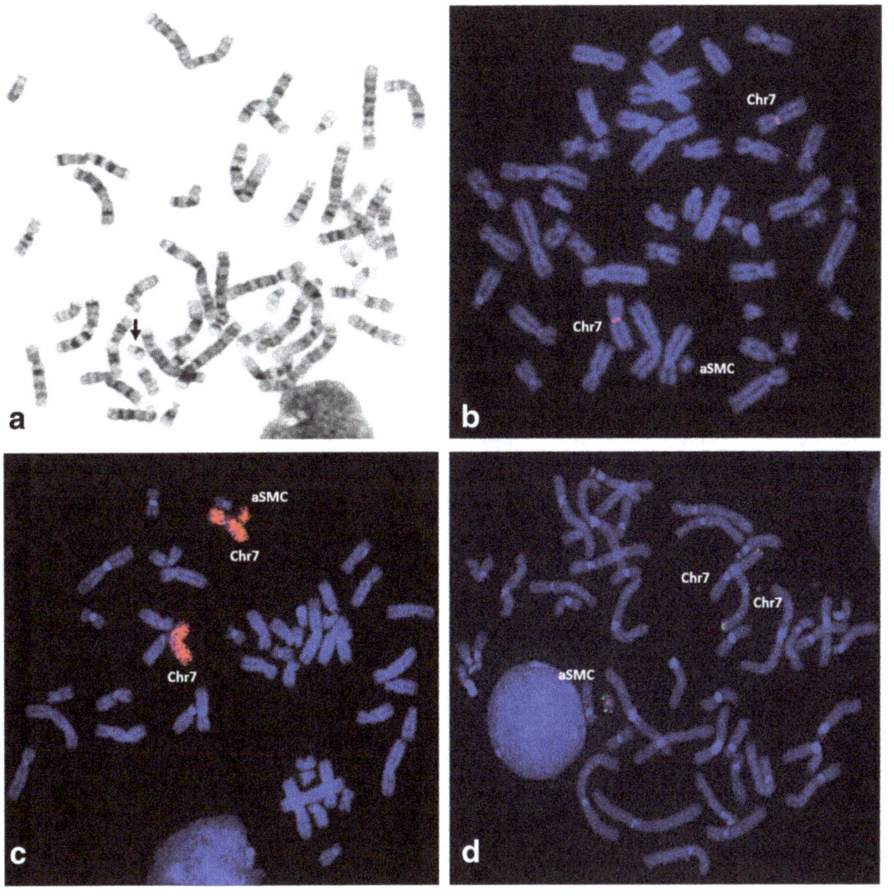


**Fig. 2** Cytogenetic and FISH investigation **a** GTL-banded chromosomes showing the aSMC (arrow); FISH with **b** α-satellite probe for chromosome 7 showing absence of signal on the aSMC; **c** WCP(7) showing the presence of chromosome 7 euchromatin in the aSMC; **d** BAC RP11-298A10 (*red*) e subtelomeric 7q (*green*) probes showing that the aSMC is a invdup involving the terminal region of chromosome 7 (7q35-qter)

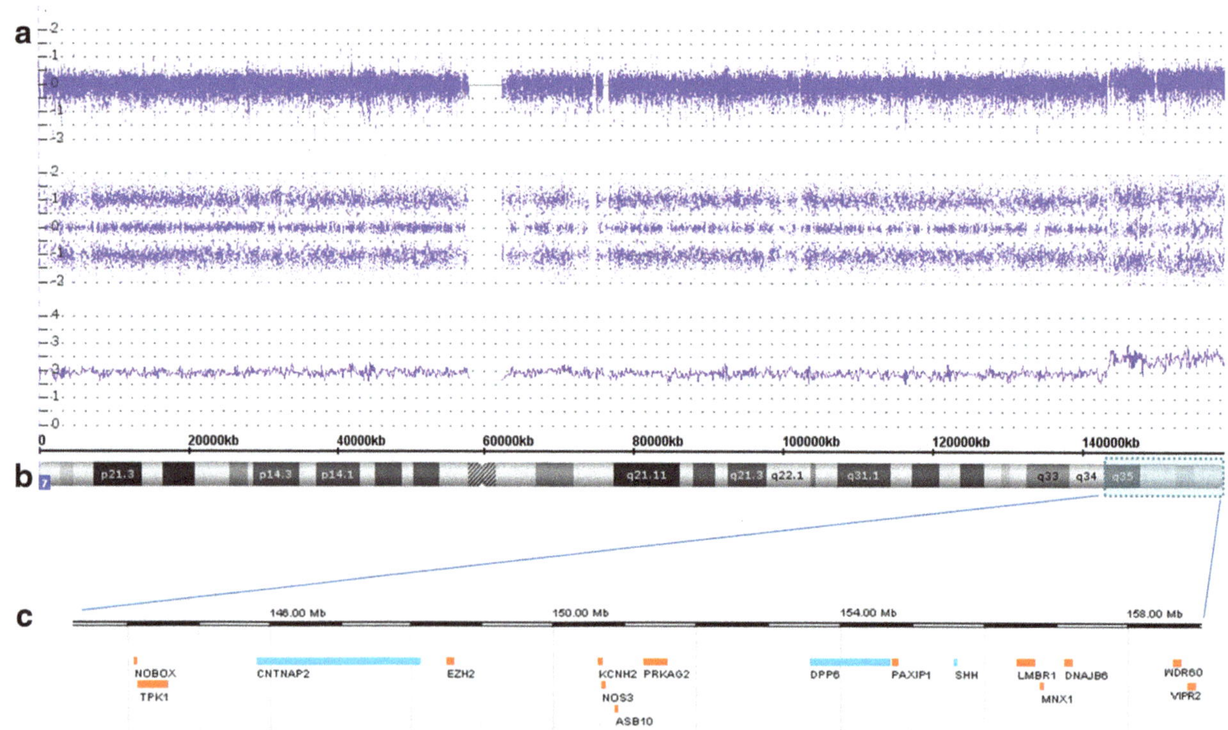


**Fig. 3** SNParray profile for chromosome 7. **a** Copy number probe intensities (log2 ratio) are represented in the upper track, allele peak tracks in the middle and smooth signal below indicating a mosaic gain. **b** Chromosome 7 ideogram showing the tetraplicated region (*blue* box); **c** OMIM genes associated to disorder present in the aSMC: In *blue* = more potentially implicated in phenotype; In *orange* = apparently not related to phenotype

which consists of an invdup(7) of maternal origin, resulting in tetrasomy of 7q35qter region, with a size of 15.42 Mb and no morbid gene disrupted at the breakpoint. It contains 67 OMIM genes, 16 of which associated to disease and therefore predicted to cause phenotypic effects.

The correlation of syndromic manifestations with specific chromosome segments duplications is not simple, since a pure 7q partial trisomy is rare. In 2008, Scelsa et al. reviewed 18 cases with apparently pure dup(7) and compared them with a patient who had trisomy of 7q32-7qter region [11]. In this study the authors classified the patients into four groups according to the size of the rearrangement. The last group, were we can include our patient, presents distal duplications and the most frequent phenotypic features are: macrocephaly, frontal bossing, small nose, low-set ears and usually severe developmental delay. However, from the seven cases reported in this group, only a tandem duplication of 7q36-qter could be considered as pure dup(7) since it does not involve another chromosome [12]. In the other six cases the duplicated material is present as part of a derivative chromosome that arises from a parent's balanced translocation, hence the contribution of an eventual positional effect or a gene regulatory disruption to the phenotype cannot be excluded [13–15]. In addition, these cases were not run through genome-wide studies so the presence of a single genomic imbalance region could not be confirmed. DECIPHER database lists 109 patients with a 7q gain that overlaps with our patient, but only 49 have a single region of imbalance [16]. There is only one patient with a small triplicate region of 354.50 Kb [DECIPHER ID 251853: arr[GRCh37] 7q36.3(157930785_158285281)×3] which was inherited from a normal parent, that comprises *PTPRN2* (OMIM*601698), and who presented with broad thumb, delayed speech and language development, hypertelorism and intellectual disability. Furthermore, seven of these patients have copy number gains of more than 1 Mb, being the biggest a *de novo* gain of 11.50 Mb [DECIPHER ID 268243: arr[GRCh37] 7q33q36.1(137914589_149415401)×3] that encompasses several genes, including *CNTNAP2* (OMIM*604569), whilst presenting with developmental delay and strabismus. Intellectual disability, delayed speech and language development are the most common phenotypic features associated with terminal 7q gains, however global development delay and specific learning disability can also be found.

The tetraplicated region of our patient encloses 16 morbid genes. The analysis of these genes permitted to highlight *CNTNAP2* (OMIM*604569), *DPP6* (OMIM*126141) *and SHH* (OMIM*600725). *CNTNAP2* and *SHH* are confirmed as causing developmental disorder in multiple unrelated cases [16]. *CNTNAP2* was linked to complex neurological disorders, including language impairment, autism, intellectual disability, schizophrenia, epilepsy, speech delay, attention deficit hyperactivity disorder, cortical dysplasia-focal epilepsy and Pitt-Hopkins-like syndrome [17–19]. *SHH* (sonic hedgehog) belongs to a family of genes that code for a class of proteins that act as signalling molecules during embryogenesis, namely for nervous and skeletal systems and formation of the testis cord [20]. *DPP6* has been related to microcephaly and mental retardation as well in the pathogenesis of autism spectrum disorder and Gilles de la Tourette syndrome [21–23]. Most of the reports associate the phenotype of patients to haploinsufficiency of these genes, resulting from deletions, mutations or disruptions, and not to overexpression. However, the overexpression of the *SHH* was suggested to be responsible for the typical facial features and profound hypotonia observed in the distal 7q duplication syndrome [24] and for the congenital muscular hypertrophy described in siblings with a 0.3 Mb duplication at 7q36.3 [25]. Recently, Wong et al. (2015) described a familial 7q36.3 duplication of 0.73 Mb involving *SHH* and *RBM33* associated with agnesia of the corpus callosum, macrocephaly, broad forehead, widely spaced eyes and mild intellectual disability [26]. On the other hand, overexpression of *PRKAG2* has been associated to cardiac problems observed in a case of partial tetrasomy of 7q35q36.3 region [27]. Marshall et al. (2008) performed genome-wide studies in 427 families with autism spectrum disorders (ASDs) using SNParray, and found that both deletions and duplications on *DPP6* are implicated as a novel locus for this disease [23]. On the other hand different expression levels of *LMBR1* (OMIM*605522), required for limb formation, were implicated in acheiropodia (ACHP, OMIM#200500) and triphalangeal thumb-polysyndactyly syndrome (TPTPS, OMIM#174500) [28]. ZRS is a long-range limb-specific *SHH* enhancer, on chromosome 7q36.3 region, which lies within intron 5 of *LMBR1* approximately 1 Mb upstream of the target gene *SHH*, and determining the identity and number of digits in early limb development [29]; duplication of this gene was proposed to originate syndactyly type IV (SD4) and TPTPS as a continuum of phenotypes [30]. Some limb abnormalities can be found in patients with 7q duplications, such as a wide space between the first and second toes [24] campodactyly with 5$^{th}$ finger clinodactyly [13], adducted thumbs [11] and short fifth fingers with clinodactyly [15]. Nevertheless, our patient has 4 copies of *PRKAG2* and *LMBR1* (and ZRS), but does not present any cardiac affectation or alteration in the number or form of fingers and toes, showing only nails hypoplasia. However, little is known about the expression of the genes involved in the tetraplicated region, and the absence of cardiac and limb abnormalities could be explained by the mosaicism and/or a possible dosage compensation mechanism.

The smaller duplication of 7q36qter region described [12] is not associated with any major malformation, but with developmental delay, particularly in speech. It is important to note that this rearrangement was characterized by cytogenetics only, and that *CNTNAP2* gene spans 2.3 Mb, between the 7q35 and 7q36 bands, and is probably disrupted in this case which reinforces the importance of this "language"gene.

## Conclusion

In summary, this is the first patient with an aSMC(7) derived from the terminal 7q region who has been fully characterized by high resolution genome-wide analysis and has also a detailed clinical description. This report confirms that euchromatic supernumerary material from distal region of 7q can cause a severe phenotype with mental retardation and dysmorphisms, being language, particularly speech, the most obviously affected areas of development. This new study contributes to the knowledge of one more aSMC(7), the sixth case reported so far, and to a better understanding of this type of chromosome rearrangements which make genetic counselling extremely challenging.

We reinforce the need for a better characterization of all new findings in this region, using more informative methods, as well as the importance of a detailed clinical description of all the patients registered in databases, in order to allow a better interpretation of genomic variants. An integrated analysis of genome-wide copy number variation and parental origin, if possible associated to FISH and gene expression studies could facilitate in the future the difficult task of establishing accurate phenotype-genotype correlations and aid in genetic counselling.

### Abbreviations

arrayCGH: Array comparative genomic hybridization; ASDs: Autism-spectrum disorders; aSMC: Analphoid supernumerary marker chromosome; BAC: Bacterial artificial chromosome; cCGH: Chromosomal comparative genomic hybridization; FISH: Fluorescent *in situ* hybridization; GTL: Giemsa-trypsin-leishman; SD4: Syndactyly type IV; SMC: Supernumerary marker chromosome; SNParray: Single nucleotide polymorphism array; TPTPS: Triphalangeal thumb-polysyndactyly syndrome; UPD 7: Uniparental disomy of chromosome 7; WCP: Whole chromosome painting probe

### Acknowledgments

We thank the family for their collaboration in this study.
MyPODFinder was developed by Paul Piccinelli and Tord Jonson at the Department of Clinical Genetics, Lund, Sweden.
This study makes use of data generated by the DECIPHER community. A full list of centres who contributed to the generation of the data is available from https://decipher.sanger.ac.uk/ and via email from decipher@sanger.ac.uk. Funding for the project was provided by the Wellcome Trust.

**Funding**
There was no funding available for this study.

**Authors' contributions**
BM contributed to FISH and cCHG studies, SNParray interpretation and figures preparation. CF contributed for the case discussion and manuscript preparation. FB and CA contributed to the cytogenetic results and SP contributed to the SNParray results. MA and TL contributed to the clinical evaluation of the patient and critically reviewed the manuscript. HC participated in the design and coordination of the study. All authors read and approved the final manuscript.

**Competing interests**
The authors declare that they have no competing interests.

**Author details**
[1]Unidade de Citogenética, Departamento de Genética Humana, Instituto Nacional de Saúde Doutor Ricardo Jorge, I.P, Avenida Padre Cruz, 1649-016 Lisboa, Portugal. [2]Serviço de Genética Médica, Hospital de Dona Estefânia, Centro Hospitalar de Lisboa Central, Rua Jacinta Marto, 1169-045 Lisboa, Portugal.

**References**
1. Liehr T. Small supernumerary marker chromosomes (sSMC): a guide for human geneticists and clinicians. 1st ed. Berlin: Springer; 2012.
2. Liehr T. Small supernumerary marker chromosomes. 2016. http://www.ssmc-tl.com/. Accessed 4 Mar 2016.
3. Lamb AN, Estabrooks LL, Legator MS, Ramakrishnan R, Poole I, Piper J, Morrison LE. Combinatorial 24 chromosome multicolour FISH for the identification of constitutional abnormalities; unbalanced translocations and analphoid markerchromosomes. (Abstract #798). Am J Hum Genet. 1998; 63(Suppl 4):A142.
4. Warburton PE. Chromosomal dynamics of human neocentromere formation. Chromosome Res. 2004;12:617–26.
5. Ebrahim SA, Jiang H, Te R, Mohamed AN. Neocentromere formation in a stable rearranged chromosome 7 with class II pericentric interstitial deletion and the formation of ring chromosome 7. Am J Hum Genet. 2008;82(Suppl 4).
6. Kumar MJ, Kumar RA, Subhashree V, Jayasudha T, Hemagowri V, Koshy T, et al. Class II analphoid chromosome in a child with aberrant chromosome 7: a rare cytogenetic association. Cytogenet Genome Res. 2015;146:120–3.
7. Louvrier C, Egea G, Labalme A, Des Portes V, Gazzo S, Callet-Bauchu E, et al. Characterization of a de novo supernumerary neocentric ring chromosome derived from chromosome 7. Cytogenet Genome Res. 2015;174(2–3):111–7.
8. Mcgowan-Jordan J, Simons A, Schmid M, editors. ISCN 2016: an international system for human cytogenomic nomenclature (2016). Basel: S. Karger; 2016.
9. David D, Cardoso J, Marques B, Marques R, Silva ED, Santos H, et al. Molecular characterization of a familial translocation implicates disruption of *HDAC9* and possible position effect on *TGFβ2* in the pathogenesis of Peters' anomaly. Genomics. 2003;81(5):489–503.
10. David D, Marques B, Ferreira C, Vieira P, Corona-Rivera A, Ferreira JC, et al. Characterization of two ectrodactyly-associated translocation breakpoints separated by 2.5 Mb on chromosome 2q14.1–q14.2. Eur J Hum Genet. 2009;17:1024–33.
11. Scelsa B, Bedeschi FM, Guerneri S, Lalatta F, Introvini P. Partial trisomy of 7q: case report and literature review. J Child Neurol. 2008;23(5):572–9.
12. Verma RS, Conte RA, Pitter JH. Tandem duplications of the terminal band of the long arm of chromosome 7 (dir dup (7) (q36 → qter)). J Med Genet. 1992;29:344–5.
13. Rodríguez L, López F, Paisán L, de la Red Mdelm P, Ruiz AM, Ruiz AM, et al. Pure partial trisomy 7q: two new patients and review. Am J Med Genet. 2002;113:218–24.
14. Bartsch O, Kalbe U, Ngo TKN, Lettau R, Schwinger E. Clinical diagnosis of partial duplication 7q. Am J Med Genet. 1990;37:254–7.
15. Romain DR, Cairney H, Stewart D, Columbano-Green LM, Garry M, Parslow MI, et al. Three cases of partial trisomy 7q owing to rare structural rearrangements of chromosome 7. J Med Genet. 1990;27:109–13.
16. DECIPHER: Database of chromosomal imbalance and phenotype in humans using ensembl resources. Firth, H.V. et al. Am j hum genet 2009;84,524-533. genome research limited web site: https://decipher.sanger.ac.uk/. Accessed 29 Mar 2016.
17. Poot M. Connecting the *CNTNAP2* networks with neurodevelopmental disorders. Mol Syndromol. 2015;6:7–22.
18. Alarcón M, Abrahams BS, Stone JL, Duvall JA, Perederity JV, Bomar JM, et al. Linkage, association, and gene-expression analyses identify *CNTNAP2* as an autism-susceptibility gene. Am J Hum Genet. 2008;82:150–9.
19. Rodenas-Cuadrado P, Ho J, Vernes SC. Shining a light on CNTNAP2: complex functions to complex disorders. Eur J Hum Genet. 2014;22:171–8.
20. Ingham PW, Mcmahon AP. Hedgehog signaking in animal development: paradigms and principles. Genes Dev. 2001;15:3059–87.
21. Liao C, Fu F, Li R, Yang W, Liao H, Yan J, et al. Loss-of-function variation in the DPP6 gene is associated with autosomal dominant microcephaly and mental retardation. Eur J Med Genet. 2013;56:484–9.
22. Prontera P, Napolioni V, Ottaviani V, Rogaia D, Fusco C, Augello B, et al. DPP6 gene disruption in a family with Gilles de la tourette syndrome. Neurogenetics. 2014;15:237–42.
23. Marshall CR, Noor A, Vincent JB, et al. Structural variation of chromosomes in autism spectrum disorder. Am J Hum Genet. 2008;82:477–88.
24. Morava E, Barstsch O, Czakó M, Frensel A, Kalscheuer V, Kárteszi J, et al. Small inherited terminal duplication of 7q with hydrocephalus, cleft palate, joint contractures, and severe hypotonia. Clin Dysmorphol. 2003;12:123–7.
25. Kroeldrup L, Kjaergaard S, Kirchhoff M, Kock K, Brasch-Andersen C, Kibaek M, et al. Duplication of 7q36.3 encompassing the sonic hedgehog (SHH) gene is associated with congenital muscular hypertrophy. Eur J Med Genet. 2012;55:557–60.
26. Wong K, Moldrich R, Hunter M, Edwards M, Finlay D, O'Donnell S, et al. A familial 7q36.3 duplication associated with agenesis of the corpus callosum. Am J Med Genet Part A. 2015;167A:2201–8.
27. Lehnen H, Maiwald R, Neyzen S, Kohlhase J, Bohm D, Ritterbach J, et al. Severe phenotype in a girl with partial tetrasomy 7, karyotype 46, XX, trp(7)(q35q36). Cytogenet Genome Res. 2009;125:248–52.
28. Clark RM, Marker PC, Roessler E, Dutra A, Schimenti JC, Muenke M, et al. Reciprocal mouse and human limb phenotypes caused by gain- and loss-of-function mutations affecting Lmbr1. Genetics. 2001;159:715–26.
29. La L, Heaney SJH, Purdie LA, Li L, de Beer P, Oostra BA, et al. A long-range Shh enhancer regulates expression in the developing limb and fin and is associated with preaxial polydactyly. Hum Mol Genet. 2003;12(14):1725–35.
30. Dai L, Hong G, Meng H, Zhan K, Hu H, Yao H, et al. Confirmation of genetic homogeneity of syndactyly type IV and triphalangeal thumb-polysyndactyly syndrome in a Chinese family and review of the literature. Eur J Pediatr. 2003;172:1467–73.

9

# Molecular and clinical characterization of new patient with 1,08 Mb deletion in 10p15.3 region

Anna Poluha[1], Joanna Bernaciak[2], Ilona Jaszczuk[1], Marta Kędzior[2] and Beata Anna Nowakowska[2*]

**Abstract**

**Background:** Three distinct contiguous gene deletion syndromes are located at 10p chromosomal region. The deletion, involving 10p15.3 region, has been characterized by (DeScipio et al., Am J Med Genet A 158A:2152-61, 2012). However, because of the variation in size of the described deletions and lack of knowledge about the involved genes, the correlation between genotypes and patients' phenotypes remains unknown.

**Case presentation:** We describe female patient with de novo 1,08 Mb deletion in 10p15.3 region, similar to the patient nr seven reported by (DeScipio et al., Am J Med Genet A 158A:2152-61, 2012) but with more severe clinical features. Our patient demonstrated speech and motor delay, dysmorphic features, brain abnormalities and Tetralogy of Fallot with pulmonary atresia.

**Conclusions:** This case shows the importance of collection of more patients with deletion in order to obtain a more precise physical map of 10p region.

**Keywords:** 10p15.3 deletion, Intellectual disability, Language impairment

## Background

Partial monosomy of 10p is a rare chromosomal aberration. Recently three distinct contiguous gene deletion syndromes, located at 10p chromosomal region, have been described. Haploinsufficiency of proximal 10p13-10p14 region, designate as DiGeorge critical region 2 (DGCR2), associated with congenital heart defect and thymus hypoplasia or T cell defect [15]. Haploinsufficiency of more distal region 10p14, responsible for hypoparathyroidism, deafness and renal anomalies (HDR Syndrome) [8, 10, 16]. And recently defined by DeScipio et al. [3] submicroscopic deletion involving 10p15.3 region, associated with intellectual disability and language impairment [3, 9, 17].

Subtelomeric deletion of 10p15.3 was up today reported in 21 unrelated patients [3, 13], two familial members of different generations [4] and one pair of monozygotic twins [17]. The first two cases were included in the large subtelomeric FISH study by Ravnan et al. [13] and the deleted region was not molecularly mapped. All other described deletions varied in size and ranged between 0,15 and 4 Mb. The size of the deletion generally does not correlate with severity of patients' phenotype and so far critical region was not determined. However, deletion is mainly associated with cognitive/developmental and speech delay, motor delay, brain anomalies and seizures [3, 17]. Two genes, *ZMYND11* and *DIP2C*, mapping within 10p15.3 were most commonly deleted in illustrated patients [3] and were suggested to be responsible for development delay and speech impairment. Recently mutations in the *ZMYND11* gene have been demonstrated by several authors to be associated with severe speech delay and language disorder, complex cognitive, behavioral and developmental difficulties as well as dysmorphic features in some of the reported patients [1, 2, 11].

Here we present clinical and molecular data of a pediatric patient with de novo 1,08 Mb deletion in 10p15.3 region and clinical features suggestive of del22q11. Our patient has similar deletion size to the patient nr 7 reported by DeScipio et al. [3], but more severe clinical phenotype, including brain malformation, and heart abnormalities observed only in 2/21 patients with 10p15.3 deletion (Table 1).

* Correspondence: beata.nowakowska@imid.med.pl
[2]Department of Medical Genetics, Cytogenetics, Institute of Mother and Child, Kasprzaka 17, A 01-211 Warsaw, Poland
Full list of author information is available at the end of the article

**Table 1** Summary of clinical features in the cohort of Vargiami et al. [17] and DeScipio et al. [3], with distinction of patient nr 7, patient with missense mutation in ZMYND11 gene [1] and our index patient

| | DeScipio et al., Varigiami et al. | Patient 7 from DeScipio et al. cohort with the closest overlapping deletion | Patient with mutation in *ZMYND11* gene described by Cobben et al. | Patient with mutation in *ZMYND11* gene described by Moskowitz et al. | Our patient |
|---|---|---|---|---|---|
| sex | Male:Female 8:6 | Male | Male | Female | Female |
| Age at report | 1y9m – 48y | 5y | 7y | 24y | 5y |
| Birth weight | < 3rd centile – 25th centile | 3402 g (25th centile) | 1867 g (<3rd centile) | 3740 g (50th centile) | 3370 g (25th centile) |
| Height | <3rd centile – 75th centile | 25th centile | < 3rd centile | Not provided | < 3rd centile |
| Weight | <3rd centile – > 95th centile | 75th centile | Not provided | Not provided | < 3rd centile |
| Head circumference | 10th - >95th centile | 75th centile | Microcephaly (<3rd centile) | Microcephaly (<3rd centile) | 25th centile |
| Cognitive/ behavioral/ developmental differences | 13/13 | Hyperactivity | Severe developmental delay | Severe global developmental delay, able to understand to some degree and can communicate using a few sings, happy disposition, smiles almost constantly | Mild ID, temper tantrums, aggression |
| Speech delay | 10/10 | Severe One or two word sentences at 5y | At the age of 7 years uses only two words | Non verbal, makes sounds | Severe Single words at 5y |
| Motor delay | 11/11 | Started to walk independently at 2,5y Unable to run well or ride a bicycle at 5y | At the age of 7 years walks behind a walking device | Severe motor delay, ataxic, wide base gait, walks only short distances with assistance. | Started to walk independently at 2y Clumsy running at 5y |
| Craniofacial dysmorphic features | 9/12 Inconsistent | Plagiocephaly, hypertelorism, prominent columella, hypoplastic alae, | Slight metopic ridge, low-set ears, hypopigmentation of the right eyebrow and eyelashes, telecanthi, epicanthic folds, slant-up and narrowing of palpebral fissures, broad nasal bridge, small nares with broad alaenasi, smooth philtrum with thin upper lip and everted lower lip, widely-spaced teeth, retrognathia. | Bulbous nose with wide base and ridge,, deep set eyes, long palpebral fissures, epicanthal fold, prominent jaw | Flat face, mild synophrys, long eyelashes, long palpebral fissures, epicanthal folds, wide nasal ridge, low set, posteriorly rotated and slightly protruding ears, underdeveloped antitargus, short chin |
| Brain abnormalities | 6/8 cortical atrophy (4), hydrocephalus (1), arachnoid cyst (1) | No | Delayed myelination | Cerebral atrophy and delayed myelination without evidence of focal abnormality | Chiari malformation type I with spinal cord edema requiring surgical decompression |
| Hypotonia | 7/13 | No | Yes | Yes | in infancy |
| Hand/ft anomalies | 5/13 | 5th finger clinodactyly, fetal pads, pes planus, clinodactyly of toes 3,4,5 | Valgus feet, short metacarpals of both hands and a brachymesophalanx V, broad hands with deep palmar creases and pillowing of the areas between the grooves, short tapering fingers and broad feet with short toes and small nails | 5th finger clinodactyly, small feet | 5th finger clinodactyly pes planus |
| Seizures | 3/9 | Partial complex | Absence seizures | Severe intractable seizures | Absence seizures |
| Cardiac anomalies | 2/11 bicuspid aortic valve, | Systolic murmur | Spontaneously closed VSD | None | Tetralogy of Fallot with pulmonary atresia |

**Table 1** Summary of clinical features in the cohort of Vargiami et al. [17] and DeScipio et al. [3], with distinction of patient nr 7, patient with missense mutation in ZMYND11 gene [1] and our index patient *(Continued)*

| | | | | | |
|---|---|---|---|---|---|
| | patent foramen ovale, murmur | | | | |
| Other features | | Diaphragmatic hernia, mildly narrow palate, shawl scrotum and wide-based gait | Feeding difficulties requiring supplementary tube feeding, fusion of the 2nd and 3rd vertebrae and compression of the myelum, pyloric stenosis non-descended testes and urethral stenosis, inverted and widely-spaced nipples, dimples on elbows and knees | Neurogenic bladder Severe eosinophilic gastroesophagitis, gastroesophageal reflux Asthma, multiple food, environmental and medication allergies Myopia Bilateral moderate hearing impairment (family history positive for hearing impairment) | wide-base gait protein C deficiency |

## Patient

Female patient was born as a third child of a healthy nonconsanguineous couple in a family without a history of congenital malformation nor intellectual disability. The pregnancy was uneventful with no confirmed teratogenic exposure and full term. Girl was born with weight 3370 g, length – 55 cm and OFC - 35 cm initially in a good condition which started to deteriorate rapidly due to severe congenital heart defect - tetralogy of Fallot with pulmonary atresia. Single stage cardiosurgery has been performed on 7th day after delivery. The postoperative period has been complicated by thrombotic events due to protein C deficiency requiring surgical clot removal. Following her initial neurologic examination at the age of 3,5 months which revealed axial hypotonia and head circumference of 38,5 cm (10th centile) with normal results of cranial ultrasound, she has been systematically evaluated by pediatric neurologist. Her developmental milestones were markedly delayed. She started to walk unaided at 24 months and she did not vocalize till 3 years of age. The results of her neuropsychologic evaluation at this time indicated mild mental retardation with difficulties in gross motor skills and socioemotional functions with relatively well visuomotor skills. At 3 years of age her parents noticed unsteady, wide-base gait and unusual behavior presenting as unprovoked temper tantrums, aggression and sudden-onset interruption of on-going activities with blank stare and impairment of consciousness. Abnormal EEG (Electroencephalography) results at that time indicated epilepsy and the antiepileptic drugs has been introduced. Additionally her brain MRI (Magnetic resonance imaging) revealed downward displacement of medullary tonsils (22 mm below foramen magnum) with spinal cord edema without syrinx, consistent with Chiari malformation type I. She underwent the posterior fossa decompression with C1 and partial C2 laminectomy accompanied by duraplasty which later required two additional surgical corrections. After last surgery, significant progression of her development was noted.

Girl was initially assessed at our Genetic Clinic at the age of three. She presented with developmental delay, mild mental retardation, severe language impairment and failure to thrive. Her height was 89 cm(< 3rd centile), weight was 12 kg(< 3rd centile) and her head circumference was 48,5 cm (25th centile). Dysmorphic features included: flat face, mild synophrys, long eyelashes, long palpebral fissures (2,8 cm >90th centile), epicanthal folds, wide nasal bridge, low set, posteriorly rotated and slightly protruding ears with underdeveloped antitargus, short chin and fifth finger clinodactyly. Dysmorphic features in combination with, short stature, developmental delay, impaired speech development and congenital heart defect were suggestive of DiGeorge syndrome (Fig. 1a–c).

## Methods

Genetic diagnostic studies were done including chromosome analysis after GTG banding with a resolution of approximately 500 bands per haploid genome.

Genomic DNA was extracted from patient's peripheral blood cells using a Genomic DNA purification kit (Puregene, Gentra Systems, Minneapolis, MN) according to the manufacturer's instruction.

MLPA (245 SALSA MLPA probemixes, MRC-Holland) analysis was performed to exclude the 22q11 deletion.

Array CGH was performed using a 180 K oligonucleotide microarray (CytoSure, ISCA v2, Oxford Gene Technology, Oxford, UK). DNA of the patient was hybridized against a female control. Labeling and hybridization were performed following the manufacturer's protocols (Invitrogene, BioPrime Array CGH, Carlsbad, CA). Briefly, 1 μg of DNA was labeled overnight by random primers. Labeled products were purified on the columns centrifugal filters (Invitrogene, BioPrime Array CGH) according to the manufacturer's instruction. After probe denaturation and prehybridization with Cot-1 DNA, hybridization was performed at 65 °C with rotation for 72 h. After washing the array was analyzed with the Agilent scanner and Feature Extraction software (Agilent Technologies, Santa Clara, CA) and text file outputs from the quantization

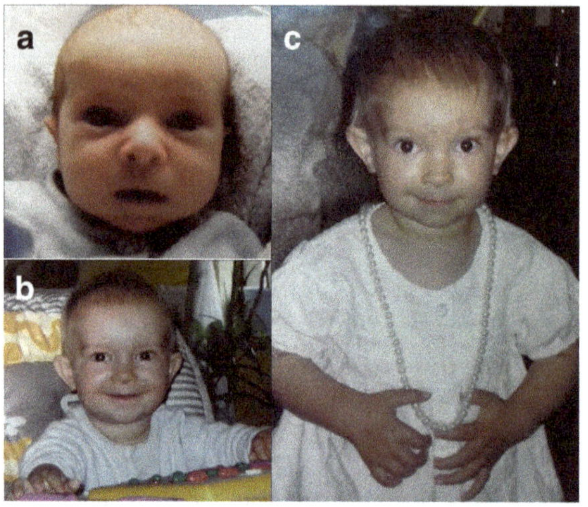


**Fig. 1** **a** Patient on the first day of life: round face, long palpebral fissures, epicanthal folds, wide nasal root and wide nasal bridge. **b** Patient at the age 8 months: round face, upstanding palpebral fissures, low set nasal root, short columella, narrow upper lip, long and protruding ears. **c** Patient at the age 2 years: frontal bossing, ocular hypertelorism, long upstanding palpebral fissures, long lashes, low set nasal root, wide nasal bridge, narrow upper lip, short chin

analysis were imported to CytoSure Interpret Software (Oxford Gene Technology) for copy number analysis.

FISH analyses of the 10p15.3 region was performed according to a standard protocol, using BAC clone RP11–62O22. Briefly, a 500 ng DNA of BAC clone was labeled with Spectrum Red dUTP by random prime method (Invitrogene, BioPrime Array CGH), according to the manufacturer's' protocol. Slides were viewed on a Zeiss Axioplan2 fluorescence microscope and images were captured and analyzed using Applied Spectral Imaging Acquisition 5.0 analysis system (Applied Spectral Imaging, Inc. Vista, CA).

## Results

Chromosome analysis revealed normal female karyotype. Also MLPA analysis for common deletions was normal.

The whole genome CGH array identified a 1,08 Mb deletion on chromosome 10p15.3 (Fig. 2a). The proximal breakpoint was mapped at the position 126,145 and the distal breakpoint at 1,204,340 (UCSC Genome Browser on Human, hg18). No other CNVs have been detected.

FISH analysis with BAC clone RP11–62O22 confirmed the deletion (Fig. 2b) and parental studies showed that deletion occurred de novo.

Deleted genomic region harbors 8 RefSeq known genes; *ZMYND11, DIP2C, RRR26, LARP4B, GTPBP4, IDI2, IDI1, WDR37*. Only 4 OMIM annotated; *ZMYND11, DIP2C, IDI1, IDI2*, and two dosage sensitive; *LARP4B (LARP5)* and *IDI1*. Happloinsufficiency score of the dosage sensitive gene is 0,601 and 0,488 for *LARP4B* and *IDI1*, respectively [5].

## Discussion

We report female patient with 1,08 Mb deletion on chromosome 10p15.3 presenting with development delay, severe language impairment, motor delay, dysmorphic features, hypotonia, seizures, brain malformations and severe congenital heart disease. To our knowledge 25 patients has been reported so far with 10p15.3 deletion and some overlap in phenotypic features. Though not for all described cases detailed clinical information is known, the patients' phenotype does not simply correlate with the size of the deletion. Our patient has similar deletion to the patient seven from DeScipio et al., [3] study, but more severe phenotype, including congenital heart condition and Chiari malformation type 1 not seen before in this patients' cohort. Cardiac anomalies have been observed only in 2 out of 25 patients with this deletion. As for the brain abnormalities, they were noted in four out of six radiologically evaluated patients reported by DeScipio et al. [3]: hydrocephalus (1 patient), small arachnoid cyst (1 patient) and cortical atrophy (2 patients). The later has also been present in the female twins reported by Vargiami et al. [17]. None of the previously described patients has been found to have structural defects of the cerebellum. It should be noted that the patient reported by DeScipio et al. [3] is a male while our patient is a female. However limited information about the deleted genes' function does not allow to determine if sex factor could contribute to the severity of our patient's clinical symptoms. None such correlation has been pointed out in the cohort of patients reported by DeScipio et al. [3] in which female to male ratio was 10:9.

Little is currently known about the genes located within 10p15.3 region, and this complicates the genotype – phenotype correlation. DeScipio et al. [3] distinguished two genes, *ZMYND11* and *DIP2C*, although no single gene was deleted in all 19 studied individuals. Several cases with a de novo mutation in *ZMYND11* gene have been reported [1, 2, 6, 11]. First case with a G > A substitution in codon 239, predicted to alter a splice site in the *ZMYND11* gene [6]. However, this patient had an autism spectrum disorder but no intellectual disability and no obvious dysmorphism. Second patient with a de novo missense mutation C > T in codon 1798 in *ZMYND11* gene presented severe developmental delay and dysmorphic feature (Table 1). This variant changed an evolutionary highly conserved, positively charged, arginine into a neutral tryptophan [1]. Coe and co-authors (2014) in their study of large cohort of patients with neurodevelopmental diseases, using integrated analysis of copy number variants and single-nucleotide variants followed by resequencing of candidate genes, identified five different truncating *ZMYND11* mutations in patients with overlapping clinical presentation including speech and motor delay, borderline

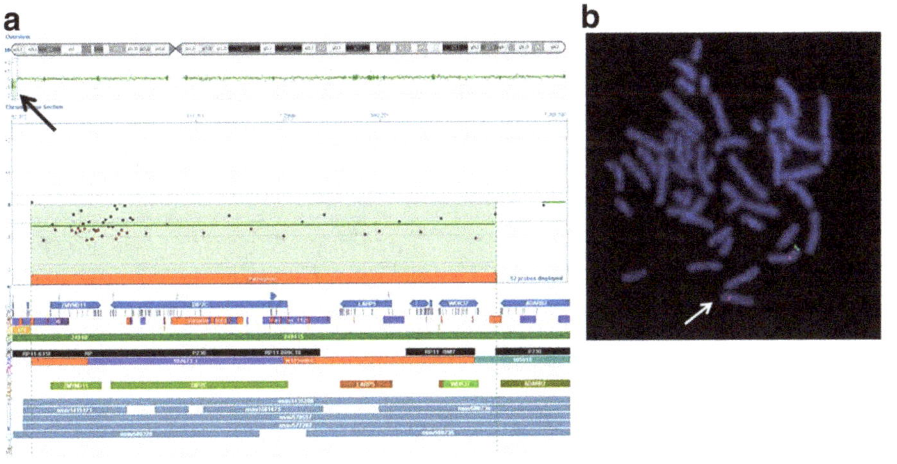

**Fig. 2 a** Array-CGH analysis showing deletion of the 10p15.3 region. **b** FISH analysis of the 10p15.3 region using BAC clone RP11–62O22 (green), confirmed deletion

IQ, mild dysmorhism as well as complex behavioral and developmental problems. They also suggested that truncating mutations in *ZMYND11* gene are likely to be associated with other more complex neuropsychiatric disorders. More recently Moskowitz et al. [11] presented a female patient with a severe global developmental delay, intractable epilepsy, hypotonia and dysmorphic features associated with a de novo missense mutation in *ZMYND11* gene.

*ZMYND11* (OMIM 608668) is located to the nucleus and regulates RNA polymerase II elongation [19]. *DIP2C* (OMIM 611380) is expressed in all adult and fetal tissues, including specific adult brain regions, but except lung and pancreas, where expression was detected at low level [12]. However two different genes are deleted in our patient and are known to be dosage sensitive: *LARP4B* and *IDI1*. *LARP4B* is not annotated in OMIM and still very little is known about its function. It belongs to an evolutionarily conserved family of factors with predicted roles in RNA metabolism. Schäffler et al. [14] demonstrated its role in bridging mRNA factors of the 3′end with initiating ribosomes. Overexpression of LARP4B stimulated protein synthesis, whereas knockdown of the factor by RNA interference impaired translation of a large number of cellular mRNAs. Additionally, Wang et al. [18] suggested that abnormal expression of Larp4b can be found in leukemia patients. *IDI1* gene (OMIM 604055) catalyzes a critical activation step in isoprenoid pathway and has a reduced activity in liver tissue from patients with the peroxisomal deficiency diseases Zellweger syndrome and neonatal adrenoleukodystrophy [7]. Based on this very limited information about the genes function it is very difficult to draw conclusion which of these genes can be crucial for observed phenotypes and how they can influence the variability in clinical features. Also, so far no patients with mutation in other genes than *ZMYND11* have been described. However, common clinical features observed in most patients with deletion of 10p15.3 and patients with mutations in *ZMYND11* suggest that haploinsufficiency of *ZMYND11* contributes to the clinical features of 10p15.3 deletions syndrome and most likely it is responsible for intellectual disability in those patients. But molecular and clinical description of new patients with deletion in 10p15 is necessary before the full gene – phenotype correlation will be established for this region.

**Acknowledgements**
We are grateful to the patient and her family for participation in these studies.

**Funding**
This work was made possible by grant from National Science Centre (OPUS NCN 2015/17/B/NZ5/01357 to BN).

**Authors' contributions**
AP and IJ described clinical features of our patient. AP made the comparison with clinical features of patients already described in literature. JB performed the FISH study. MK performed MLPA study. BN performed array and was a major contributor in writing the manuscript. All authors read and approved the final manuscript.

**Competing interests**
The authors declare that they have no competing interests.

**Author details**
[1]Department of Pediatric Hematology, Oncology and Transplantation Children's University Hospital, Lublin, Poland. [2]Department of Medical Genetics, Cytogenetics, Institute of Mother and Child, Kasprzaka 17, A 01-211 Warsaw, Poland.

**References**

1. Cobben JM, Weiss MM, van Dijk FS, De Reuver R, de Kruiff C, Pondaag W, Hennekam RC, Yntema HG. A de novo mutation in ZMYND11, a candidate gene for 10p15.3 deletion syndrome, is associated with syndromic intellectual disability. Eur J Med Genet. 2014;57(11-12):636–8.

2. Coe BP, Witherspoon K, Rosenfeld JA, van Bon BWM, Vulto-van Silfhout AT, Bosco P, Friend KL, Baker C, Buono S, Vissers LELM, Schuurs-Hoeijmakers JH, Hoischen A, Pfundt R, Krumm N, Carvill GL, Li D, Amaral D, Brown N, Lockhart PJ, Scheffer IE, Alberti A, Shaw M, Pettinato R, Tervo R, de Leeuw N, Reijnders MRF, Torchia BS, Peeters H, O'Roak BJ, Fichera M, Hehir-Kwa JY, Shendure J, Mefford HC, Haan E, Gécz J, de Vries BBA, Romano C, Eichler EE. Refining analyses of copy number variation identifies specific genes associated with developmental delay. Nat Genet. 2014;46(10):1063–71.
3. DeScipio C, Conlin L, Rosenfeld J, Tepperberg J, Pasion R, Patel A, McDonald MT, Aradhya S, Ho D, Goldstein J, McGuire M, Mulchandani S, Medne L, Rupps R, Serrano AH, Thorland EC, Tsai AC, Hilhorst-Hofstee Y, Ruivenkamp CA, Van Esch H, Addor MC, Martinet D, Mason TB, Clark D, Spinner NB, Krantz ID. Subtelomeric deletion of chromosome 10p15.3: clinical findings and molecular cytogenetic characterization. Am J Med Genet A. 2012; 158A(9):2152–61.
4. Fernández RM, Sánchez J, García-Díaz L, Peláez-Nora Y, González-Meneses A, Antiñolo G, Borrego S. Interstitial 10p deletion derived from a maternal ins (16;10)(q22;p13p15.2): report of the first familial case of 10p monosomy affecting to two familial members of different generations. Am J Med Genet A. 2016;170A(5):1268–73.
5. Huang N, Lee I, Marcotte EM, Hurles ME. Characterising and predicting haploinsufficiency in the human genome. PLoS Genet. 2010;6(10):e1001154.
6. Iossifov I, Ronemus M, Levy D, Wang Z, Hakker I, Rosenbaum J, Yamrom B, Lee YH, Narzisi G, Leotta A, Kendall J, Grabowska E, Ma B, Marks S, Rodgers L, Stepansky A, Troge J, Andrews P, Bekritsky M, Pradhan K, Ghiban E, Kramer M, Parla J, Demeter R, Fulton LL, Fulton RS, Magrini VJ, Ye K, Darnell JC, Darnell RB, Mardis ER, Wilson RK, Schatz MC, McCombie WR, Wigler M. De novo gene disruptions in children on the autistic spectrum. Neuron. 2012;74(2):285–99.
7. Krisans SK, Ericsson J, Edwards PA, Keller GA. Farnesyl-diphosphate synthase is localized in peroxisomes. J Biol Chem. 1994;269:14165–9.
8. Lichtner P, König R, Hasegawa T, Van Esch H, Meitinger T, Schuffenhauer S. An HDR (hypoparathyroidism, deafness, renal dysplasia) syndrome locus maps distal to the DiGeorge syndrome region on 10p13/14. J Med Genet. 2000;37(1):33–7.
9. Lindstrand A, Malmgren H, Verri A, Benetti E, Eriksson M, Nordgren A, Anderlid BM, Golovleva I, Schoumans J, Blennow E. Molecular and clinical characterization of patients with overlapping 10p deletions. Am J Med Genet A. 2010;152A(5):1233–43.
10. Melis D, Genesio R, Boemio P, Del Giudice E, Cappuccio G, Mormile A, Ronga V, Conti A, Imperati F, Nitsch L, Andria G. Clinical description of a patient carrying the smallest reported deletion involving 10p14 region. Am J Med Genet A. 2012;158A(4):832–5.
11. Moskowitz AM, Belnap N, Siniard AL, Szelinger S, Claasen AM, Richholt RF, De Both M, Corneveaux JJ, Balak C, Piras IS, Russell M, Courtright AL, Rangasamy S, Ramsey K, Craig DW, Narayanan V, Huentelman MJ, Schrauwen I. A de novo missense mutation in ZMYND11 is associated with global developmental delay, seizures, and hypotonia. Cold Spring Harb Mol Case Stud. 2016;2(5):a000851.
12. Nagase T, Ishikawa K, Suyama M, Kikuno R, Hirosawa M, Miyajima N, Tanaka A, Kotani H, Nomura N, Ohara O. Prediction of the coding sequences of unidentified human genes. XIII. The complete sequences of 100 new cDNA clones from brain which code for large proteins in vitro. DNA Res. 1999;6: 63–70.
13. Ravnan JB, Tepperberg JH, Papenhausen P, Lamb AN, Hedrick J, Eash D, Ledbetter DH, Martin CL. Subtelomere FISH analysis of 11 688 cases: an evaluation of the frequency and pattern of subtelomere rearrangements in individuals with developmental disabilities. J Med Genet. 2006;43(6):478–89.
14. Schäffler K, Schulz K, Hirmer A, Wiesner J, Grimm M, Sickmann A, Fischer U. A stimulatory role for the la-related protein 4B in translation. RNA. 2010; 16(8):1488–99.
15. Schuffenhauer S, Lichtner P, Peykar-Derakhshandeh P, Murken J, Haas OA, Back E, Wolff G, Zabel B, Barisic I, Rauch A, Borochowitz Z, Dallapiccola B, Ross M, Meitinger T. Deletion mapping on chromosome 10p and definition of a critical region for the second DiGeorge syndrome locus (DGS2). Eur J Hum Genet. 1998;6(3):213–25.
16. Van Esch H, Groenen P, Nesbit MA, Schuffenhauer S, Lichtner P, Vanderlinden G, Harding B, Beetz R, Bilous RW, Holdaway I, Shaw NJ, Fryns JP, Van de Ven W, Thakker RV, Devriendt K. GATA3 haplo-insufficiency causes human HDR syndrome. Nature. 2000;406(6794):419–22.
17. Vargiami E, Ververi A, Kyriazi M, Papathanasiou E, Gioula G, Gerou S, Al-Mutawa H, Kambouris M, Zafeiriou DI. Severe clinical presentation in monozygotic twins with 10p15.3 microdeletion syndrome. Am J Med Genet A. 2014;164A(3):764–8.
18. Wang XJ, Pang YK, Cheng H, Dong F, Liang HY, Zhang YC, Wang XM, Xu J, Cheng T, Yuan WP. Knockdown of Larp4b in Lin(−) cells does not affect the colony forming ability of mouse hematopoietic cells. Zhongguo Shi Yan Xue Ye Xue Za Zhi. 2013;21(3):735–40.
19. Wen H, Li Y, Xi Y, Jiang S, Stratton S, Peng D, Tanaka K, Ren Y, Xia Z, Wu J, Li B, Barton MC, Li W, Li H, Shi X. ZMYND11 links histone H3.3K36me3 to transcription elongation and tumour suppression. Nature. 2014;508:263–8.

# 10

# The presence of two rare genomic syndromes, 1q21 deletion and Xq28 duplication, segregating independently in a family with intellectual disability

Kyungsoo Ha[1,2], Yiping Shen[3], Tyler Graves[2], Cheol-Hee Kim[4] and Hyung-Goo Kim[2,5*]

**Abstract**

**Background:** 1q21 microdeletion syndrome is a rare contiguous gene deletion disorder with *de novo* or autosomal dominant inheritance patterns and its phenotypic features include intellectual disability, distinctive facial dysmorphism, microcephaly, cardiac abnormalities, and cataracts. *MECP2* duplication syndrome is an X-linked recessive neurodevelopmental disorder characterized by intellectual disability, global developmental delay, and other neurological complications including late-onset seizures. Previously, these two different genetic syndromes have not been reported segregating independently in a same family.

**Case presentation:** Here we describe two siblings carrying either a chromosome 1q21 microdeletion or a chromosome Xq28 duplication. Using a comparative genomic hybridization (CGH) array, we identified a 1.24 Mb heterozygous deletion at 1q21 resulting in the loss of 9 genes in a girl with learning disability, hypothyroidism, short stature, sensory integration disorder, and soft dysmorphic features including cupped ears and a unilateral ear pit. We also characterized a 508 kb Xq28 duplication encompassing *MECP2* in her younger brother with hypotonia, poor speech, cognitive and motor impairment. The parental CGH and quantitative PCR (qPCR) analyses revealed that the 1q21 deletion in the elder sister is *de novo*, but the Xq28 duplication in the younger brother was originally inherited from the maternal grandmother through the mother, both of whom are asymptomatic carriers. RT-qPCR assays revealed that the affected brother has almost double the amount of *MECP2* mRNA expression compared to other family members of both genders including maternal grandmother and mother who have the same Xq28 duplication with no phenotype. This suggests the X chromosome with an Xq28 duplication in the carrier females is preferentially silenced.

**Conclusion:** From our understanding, this would be the first report showing the independent segregation of two genetically unrelated syndromes, 1q21 microdeletion and Xq28 duplication, in a same family, especially in siblings. Although these two chromosomal abnormalities share some similar phenotypes such as intellectual disability, mild dysmorphic features, and cardiac abnormalities, the presence of two unrelated and rare syndromes in siblings is very unusual. Therefore, further comprehensive investigations in similar cases are required for future studies.

**Keywords:** Intellectual disability, 1q21 microdeletion, MECP2, Xq28 duplication, X chromosome inactivation, Segregation of two rare syndromes

* Correspondence: hkim@augusta.edu
[2]Section of Reproductive Endocrinology, Infertility & Genetics, Department of Obstetrics & Gynecology, Augusta University, Augusta, GA 30912, USA
[5]Department of Neuroscience and Regenerative Medicine, Augusta University, 1120 15th Street, Augusta, GA 30912, USA
Full list of author information is available at the end of the article

## Background

The 1q21 microdeletion (MIM 612474) is a very rare genetic disorder with the deleted region spanning from 145.4 Mb to 147.8 Mb (hg19) on chromosome 1. 1q21 microdeletion can occur *de novo*, but the majority of microdeletions are inherited from either parent in an autosomal dominant manner [1–3]. Haploinsufficiency of the genes deleted at 1q21 likely contribute to the clinical phenotypes associated with this microdeletion. A parent with the same microdeletion generally shows a normal phenotype, or very mild phenotype that is similar to or less severe than that of their child [1]. This suggests the possibility of parental imprinting, reduced penetrance, or variable expressivity. The phenotypic features prompting diagnosis of 1q21 microdeletion include mild to moderate intellectual disability, learning disability, microcephaly, mildly dysmorphic facial features and skeletal malformations [1–4], cataracts [2, 5] and heart abnormalities [5, 6]. Because these clinical features are also seen in other genetic disorders, 1q21 microdeletion is difficult to be diagnosed clinically and more often molecularly diagnosed by chromosomal microarray analysis [1, 2, 4].

Xq28 duplication syndrome (MIM 300815) resulting in functional disomy of Xq28 has been predominantly described in male patients with syndromic intellectual disability including infantile hypotonia, poor or absent speech, and recurrent pulmonary infections [7, 8]. The clinical features of Xq28 duplications differ, dependent on the location and the size ranging typically from 0.3 to 2 Mb [9–12]. One of the multiple genes duplicated in this intellectual disability syndrome is methyl CpG-binding protein 2 (*MECP2*; MIM 300005), a chromosomal protein that binds specifically to methylated DNA [13]. Early studies demonstrated that MECP2 represses transcription from methylated promoters [14] and is subject to X chromosome inactivation in both mouse and human [15, 16]. Furthermore, MECP2 is an essential regulator in postnatal brain development and a critical dosage-sensitive gene involved in neurological abnormalities [17, 18]. In the inherited cases, the disorder almost exclusively affects males, and the MECP2 duplication in a carrier mother with favorable skewing of X-chromosome inactivation results in minimal to no clinical findings [8] But rarely, females who carry the same duplication on one X chromosome may exhibit mild to severe clinical features seen in affected males [12, 19]. In some cases, the duplication occurs *de novo* [12, 20].

Here we report two genetically unrelated rare syndromes in a family. A deletion in a girl and one duplication inherited in her brother. The first chromosomal aberration is a *de novo* 1q21 microdeletion involving 9 genes. The other chromosomal anomaly, Xq28 duplication encompassing 15 genes including *MECP2*, is inherited from the asymptomatic mother. We performed qPCR to further confirm the CNVs and familial inheritance patterns of these chromosome rearrangements, and quantified the mRNA expression levels of *MECP2* using RT-qPCR. In addition, we discussed genotype-phenotype correlations in patients with these two rare syndromes.

## Methods

### Cell culture

Lymphoblastoid cell lines (LCLs) were established from blood samples obtained from patients and their family members and maintained as previously described [21].

### Comparative genomic hybridization (CGH) array

Genomic DNA (gDNA) was extracted from peripheral blood lymphocytes using standard phenol/chloroform extraction method [21]. The isolated genomic DNAs were examined for copy number variations (CNVs) using the Agilent 244 K Agilent comparative genomic hybridization (CGH) array (Agilent Technologies).

### Quantitative polymerase chain reaction (qPCR) for the confirmation of deletion and duplication

Primers used for the confirmation of the 1q21 and 7q11 deletion and Xq28 duplication are listed in Table 1. A primer set amplifying the exon 8 of *GAPDH* was used as an internal control. Total 10 ng of gDNA was mixed with Power SYBR Green PCR Master Mix (Applied Biosystems, Carlsbad, CA) and the primers, according to the manufacturer's protocol. Quantitative PCR (qPCR) was performed for the amplification of the targeted

**Table 1** Primers used for qPCR in this study

| Name | Primer sequence (5′ → 3′) | |
|---|---|---|
| | Forward | Reverse |
| chr1q21.1 #1 | TGAGCAGTTCAAAGGAGTGTAG | ATGACCCACAAAGTGAGAGAAA |
| chr1q21.1 #2 | AAGGCTGTGAAGGAGGAAATC | CTGACCAGGCAGAAGACATAAA |
| chr7q11 | GGAGCACAAAGCAACTGAATG | AGACAGCAATGCAGAGGAA |
| chrXq28 #1 | AGAGCTCGGACTCCATCTAAT | CCTTCCCATGTCAGTGTGTTAT |
| chrXq28 #2 | CTCACTTCTGGGTCTCACATTC | AATCCCAAGTGACTTCCAAGG |
| GAPDH | GATCATCAGCAATGCCTCCT | ATGGCATGGACTGTGGTCAT |

region utilizing a 7500 Real-Time PCR system (Applied Biosystems, Carlsbad, CA). The PCR reactions were cycled 40 times after initial denaturation (95 °C, 10 min) with the following parameters: denaturation at 95 °C for 15 s; annealing at 60 °C for 1 min. The amplification levels of *GAPDH* exon 8 were used to normalize relative levels of DNA.

### Reverse transcription-quantitative polymerase chain reaction (RT-qPCR)

Total RNA was extracted from the lymphocyte cell lines using RNeasy Mini Kit (Qiagen, Valencia, CA) according to the instructions of the manufacturer. Total RNA 2 μg was reverse transcribed and converted into complementary DNA (cDNA) using the RevertAid First Strand cDNA synthesis kit (Thermo Scientific, Waltham, MA). The following are primer sequences used for amplification of *MECP2* (NM_004992.3) and *GAPDH* (NM_002046.4); *MECP2 #1* forward 5' – CTCAGGCCATTCCCAAGAAA – 3' and reverse 5' – TCCTGCACAGATCGGATAGA – 3'; *MECP2 #2* forward 5' – CTCTGCTGGGAAGTATGAT GTG – 3' reverse 5' – TCATTAGGGTCCAGGGATGT – 3'; *GAPDH* forward 5' – GATCATCAGCAATGCCTCCT – 3' and reverse 5' – ATGGCATGGACTGTGGTCAT – 3'. The cDNAs were mixed with Power SYBR Green PCR Master Mix (Applied Biosystems, Carlsbad, CA) and primers. All samples and loading controls were plated in triplicate and centrifuged briefly. RT-qPCR was performed for the amplification of *MECP2* and *GAPDH* utilizing a 7500 Real-Time PCR system (Applied Biosystems, Carlsbad, CA). The PCR reactions were cycled 40 times after initial denaturation (95 °C, 10 min) with the following parameters: denaturation at 95 °C for 15 s; annealing at 60 °C for 1 min. Expression of *GAPDH* was used to normalize relative expression of *MECP2* mRNA.

## Case presentation

Our proband 1 is a 10 and half-year old Caucasian female with learning disability, significant growth retardation, microcephaly and speech delay. She was born at a full term after a normal pregnancy and delivery with average birth weight (3.27 kg, 50 percentile) and length (49.5 cm, 50 percentile). No jaundice, hypotonia or problems with feeds was observed during newborn period. However, her weight was 25th percentile at 2 months, and less than 3rd percentile from age 8 months. Although both her weight and length has been below 3rd percentile from age of 9 months, she has not shown any sign of delayed milestones. At the age of seven months, she developed oral thrush and began to demonstrate decreased development and feeding. She became a poor eater and tended to only drink water and breastfeed for liquids. She had failure to thrive partly because of her swallowing problem and tongue thrust. Since 6 months old, she continues to have constipation with bowel movement every 3–5 days. It has not improved with thyroid treatment and enema was required at times. At 1 year and 10 months, she had laboratory evidence of compensated hypothyroidism with normal thyroid levels and elevated thyroid stimulating hormone, on Synthroid treatment for symptomatic control. She has soft dysmorphic features including cupped ears and a unilateral ear pit in her right ear (Fig. 1a, b). Her length was below the 3rd percentile, but her weight to length curve was normal in the 22nd percentile (Fig. 1c). Brain MRI, performed at 2 years and 3 months of age,

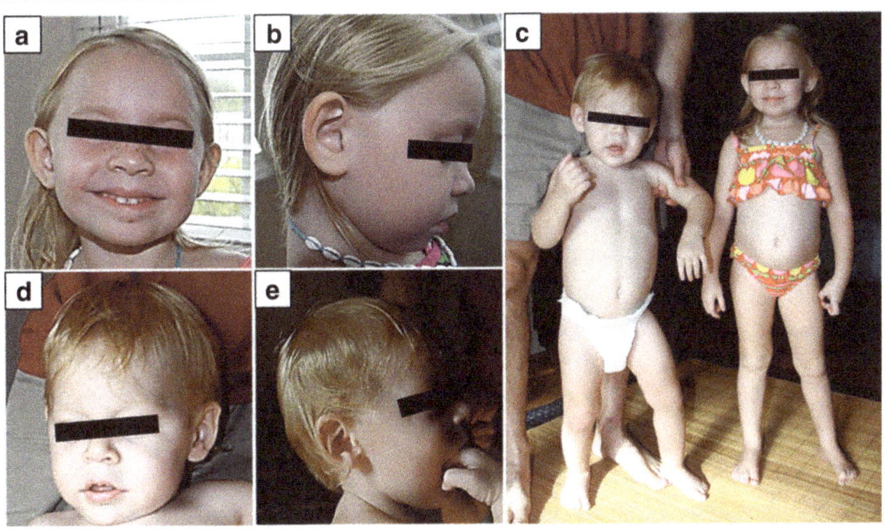


**Fig. 1** Facial and whole body photographs of two affected children in our study. **a**, **b** Proband 1 at age of 4 years and 8 months has cupped ears as well as a unilateral ear pit in her right ear. **c** Proband 1 at age of 4 years and 8 months shows similar length with her younger brother, proband 2 at 2 years and 2 months. **d**, **e** Proband 2 at age of 2 years and 2 months has mild craniofacial dysmorphisms with bilateral epicanthal folds and periorbital swelling

showed normal. She presents significant overall sensory regulation issues. For instance, she seeks movement and touch constantly and has inconsistent sleep patterns as well. She demonstrates behaviors consistent with anxiety and high arousal state. She seeks specific oral motor input and prefers to have crunch and/or chewy textures. Her behavioral studies revealed the auditory processing concerns with difficulty processing specific directions, which are consistent with a system that is high in adrenaline and low in serotonin and dopamine. She has a learning disability, struggling in math at the school, and is seeing a speech therapist for reading difficulties. At 10.5 years of age, her cognitive function is at the level of 8.5 years.

A 244K Agilent CGH array revealed a deletion of 1q21.1-1q21.2 spanning about 1.24 Mb of genomic DNA with the genome coordinates from 146,542,843 to147,786,706 (GRCh37/hg19), resulting in the loss of 9 genes including *PRKAB2, FMO5, CDH1L, BCL9, ACP6, GJA5, GJA8, GPR89B, and NBPF11* (Figs. 2a and 3a, Table 2). This deletion has been reported to be causative for the 1q21 recurrent microdeletion syndrome [2]. The results of CGH array in both parents demonstrated that this del(1)(q21.1q21.2) in proband 1 occurred *de novo* and this result was also confirmed by qPCR (Fig. 4a). Another deletion identified in proband 1 was a 68 Kb deletion within intron 2 of *AUTS2* gene at 7q11.22 (Figs. 2b and 3b). The qPCR results showed that the intronic deletion in AUTS2 in proband 1 was inherited from the healthy father suggesting that this deletion is a polymorphism with no clinical effect (Fig. 4b).

Proband 2 is a 8-year old Caucasian male with developmental delays, hypotonia, speech delay as well as cognitive and motor impairment. He was born at full term following a normal pregnancy, labor and delivery with appropriate growth parameters, birth weight 3.92 Kg and length 51 cm. He remained in a hospital for three days due to a detected ventricular septal defect (VSD) and breathing problems. Later, he was admitted two times at the ages of four months and then fourteen months for enlarged heart and cyanotic changes, but VSD subsequently closed spontaneously. At the age of

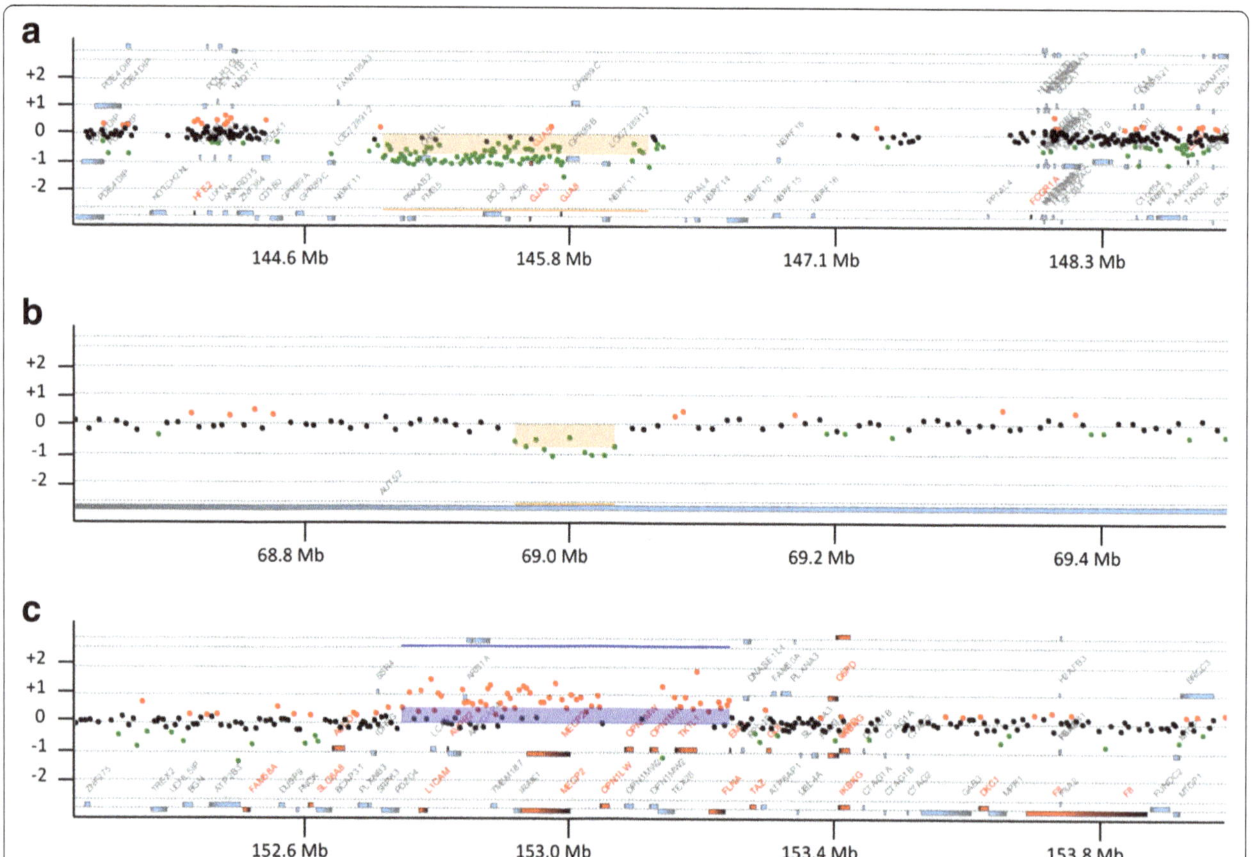


**Fig. 2** The relevant section of copy number variants (CNVs) by array comparative genomic hybridization with the use of Agilent 244 K arrays. Please note that the coordinates shown in Fig. 2 are based on NCBI36/hg18 of the Human Genome Browser, which were translated into GRCh37/hg19 in the Case Presentation section. **a** 1q21 deletion in proband 1. **b** 7q11.22 deletion in proband 1. **c** Xq28 duplication in proband 2. On the scale of deviation from the normal diploid genotype, −2 indicates a homozygous deletion, −1 indicates a haploid deletion, 0 indicates no deviation, 1 indicates a duplication, and 2 indicates a triplication. X axis indicates the location of CNVs on chromosomes (hg18)

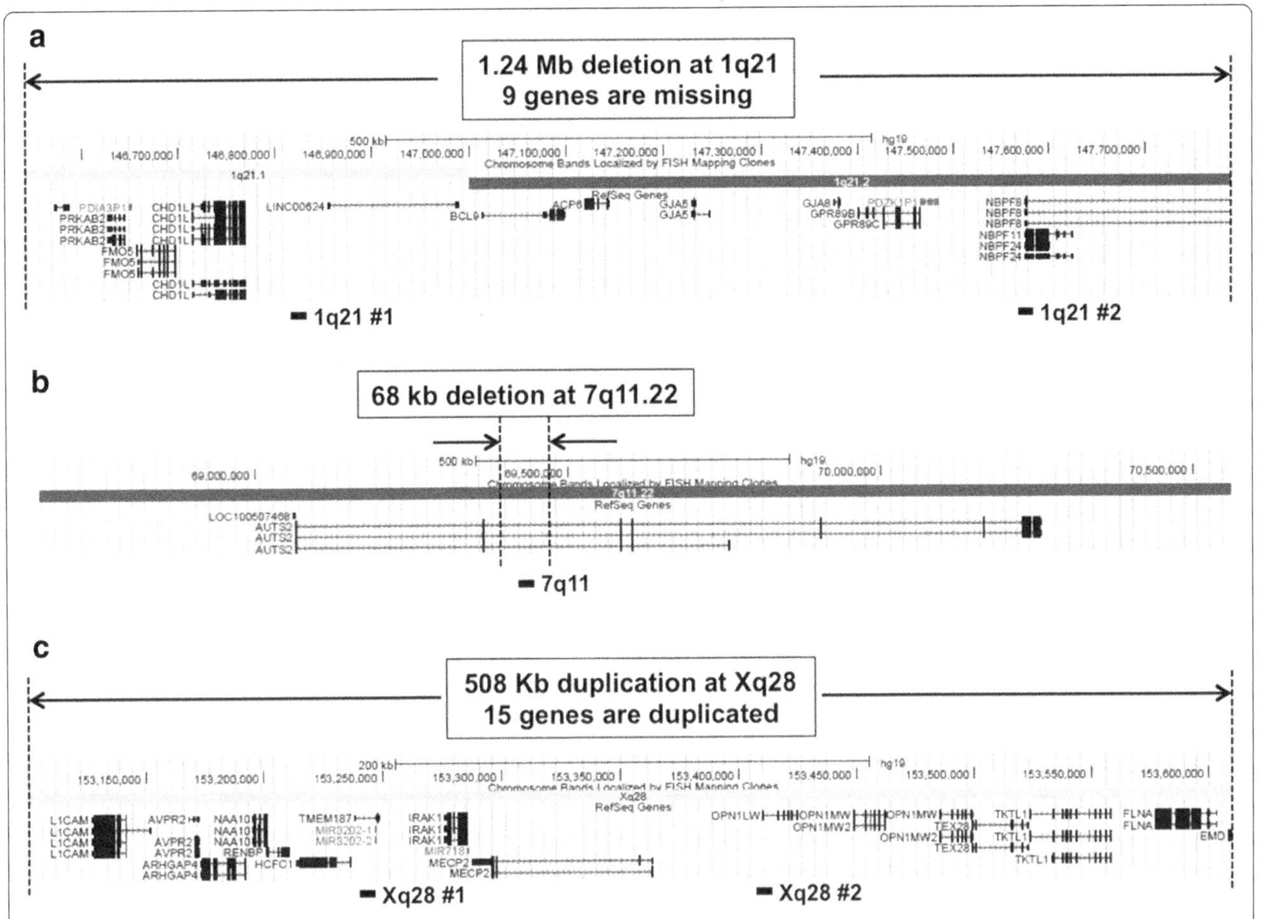


**Fig. 3** Genome view of deletion and duplication regions in proband 1 (**a** and **b**) and 2 (**c**) exported from Human Genome Browser (Build 37/hg19). RefSeq genes are described in http://www.genome.ucsc.edu/. Black boxes under browser maps show approximate locations of loci where primers were designed for qPCR

eleven months, he had pressure equalization tubes and was diagnosed with juvenile idiopathic arthritis. His developmental delay particularly regarding his motor milestones was observed from 6 months of age; rolling from front to back and back to front at 3 months of age; pulling to stand at 10 months; sitting at 11 months; crawling in reciprocal fashion by 13 months of age and walking with support at 20 months. However, muscle mass, strength and muscle stretch reflexes were within normal limits. There is no history of seizures or periodic breathing, and no major difficulties with constipation or teeth grinding. In the developmental test performed at the age of 2 years, he demonstrated severe delays across all areas consistent with overall cognitive and motor impairment as well as craniofacial dysmorphisms with bilateral epicanthal folds and periorbital swelling (Fig. 1d, e). He had a few mild behaviors consistent with an autistic spectrum disorder such as lack of pointing, limited play skills and poor eye contact, but generally seems to interact at a level consistent with his developmental level. His poor eye contact also seems more a symptom of overall poor attention span, and visual inattentiveness, as opposed to lack of social awareness. He also displayed limited integration of social communication behaviors (gaze, sounds, gestures and facial expressions) and difficulty initiating and sustaining social interactions.

A CGH array result demonstrated that proband 2 has 508 Kb duplication at Xq28 with the genome coordinates from 153,101,077 to 153,609,163 (GRCh37/hg19) encompassing 15 genes including *MECP2*, one of responsible genes for Xq28 duplication syndrome (Figs. 2c and 3c, Table 2). Parental CGH array results revealed that this Xq28 duplication was inherited from mother. The qPCR results using two different primers amplifying regions within the known duplicated region revealed that Xq28 duplication was originally inherited from maternal grandmother who inherited it to mother, a carrier with a normal phenotype (Fig. 4c). We performed qRT-PCR to compare the mRNA expression levels of *MECP2* in proband 2 with those in other family members whose blood samples were available. Figure 4d shows proband 2 has almost double amount of *MECP2* mRNA expression

**Table 2** List of affected genes in probands 1 and 2

| Gene symbol | Gene name | OMIM # | Function |
|---|---|---|---|
| Proband 1 with 1.24 Mb deletion at 1q21 | | | |
| *PRKAB2* | AMP-activated kinase complex noncatalytic beta-2 | 602741 | Maintains systemic and cellular energy homeostasis |
| *FMO5* | Flavin-containing monooxygenase 5 | 603957 | Involved in the metabolic activation of drugs and xenobiotic compounds |
| *CHD1L* | Chromodomain helicase DNA-binding protein 1-like | 613039 | Has a role in chromatin modification and DNA damage response |
| *BCL9* | B-cell CLL/lymphoma 9 | 602597 | A signal transduction protein required for efficient beta-catenin-mediated transcription in Wnt signaling pathway |
| *ACP6* | Acid phosphatase 6 | 611471 | Hydrolyzes lysophosphatidic acid containing fatty acid |
| *GJA5* | Gap junction protein, alpha-5 | 121013 | A cardiac gap junction protein connexin 40 that facilitates cell-to-cell adhesion and intercellular communication |
| *GJA8* | Gap junction protein, alpha-8 | 600897 | A transmembrane connexin protein that is necessary for lens growth and maturation of lens fiber cells |
| *GPR89B* | G protein-coupled receptor 89B | 612806 | Voltage dependent anion channel regulating the acidification and function of Golgi apparatus |
| *NBPF11* | Neuroblastoma breakpoint family, member 11 | 614001 | A member of the NBPF family and diseases associated with *NBPF11* include neuroblastoma |
| Proband 2 with 508 kb duplication at Xq28 | | | |
| L1CAM | L1 cell adhesion molecule | 308840 | Belongs to immunoglobulin superfamily cell adhesion molecules and has a role in neuronal migration and survival |
| AVPR2 | arginine vasopressin receptor 2 | 300538 | G protein-coupled receptor involved in the regulation of the urine and water homeostasis in kidney |
| ARHGAP4 | Rho GTPase activating protein 4 | 300023 | Regulates the function of small GTP-binding proteins belonging to the RAS superfamily |
| NAA10 | N(alpha)-acetyltransferase 10, NatA catalytic subunit | 300013 | Catalytic subunit of the N-terminal acetyltransferase A complex, which transfers an acetyl group from acetyl-coenzyme A to the alpha-amino group on a nascent polypeptide |
| RENBP | renin binding protein | 312420 | Inhibits renin by forming a dimer with renin and involved in transport to the Golgi and synthesis of substrates in N-glycan biosynthesis |
| HCFC1 | host cell factor C1 | 300019 | Involved in cell cycle regulation and functions as a transcription repressor by inhibiting the recruitment of p300 to promoter. Mutations of this gene cause non-syndromic X-linked intellectual disability and X-linked cobalamin disorder. |
| TMEM187 | transmembrane protein 187 | 300059 | A multi-pass membrane protein, but its biological function is not determined |
| IRAK1 | interleukin 1 receptor associated kinase 1 | 300283 | A putative serine/threonine kinase that plays a critical role in immune response and become associated with the IL-1 receptor |
| MECP2 | methyl-CpG binding protein 2 | 300005 | Specifically binds to a single methyl-CpG pair and mediates transcriptional repression through interaction with histone deacetylase and a corepressor |
| OPN1LW | opsin 1 (cone pigments), long-wave-sensitive | 300822 | Long-wavelength sensitive opsin, transmembrane receptor protein with a visual pigment, which is a light-absorbing molecules that mediate vision |
| OPN1MW | opsin 1 (cone pigments), medium-wave-sensitive | 300821 | Medium-wavelength sensitive opsin, transmembrane receptor protein with a visual pigment, which is a light-absorbing molecules that mediate vision |
| TEX28 | testis expressed 28 | 300092 | A member of the red/green cone visual pigment gene family |
| TKTL1/TKT2 | transketolase-like 1/transketolase 2 | 300044 | A thiamine-dependent enzyme that links the pentose phosphate pathway with the glycolytic pathway. |
| FLNA | Filamin A | 300017 | An actin-binding protein involved in the reorganization of cytoskeleton to effect in cell migration |
| EMD | emerin | 300384 | A nuclear membrane protein that associates with the nuclear membrane lamina and mediates membrane anchorage to the cytoskeleton |

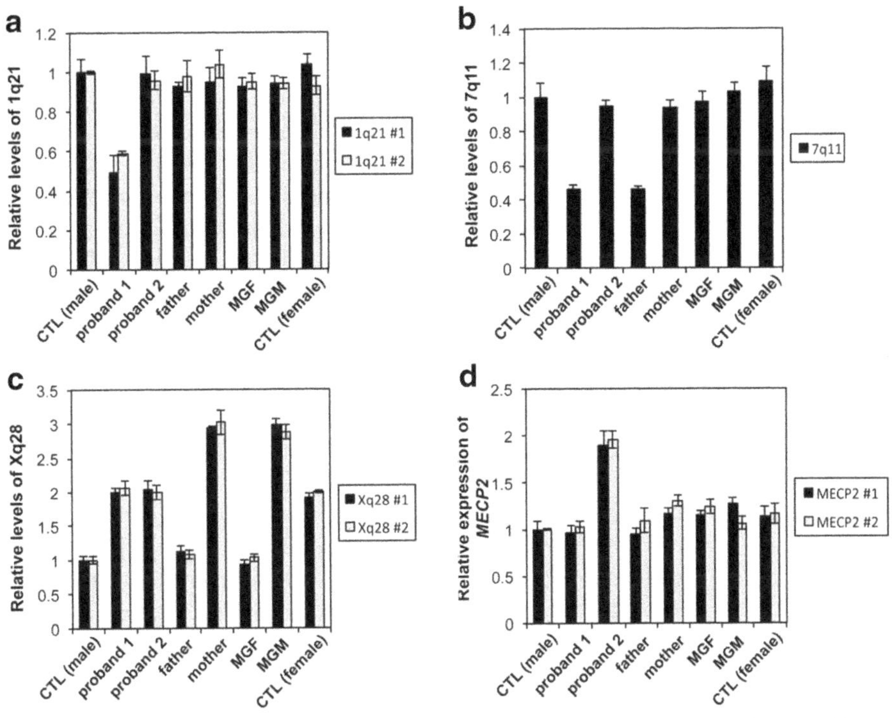


**Fig. 4** Quantitative PCR results of deletions and duplication in our family members. **a** qPCR results showing the 1q21 deletion using 2 different set of primers amplifying the regions within the known deleted region in proband 1. Deletion was detected only in proband 1. A value close to 0.5 indicates deletion on one chromosome 1, but a value close 1 indicates no deletion. **b** qPCR results showing the 7q11 deletion in both father and proband 1. Deletion in proband 1 was inherited from healthy father suggesting that this deletion is polymorphism. A value close to 0.5 indicates deletion on one chromosome 7, but a value close 1 indicates no deletion. **c** qPCR results showing duplication of Xq28 in proband 2, mother and MGM. Xq28 duplication in proband 2 is originally inherited from the maternal grandmother. Values indicate that: 1 (no deletion on chromosome X in male); 2 (duplication on chromosome X in male, no duplication in female); 3 (duplication on chromosome X in female). The amplification levels of *GAPDH* exon 8 were used to normalize relative levels of DNA. **d** The mRNA expression levels of *MECP2* in the family members. Quantitative RT-PCR was performed to measure the mRNA levels of *MECP2* using 2 different sets of primers specific to *MECP2* mRNA (NM_004992.3). Expression of *GAPDH* was used to normalize relative expression of *MECP2* mRNA. Error bars represent standard errors. Proband 1: a 10-year old Caucasian female with 1q21 microdeletion; Proband 2: an 8-year old Caucasian male with Xq28 duplication; MGF: maternal grandfather; MGM: maternal grandmother

compared to other family members. However, both maternal grandmother and mother have normal expression levels of *MECP2*, even though they both have same duplication.

## Discussion

In this study, we report two genetically unrelated disorders, 1q21 microdeletion and Xq28 duplication in siblings with intellectual disability. Microarray analysis revealed that the sister, our proband 1, carries 1.24-Mb heterozygous deletion at 1q21.1-1q21.2 region involving 9 genes (Fig. 3a, Table 2) and a 68 Kb deletion within intron 2 of *AUTS2* gene at 7q11.22 (Fig. 2b). 1q21 microdeletion is a contiguous gene deletion syndrome caused by the recurrent distal 1.35-Mb heterozygous deletion in the 1q21 region and characterized by dysmorphic facial features, mild-moderate developmental delay, intellectual disability, microcephaly and short stature [1, 2, 4]. In rare cases, individuals with the deletion may have autism [22], schizophrenia [23], cataracts [2, 5] and isolated heart defects [6]. It is also possible that apparently unaffected patients with 1q21 deletion could have subtle phenotypic features that are highly variable and therefore not easily recognizable. A previous study stated that subtle cataracts and patent ductus arteriosus were detected from one of their patients after directive studies were performed upon discovery of the 1q21 deletion [2]. Although our proband 1 did not have cardiac anomalies and eye problems, a lot of phenotypes detected in proband 1 overlap the common characteristic features of 1q21 deletion syndrome such as microcephaly, developmental delay, mild facial dysmorphism and short stature, suggesting that it is likely that some of the missing genes in chromosome 1 would be the causative genes for her phenotypes, because the deletion in the intron 2 of *AUTS2* gene at 7q11.22 is found in her healthy father as well as the healthy population.

Haploinsufficiency or pathogenic variants of some genes of interest such as *PRKAB2*, *CDH1L*, *BCL9*, *GJA5* and *GJA8* within the region of 1q21 microdeletion likely contributes to the recognizable phenotpyes associated with 1q21 microdeletion. *PRKAB2* is a member of the AMP kinase complex, which maintains systemic and cellular energy homeostasis [24], while *CHD1L* is an enzyme with a role in chromatin modification and DNA damage response [25]. The protein levels of both PRKAB2 and CHD1L were decreased in lymphoblastoid cell lines from persons with 1q21 deletion and AMP kinase function in those LCLs was highly attenuated [26]. In addition, LCLs showed significant reduction in DNA damage repair following treatment with a topoisomerase II inhibitor [26]. These results would support the pathological roles for *PRKAB2* and *CDH1L* in 1q21 microdeletion. Furthermore, the fact that *PRKAB2* is highly expressed in skeletal muscle [27] may explain the short stature and skeletal malformations in patients with 1q21 microdeletion as well as our proband 1. *BCL9* is required for efficient beta-catenin-mediated transcription in Wnt signaling pathway [28], influencing neuroplasticity, adult neurogenesis and mental disorders [29–31]. Therefore, *BCL9* may have contributed to phenotypes including neurological defects and mild intellectual disability in 1q21 microdeletion. Two different gap junction proteins, GJA5 and GJA8 are also associated with phenotypic features in patients with 1q21 microdeletion. GJA5 and GJA8 encode for the cardiac gap junction protein connexin 40 [32] and a transmembrane connexin protein that is necessary for lens growth and maturation of lens fiber cells [33], respectively. Although our proband 1 has neither cardiac abnormalities nor cataract, in many different cases, the phenotypes related with mutations in these two genes have already been reported. GJA5 is thought to be a susceptibility gene for cardiac abnormalities, because one heterozygous nonsense mutation and three missense mutations segregating with this phenotype were found in one and three unrelated families, respectively [34, 35]. Mutations in the GJA8 gene have been found to cause several types of autosomal dominant cataract [36], which have been described as congenital nuclear [37], nuclear pulverulent [38], zonular pulverulent [39], stellate nuclear [39] and posterior subcapsular [40]. Therefore, the most common clinical features of 1q21 microdeletion would have been associated with haploinsufficiency of multiple genes located in the deleted region.

We also describe another individual in the same family, who carries duplication in Xq28 region involving 15 genes and including *MECP2* gene that has been associated with Rett syndrome (Fig. 3c, Table 2). Unlike *MECP2* duplication syndrome, Rett syndrome is caused by the pathogenic *MECP2* variants such as missense mutations and intragenic rearrangements of *MECP2* gene. The pathogenic variants of *MECP2* gene were detected in approximately 80 % of individuals with classic Rett syndrome [41–43] and 40 % of individuals with atypical Rett syndrome [41, 42, 44]. Our proband 2 does not meet clinical criteria for Rett syndrome, but does reflect the clinical features described previously in males with duplication of *MECP2* [45–47]. Among the criteria for the diagnosis of Rett syndrome [48], he only meets evidence of an acquired deceleration in head growth and absent gait. He has lost no skills but is delayed in communication and fine motor skills as well. Among the supportive criteria [48], he has had some falloff in linear growth over the last several months, but otherwise fulfills none of these.

Autism like phenotypes are reported in some cases with Xq28 duplication syndrome [49, 50], and it is very hard to distinguish between Xq28 duplication syndrome and autism, especially children in very young age. Our proband 2, an 8-year old boy, also has a social communication delay and reciprocal behaviors including lack of response to contextual cues, lack of showing and sharing interest, lack of communicative vocalizations with consonant, and repetitive movements with object and body associated with the criteria for autism spectrum disorder [49]. However, the pattern of delays is inconsistent with an autistic spectrum disorder, and his social skills are commensurate with his language and cognitive development whereas autism typically results in more severely delayed social skills versus other areas of development. Although his pattern of behaviors may be characteristic of autism spectrum disorder, it is felt that these behaviors reflect his significant developmental delay and that these characteristics are better accounted for by his developmental delays associated with *MECP2* duplication syndrome.

The *MECP2* gene encodes for MECP2, a chromatin-associated protein that regulates transcription of genes [13, 14]. It is required for maturation of neurons [51] and critical for normal brain function [18]. The presence of an extra copy of the *MECP2* gene is believed to improperly regulate the expression of other genes and this misregulation of gene expression in the brain results in abnormal neuronal function [17, 18], leading to the signs and symptoms of *MECP2* duplication syndrome. Indeed, mild overexpression of Mecp2 in mice causes a progressive neurological disorder including seizures, spasticity and akinesis [17, 52], that are frequently observed in individuals with Xq28 duplication. In addition to *MECP2*, this duplication encompassed several other genes of interest including *L1CAM*, *FLNA* and *HCFC1* that previously reported in other patients with a Xq28 duplication. L1CAM, a cell-to-cell adhesion molecule, is primarily found in the nervous system and functions in neuronal cell migration and survival [53]. Mutations in *L1CAM* gene are responsible for an X-linked recessive neurological disorder that has been described as X-linked hydrocephalus [54], MASA syndrome [55] or spastic paraplegia type I (SPG1) [56]. FLNA encodes filamin A, an actin-binding protein involved in the reorganization of cytoskeleton to effect in cell migration [57]. Mutations in the X-linked FLNA gene can cause the multiple malformation [58] and neurologic disorder periventricular heterotopia mediated by a failure in neuronal migration into the cerebral cortex [57]. Mutations in the *HCFC1* gene have been found in males with X-linked cobalamin disorder characterized by severe neurological symptoms including intractable epilepsy, seizures and profound development delay, along with variable biochemical manifestations [59]. Another mutation in the 5' UTR region of the *HCFC1* gene that leads to overexpression of HCFC1 was identified in affected members of a family with X-linked intellectual disability (MRX3, MIM 309541) [60], suggesting that HCFC1 gene may be responsible for some phenotypes, especially intellectual disability, in Xq28 duplication.

Xq28 duplication syndrome predominantly affects males and in most cases, it is inherited from a carrier mother, who has favorable skewing of X chromosome inactivation and no symptoms [8]. Using qPCR analysis, the screening of familial inheritance in our study demonstrated that Xq28 duplication in proband 2 was passed down through his mother and maternal grandmother, a carrier with a normal phenotype (Fig. 4c). The RT-qPCR analysis of *MECP2* expression levels revealed that proband 2 has almost double amount of *MECP2* mRNA expression compared to other family members including maternal grandmother and mother who have the same *MECP2* duplication, further suggesting that the skewed inactivation of X chromosome with *MECP2* duplication in two female carriers. This suggests that *MECP2* duplicated on the inactive X chromosome in the asymptomatic carrier females is completely silenced without escaping inactivation. Given that both microdeletion and microduplication of Xq28 encompassing *MECP2* cause common phenotypic features such as intellectual disability, infantile hypotonia, absent speech and developmental regression [18, 45, 47, 61], the dosage of MECP2 is likely stringently regulated, because both decreased and increased amount of MECP2 cause distinct clinical phenotypes. Importantly, proband 2's maternal uncle who died at 11 years old in a drowning accident had significant intellectual disability and similar phenotypes with proband 2, indicating that maternal uncle was likely affected with the same Xq28 duplication detected in his mother and sister as well as proband 2. Pedigree analysis indicates X-linked recessive inheritance of Xq28 duplication (Fig. 5).

Although patients with 1q21 deletion and *MECP2* duplication syndromes share some phenotypes such as mild dysmorphic features, cardiac abnormalities and mental retardation, it has not been reported for these two genetically unrelated syndromes to occur in the same family, especially in siblings like our case. Therefore, the presence of two seemingly unrelated and rare chromosome abnormalities in siblings is provocative, unusual and calls for further investigations.

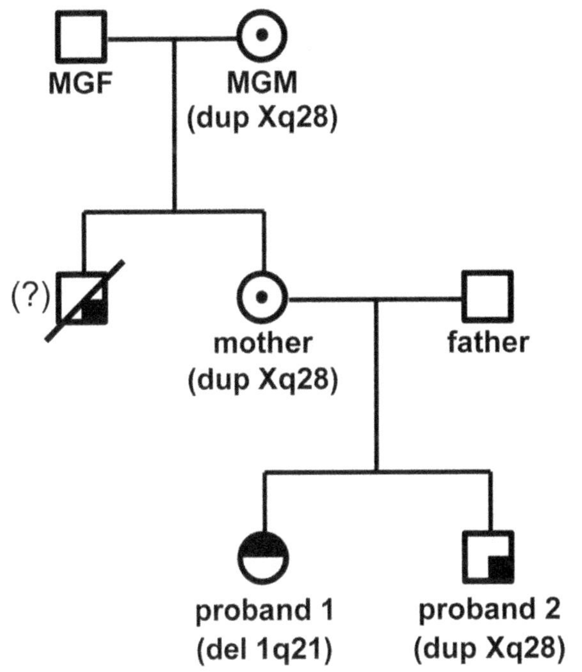


**Fig. 5** Pedigree of three generations showing the inheritance of 1q21 deletion and Xq28 duplication in the family. 1q21 deletion in proband 1 occurred *de novo* and Xq28 duplication in proband 2 was originally inherited from the maternal grandmother, a carrier who inherited it to his mother, a carrier. The maternal uncle who died at 11 years old from an accident also suffered from a similar phenotype as his nephew. This indicates that the uncle and the nephew might have had the same Xq28 duplication

## Conclusions

In conclusion, we report on two siblings with genetically unrelated rare syndromes, 1q21 microdeletion or Xq28 duplication. The results of parental CGH and qPCR analyses reveal that the 1q21 microdeletion in the elder sister is *de novo*, and the Xq28 duplication in the younger brother is inherited from the maternal grandmother through the mother. RT-qPCR results revealed that the affected brother has almost double the amount of *MECP2* mRNA expression compared to other family members, including the maternal grandmother and mother with no phenotypes. This indicates the favorable skewing of X-chromosome inactivation in female carriers. Given that the segregation of two rare genetic syndromes in siblings is very unusual, our report draws an attention to the presence of two genetically unrelated syndromes in a same family and further investigations in similar cases would be highly informative for future studies.

### Abbreviations

*ACP6*: Acid phosphatase 6; *AUTS2*: Autism susceptibility candidate 2; *BCL9*: B-cell CLL/lymphoma 9; *CDH1L*: Chromodomain helicase DNA binding protein 1-like; CGH array: Comparative genomic hybridization (CGH) array; CNV: Copy number variation; *FLNA*: Filamin A, alpha; *FMO5*: Flavin Containing Monooxygenase 5; *GJA5*: Gap junction protein, alpha 5; *GJA8*: Gap junction protein, alpha 8; *GPR89B*: G protein-coupled receptor 89B; *HCFC1*: Host cell factor C1; *L1CAM*: L1 cell adhesion molecule; MASA syndrome: Mental retardation, aphasia, spastic paraplegia adducted thumbs syndrome; *MECP2*: Methyl CpG-binding protein 2; *NBPF11*: Neuroblastoma breakpoint family, member 11; *PRKAB2*: Protein Kinase, AMP-Activated, Beta 2 Non-Catalytic Subunit; RT-qPCR: Reverse transcription-quantitative polymerase chain reaction; SPG1: Spastic paraplegia type I; VSD: Ventricular septal defect

### Acknowledgements

We would like to thank DGDP041 family members who kindly agreed to participate in this study.

### Funding

KH is supported by a postdoctoral training grant from NIH (T32HL07676). CK was supported by the Bio & Medical Technology Development Program of the National Research Foundation (NRF) funded by the Ministry of Science, ICT & Future (NRF-2015M3A9A8029261) and the National Research Foundation of Korea (NRF) grant funded by the Korean government Ministry of Science, ICT and Future Planning (MSIP) (2014R1A2A1A11053562). We are also grateful for the funding support provided by Caroline Jones-Carrick and Collin Carrick.

### Authors' contributions

KH was responsible for data collection and drafted the manuscript, and HK conceived the project, analyzed and interpreted the data, and revised the manuscript. YS performed CGH array analysis, and TG did cell culture, cell transformation, and DNA extraction. CK analyzed and interpreted the data. All authors read and approved the final manuscript.

### Competing interests

The authors declare that they have no competing interests.

### Author details

[1]Department of Molecular Physiology and Biophysics, Baylor College of Medicine, Houston, TX 77030, USA. [2]Section of Reproductive Endocrinology, Infertility & Genetics, Department of Obstetrics & Gynecology, Augusta University, Augusta, GA 30912, USA. [3]Department of Neurology, Massachusetts General Hospital, Harvard Medical School, Boston, MA 02114, USA. [4]Department of Biology, Chungnam National University, Daejeon 34134, South Korea. [5]Department of Neuroscience and Regenerative Medicine, Augusta University, 1120 15th Street, Augusta, GA 30912, USA.

### References

1. Brunetti-Pierri N, Berg JS, Scaglia F, Belmont J, Bacino CA, Sahoo T, et al. Recurrent reciprocal 1q21.1 deletions and duplications associated with microcephaly or macrocephaly and developmental and behavioral abnormalities. Nat Genet. 2008;40(12):1466–71. doi:10.1038/ng.279.
2. Mefford HC, Sharp AJ, Baker C, Itsara A, Jiang Z, Buysse K, et al. Recurrent rearrangements of chromosome 1q21.1 and variable pediatric phenotypes. N Engl J Med. 2008;359(16):1685–99. doi:10.1056/NEJMoa0805384.
3. Mefford HC, Eichler EE. Duplication hotspots, rare genomic disorders, and common disease. Curr Opin Genet Dev. 2009;19(3):196–204. doi:10.1016/j.gde.2009.04.003.
4. Bernier R, Steinman KJ, Reilly B, Wallace AS, Sherr EH, Pojman N, et al. Clinical phenotype of the recurrent 1q21.1 copy-number variant. Genet Med. 2015. doi:10.1038/gim.2015.78.
5. Redon R, Ishikawa S, Fitch KR, Feuk L, Perry GH, Andrews TD, et al. Global variation in copy number in the human genome. Nature. 2006;444(7118):444–54. doi:10.1038/nature05329.
6. Christiansen J, Dyck JD, Elyas BG, Lilley M, Bamforth JS, Hicks M, et al. Chromosome 1q21.1 contiguous gene deletion is associated with congenital heart disease. Circ Res. 2004;94(11):1429–35. doi:10.1161/01.RES.0000130528.72330.5c.
7. Sanlaville D, Schluth-Bolard C, Turleau C. Distal Xq duplication and functional Xq disomy. Orphanet J Rare Dis. 2009;4:4. doi:10.1186/1750-1172-4-4.
8. Ramocki MB, Tavyev YJ, Peters SU. The MECP2 duplication syndrome. Am J Med Genet A. 2010;152A(5):1079–88. doi:10.1002/ajmg.a.33184.
9. El-Hattab AW, Fang P, Jin W, Hughes JR, Gibson JB, Patel GS, et al. Int22h-1/int22h-2-mediated Xq28 rearrangements: intellectual disability associated with duplications and in utero male lethality with deletions. J Med Genet. 2011;48(12):840–50. doi:10.1136/jmedgenet-2011-100125.
10. Vandewalle J, Van Esch H, Govaerts K, Verbeeck J, Zweier C, Madrigal I, et al. Dosage-dependent severity of the phenotype in patients with mental retardation due to a recurrent copy-number gain at Xq28 mediated by an unusual recombination. Am J Hum Genet. 2009;85(6):809–22. doi:10.1016/j.ajhg.2009.10.019.
11. Vanmarsenille L, Giannandrea M, Fieremans N, Verbeeck J, Belet S, Raynaud M, et al. Increased dosage of RAB39B affects neuronal development and could explain the cognitive impairment in male patients with distal Xq28 copy number gains. Hum Mutat. 2014;35(3):377–83. doi:10.1002/humu.22497.
12. Bijlsma EK, Collins A, Papa FT, Tejada MI, Wheeler P, Peeters EA, et al. Xq28 duplications including MECP2 in five females: Expanding the phenotype to severe mental retardation. Eur J Med Genet. 2012;55(6–7):404–13. doi:10.1016/j.ejmg.2012.02.009.
13. Nan X, Meehan RR, Bird A. Dissection of the methyl-CpG binding domain from the chromosomal protein MeCP2. Nucleic Acids Res. 1993;21(21):4886–92.
14. Nan X, Campoy FJ, Bird A. MeCP2 is a transcriptional repressor with abundant binding sites in genomic chromatin. Cell. 1997;88(4):471–81.
15. Adler DA, Quaderi NA, Brown SD, Chapman VM, Moore J, Tate P, et al. The X-linked methylated DNA binding protein, Mecp2, is subject to X inactivation in the mouse. Mamm Genome. 1995;6(8):491–2.
16. D'Esposito M, Quaderi NA, Ciccodicola A, Bruni P, Esposito T, D'Urso M, et al. Isolation, physical mapping, and northern analysis of the X-linked human gene encoding methyl CpG-binding protein, MECP2. Mamm Genome. 1996;7(7):533–5.
17. Collins AL, Levenson JM, Vilaythong AP, Richman R, Armstrong DL, Noebels JL, et al. Mild overexpression of MeCP2 causes a progressive neurological disorder in mice. Hum Mol Genet. 2004;13(21):2679–89. doi:10.1093/hmg/ddh282.
18. Gonzales ML, LaSalle JM. The role of MeCP2 in brain development and neurodevelopmental disorders. Curr Psychiatry Rep. 2010;12(2):127–34. doi:10.1007/s11920-010-0097-7.
19. Mayo S, Monfort S, Rosello M, Orellana C, Oltra S, Armstrong J, et al. De novo interstitial triplication of MECP2 in a girl with neurodevelopmental disorder and random X chromosome inactivation. Cytogenet Genome Res. 2011;135(2):93–101. doi:10.1159/000330917.
20. Fieremans N, Bauters M, Belet S, Verbeeck J, Jansen AC, Seneca S, et al. De novo MECP2 duplications in two females with intellectual disability and unfavorable complete skewed X-inactivation. Hum Genet. 2014;133(11):1359–67. doi:10.1007/s00439-014-1469-6.
21. Nishimoto HK, Ha K, Jones JR, Dwivedi A, Cho HM, Layman LC, et al. The historical Coffin-Lowry syndrome family revisited: identification of two novel mutations of RPS6KA3 in three male patients. Am J Med Genet A. 2014;164A(9):2172–9. doi:10.1002/ajmg.a.36488.
22. Autism Genome Project C, Szatmari P, Paterson AD, Zwaigenbaum L, Roberts W, Brian J, et al. Mapping autism risk loci using genetic linkage and chromosomal rearrangements. Nat Genet. 2007;39(3):319–28. doi:10.1038/ng1985.
23. Stefansson H, Rujescu D, Cichon S, Pietilainen OP, Ingason A, Steinberg S, et al. Large recurrent microdeletions associated with schizophrenia. Nature. 2008;455(7210):232–6. doi:10.1038/nature07229.
24. Ronnett GV, Ramamurthy S, Kleman AM, Landree LE, Aja S. AMPK in the brain: its roles in energy balance and neuroprotection. J Neurochem. 2009;109 Suppl 1:17–23. doi:10.1111/j.1471-4159.2009.05916.x.
25. Ahel D, Horejsi Z, Wiechens N, Polo SE, Garcia-Wilson E, Ahel I, et al. Poly(ADP-ribose)-dependent regulation of DNA repair by the chromatin remodeling enzyme ALC1. Science. 2009;325(5945):1240–3. doi:10.1126/science.1177321.
26. Harvard C, Strong E, Mercier E, Colnaghi R, Alcantara D, Chow E, et al. Understanding the impact of 1q21.1 copy number variant. Orphanet J Rare Dis. 2011;6:54. doi:10.1186/1750-1172-6-54.

27. Thornton C, Snowden MA, Carling D. Identification of a novel AMP-activated protein kinase beta subunit isoform that is highly expressed in skeletal muscle. J Biol Chem. 1998;273(20):12443–50.
28. de la Roche M, Worm J, Bienz M. The function of BCL9 in Wnt/beta-catenin signaling and colorectal cancer cells. BMC Cancer. 2008;8:199. doi:10.1186/1471-2407-8-199.
29. Lambert C, Cisternas P, Inestrosa NC. Role of Wnt Signaling in Central Nervous System Injury. Mol Neurobiol. 2015. doi:10.1007/s12035-015-9138-x.
30. Inestrosa NC, Varela-Nallar L. Wnt signaling in the nervous system and in Alzheimer's disease. J Mol Cell Biol. 2014;6(1):64–74. doi:10.1093/jmcb/mjt051.
31. Okerlund ND, Cheyette BN. Synaptic Wnt signaling-a contributor to major psychiatric disorders? J Neurodev Disord. 2011;3(2):162–74. doi:10.1007/s11689-011-9083-6.
32. Lin X, Gemel J, Glass A, Zemlin CW, Beyer EC, Veenstra RD. Connexin40 and connexin43 determine gating properties of atrial gap junction channels. J Mol Cell Cardiol. 2010;48(1):238–45. doi:10.1016/j.yjmcc.2009.05.014.
33. White TW, Goodenough DA, Paul DL. Targeted ablation of connexin50 in mice results in microphthalmia and zonular pulverulent cataracts. J Cell Biol. 1998;143(3):815–25.
34. Yang YQ, Zhang XL, Wang XH, Tan HW, Shi HF, Jiang WF, et al. Connexin40 nonsense mutation in familial atrial fibrillation. Int J Mol Med. 2010;26(4):605–10.
35. Yang YQ, Liu X, Zhang XL, Wang XH, Tan HW, Shi HF, et al. Novel connexin40 missense mutations in patients with familial atrial fibrillation. Europace. 2010;12(10):1421–7. doi:10.1093/europace/euq274.
36. Shiels A, Mackay D, Ionides A, Berry V, Moore A, Bhattacharya S. A missense mutation in the human connexin50 gene (GJA8) underlies autosomal dominant "zonular pulverulent" cataract, on chromosome 1q. Am J Hum Genet. 1998;62(3):526–32. doi:10.1086/301762.
37. Willoughby CE, Arab S, Gandhi R, Zeinali S, Arab S, Luk D, et al. A novel GJA8 mutation in an Iranian family with progressive autosomal dominant congenital nuclear cataract. J Med Genet. 2003;40(11):e124.
38. Berry V, Mackay D, Khaliq S, Francis PJ, Hameed A, Anwar K, et al. Connexin 50 mutation in a family with congenital "zonular nuclear" pulverulent cataract of Pakistani origin. Hum Genet. 1999;105(1–2):168–70.
39. Polyakov AV, Shagina IA, Khlebnikova OV, Evgrafov OV. Mutation in the connexin 50 gene (GJA8) in a Russian family with zonular pulverulent cataract. Clin Genet. 2001;60(6):476–8.
40. Devi RR, Vijayalakshmi P. Novel mutations in GJA8 associated with autosomal dominant congenital cataract and microcornea. Mol Vis. 2006;12:190–5.
41. Fukuda T, Yamashita Y, Nagamitsu S, Miyamoto K, Jin JJ, Ohmori I, et al. Methyl-CpG binding protein 2 gene (MECP2) variations in Japanese patients with Rett syndrome: pathological mutations and polymorphisms. Brain Dev. 2005;27(3):211–7. doi:10.1016/j.braindev.2004.06.003.
42. Li MR, Pan H, Bao XH, Zhang YZ, Wu XR. MECP2 and CDKL5 gene mutation analysis in Chinese patients with Rett syndrome. J Hum Genet. 2007;52(1):38–47. doi:10.1007/s10038-006-0079-0.
43. Zahorakova D, Rosipal R, Hadac J, Zumrova A, Bzduch V, Misovicova N, et al. Mutation analysis of the MECP2 gene in patients of Slavic origin with Rett syndrome: novel mutations and polymorphisms. J Hum Genet. 2007;52(4):342–8. doi:10.1007/s10038-007-0121-x.
44. Kammoun F, de Roux N, Boespflug-Tanguy O, Vallee L, Seng R, Tardieu M, et al. Screening of MECP2 coding sequence in patients with phenotypes of decreasing likelihood for Rett syndrome: a cohort of 171 cases. J Med Genet. 2004;41(6):e85.
45. Van Esch H, Bauters M, Ignatius J, Jansen M, Raynaud M, Hollanders K, et al. Duplication of the MECP2 region is a frequent cause of severe mental retardation and progressive neurological symptoms in males. Am J Hum Genet. 2005;77(3):442–53. doi:10.1086/444549.
46. del Gaudio D, Fang P, Scaglia F, Ward PA, Craigen WJ, Glaze DG, et al. Increased MECP2 gene copy number as the result of genomic duplication in neurodevelopmentally delayed males. Genet Med. 2006;8(12):784–92.
47. Friez MJ, Jones JR, Clarkson K, Lubs H, Abuelo D, Bier JA, et al. Recurrent infections, hypotonia, and mental retardation caused by duplication of MECP2 and adjacent region in Xq28. Pediatrics. 2006;118(6):e1687–95. doi:10.1542/peds.2006-0395.
48. Neul JL, Kaufmann WE, Glaze DG, Christodoulou J, Clarke AJ, Bahi-Buisson N, et al. Rett syndrome: revised diagnostic criteria and nomenclature. Ann Neurol. 2010;68(6):944–50. doi:10.1002/ana.22124.
49. Peters SU, Hundley RJ, Wilson AK, Warren Z, Vehorn A, Carvalho CM, et al. The behavioral phenotype in MECP2 duplication syndrome: a comparison with idiopathic autism. Autism Res. 2013;6(1):42–50. doi:10.1002/aur.1262.
50. Ramocki MB, Peters SU, Tavyev YJ, Zhang F, Carvalho CM, Schaaf CP, et al. Autism and other neuropsychiatric symptoms are prevalent in individuals with MeCP2 duplication syndrome. Ann Neurol. 2009;66(6):771–82. doi:10.1002/ana.21715.
51. Nguyen MV, Du F, Felice CA, Shan X, Nigam A, Mandel G, et al. MeCP2 is critical for maintaining mature neuronal networks and global brain anatomy during late stages of postnatal brain development and in the mature adult brain. J Neurosci. 2012;32(29):10021–34. doi:10.1523/JNEUROSCI.1316-12.2012.
52. Bodda C, Tantra M, Mollajew R, Arunachalam JP, Laccone FA, Can K, et al. Mild overexpression of Mecp2 in mice causes a higher susceptibility toward seizures. Am J Pathol. 2013;183(1):195–210. doi:10.1016/j.ajpath.2013.03.019.
53. Kenwrick S, Watkins A, De Angelis E. Neural cell recognition molecule L1: relating biological complexity to human disease mutations. Hum Mol Genet. 2000;9(6):879–86.
54. Schrander-Stumpel C, Fryns JP. Congenital hydrocephalus: nosology and guidelines for clinical approach and genetic counselling. Eur J Pediatr. 1998;157(5):355–62.
55. Kenwrick S, Jouet M, Donnai D. X linked hydrocephalus and MASA syndrome. J Med Genet. 1996;33(1):59–65.
56. Fransen E, Van Camp G, Vits L, Willems PJ. L1-associated diseases: clinical geneticists divide, molecular geneticists unite. Hum Mol Genet. 1997;6(10):1625–32.
57. Fox JW, Lamperti ED, Eksioglu YZ, Hong SE, Feng Y, Graham DA, et al. Mutations in filamin 1 prevent migration of cerebral cortical neurons in human periventricular heterotopia. Neuron. 1998;21(6):1315–25.
58. Robertson SP, Twigg SR, Sutherland-Smith AJ, Biancalana V, Gorlin RJ, Horn D, et al. Localized mutations in the gene encoding the cytoskeletal protein filamin A cause diverse malformations in humans. Nat Genet. 2003;33(4):487–91. doi:10.1038/ng1119.
59. Yu HC, Sloan JL, Scharer G, Brebner A, Quintana AM, Achilly NP, et al. An X-linked cobalamin disorder caused by mutations in transcriptional coregulator HCFC1. Am J Hum Genet. 2013;93(3):506–14. doi:10.1016/j.ajhg.2013.07.022.
60. Huang L, Jolly LA, Willis-Owen S, Gardner A, Kumar R, Douglas E, et al. A noncoding, regulatory mutation implicates HCFC1 in nonsyndromic intellectual disability. Am J Hum Genet. 2012;91(4):694–702. doi:10.1016/j.ajhg.2012.08.011.
61. Lugtenberg D, Kleefstra T, Oudakker AR, Nillesen WM, Yntema HG, Tzschach A, et al. Structural variation in Xq28: MECP2 duplications in 1 % of patients with unexplained XLMR and in 2 % of male patients with severe encephalopathy. Eur J Hum Genet. 2009;17(4):444–53. doi:10.1038/ejhg.2008.208.

# A novel BCR-ABL1 fusion gene identified by next-generation sequencing in chronic myeloid leukemia

Xiaodong Lyu[1,2†], Jingke Yang[3†], Xianwei Wang[2], Jieying Hu[2], Bing Liu[2], Yu Zhao[2], Zhen Guo[2], Bingshan Liu[1], Ruihua Fan[2] and Yongping Song[3*]

## Abstract

**Background:** *BCR-ABL1* fusion proteins contain constitutively active tyrosine kinases that are potential candidates for targeted therapy with tyrosine kinase inhibitors such as imatinib in chronic myeloid leukemia (CML). However, uncharacterized *BCR-ABL1* fusion genes can be missed by quantitative RT-PCR (qRT-PCR)-based routine screening methods, causing adverse effect on drug selection and treatment outcome.

**Case presentation:** In this study, we demonstrated that the next-generation sequencing (NGS) can be employed to overcome this obstacle. Through NGS, we identified a novel *BCR-ABL1* fusion gene with breakpoints in the *BCR* intron 14 and the *ABL1* intron 2, respectively, in a rare case of CML. Its mRNA with an e14a3 junction was then detected using customized RT-PCR followed by Sanger sequencing. Subsequently, the patient received targeted medicine imatinib initially at 400 mg/day, and later 300 mg/day due to intolerance reactions. With this personalized treatment, the patient's condition was significantly improved. Interestingly, this novel fusion gene encodes a fusion protein containing a compromised SH3 domain, which is usually intact in the majority of CML cases, suggesting that dysfunctional SH3 domain may be associated with altered drug response and unique clinicopathological manifestations observed in this patient.

**Conclusion:** We identified a novel *BCR-ABL1* fusion gene using NGS in a rare case of CML while routine laboratory procedures were challenged, demonstrating the power of NGS as a diagnostic tool for detecting novel genetic mutations. Moreover, our new finding regarding the novel fusion variant will provide useful insights to improve the spectrum of the genomic abnormalities recognizable by routine molecular screening.

**Keywords:** BCR-ABL1, Next-generation sequencing, Chronic myeloid leukemia, SH3 domain, Tyrosine kinase, Imatinib

## Background

Philadelphia translocation, the recurrent genomic rearrangement between chromosome 22q11 and 9q34, is a cytogenetic hallmark of Chronic myeloid leukemia (CML) [1]. It usually arises between genes *BCR* and *ABL1* in the intron regions, resulting in the formation of *BCR-ABL1* fusion genes and accordingly in the expression of chimeric gene transcripts with a juxtaposition of e13-a2, e14-a2, e19-a2, or e1-a2 [1]. These well characterized mRNA molecules, existed in three principal forms (p210, p190, and p230), have been screened routinely by multiplex quantitative RT-PCR (qRT-PCR) assays for diagnostic purpose in CML patients. However, these screening procedures have limitations as they were designed for detecting those previously characterized BCR-ABL1 fusion transcripts [2–14]. A false negative result may occur if a novel fusion mRNA does not contain sequences recognizable by primers within commercial or laboratory-developed screening kits, conferring a negative impact in treatment selection and therapeutic outcome.

To overcome these challenges, new technologies are in debt to be developed. The next-generation sequencing

* Correspondence: songyongping001@126.com
†Equal contributors
3Department of Hematology, the Affiliated Cancer Hospital of Zhengzhou University; Henan Cancer Hospital, Zhengzhou, Henan 450000, China
Full list of author information is available at the end of the article

(NGS) is a powerful tool for detecting genomic abnormalities that are both known and previously uncharacterized [15, 16]. Due to improved efficiency and affordability, both whole genome sequencing (WGS) and whole exome sequencing (WES) in NGS platforms have become increasingly popular as alternative methods for detecting unknown and complex pathogenic mutations in cancer and other diseases [17, 18]. Additionally, targeted NGS applications have also been developed for known mutations, further facilitating NGS as a diagnostic tool for daily practice [18].

A CML case was presented in the current study. While both cytogenetic analysis and Fluorescent In-Situ Hybridization (FISH) suggested a Philadelphia translocation, Fluorescence one-step multiplex qRT-PCR, a routinely used screening method, failed to identify any *BCR-ABL1* transcripts. To resolve the discrepancy, we performed genomic sequencing using a WGS in a NGS platform and identified a novel *BCR-ABL1* fusion gene variant. The related transcript was then detected using RT-PCR with customized primers followed by Sanger sequencing. Our result should provide novel insights in BCR-ABL1 diagnosis and facilitate the utilization of NGS as an alternative or daily diagnostic tool in leukemia.

## Methods

### Detection of BCR-ABL1 gene rearrangement

Fluorescence one-step RT-PCR was performed as described previously [19]. In brief, total RNA was extracted from bone marrow aspiration samples with RNeasy Kit (Qiagen, CA, USA) according to vendor's instruction and then treated with DNase I (DNA-*free*; Applied Biosystems-Ambion, TX, USA) to remove any DNA contamination. The one-step RT-PCR was then performed using Leukemia Related Fusion Gene Detection Kit for *BCR-ABL* p210, p190, or p230 (Yuanqi Bio-Pharmaceutical, Shanghai, China). For each reaction, 3 μl total RNA was mixed with 20 μl multiplex RT-PCR Buffer and 2 μl multiplex Enzyme mix in a total volume of 25 μl. The RT-PCR was conducted at 42 °C for 30 min, 94 °C for 5 min, and followed by 40 cycles 94 °C for 15 s and 60 °C for 1 min on a 7300 Real Time PCR System (ABI, USA).

### FISH analysis detecting BCR-ABL fusion

We conducted FISH analysis on patient's bone marrow aspiration sample using *BCR-ABL* FISH Probe kit (GP Medical, Beijing, China) per vender's instruction. Two DNA probes targeting the 5′ end of *BCR* and the 3′ end of *ABL1* were labeled with green and red fluorescent dye, respectively. In a normal nucleus, the probe-targeted sequences were located on different chromosomes as indicated as separated green and red signals. However, when fusion occurs in a tumor cell, a yellowish signal should be observed due to the fusion of *BCR* and *ABL1* genes, resulting in the colocalization of the green and red fluorescent signals.

### Whole genome sequencing in a next-generation sequencing platform

Genomic DNA (gDNA) library for next-generation sequencing was prepared using TruSeq Nano DNA Library Preparation Kit (Illumina, San Diego, CA). The gDNAs were shared into fragments using Covaris and ligated at both ends with indexed paired-end adaptors (Covaris, Woburn, MA, USA). The adapter-ligated gDNAS were purified and then used as templates in a ligation-mediated PCR for 8 cycles. The PCR amplicons were quantitated using Qubit 3.0 Fluorometer (Life Technologies) after removing primers, and then diluted into solutions at 0.75 ng/ul. The magnitude of enrichment were subsequently estimated using an Agilent 2100 Bioanalyzer (Agilent Technologies). Paired-end DNA sequencing was performed on a HiSeq X (Illumina, San Diego, CA). Illumina bcl2fastq software version 2.15 was used for base calling analysis.

## Case presentation

### Patient

A 24-year-old male patient presented to the hospital with significant bilateral cervical lymphadenopathy in February 2015. Multiple large necrotic lymph nodes was increased in size from 1 × 1.5 cm to 5 × 3 cm within 10 days. Thoracic computed tomography (CT) detected additional bilateral axillary lymphadenopathy. The patient also showed symptoms including constant low fever, red and swollen gums, and splenomegaly. The patient was diagnosed as CML upon the completion of blood and bone marrow examininations. The full blood count indicated leukocytosis with elevated level of white blood cells (WBCs, $222 \times 10^9$/L), neutrophils ($95.3 \times 10^9$/L), platelet ($938 \times 10^9$/L), and normal level of hemoglobin (116 g/L). Periphery blood smear analysis suggested granulocytosis with the presence of circulating myeloblasts (6 %) and immature granulocytes at various stages (Table 1). Bone marrow aspiration analysis indicated hypercellularity with prominent eosinophilia, basophilia, and elevated level of myeloblasts (5.4 %) and promyelocytes (8 %) (Table 1 and Fig. 1). A decreased level of lymphocytes with normal morphology was also observed. The myeloid/erythroid (M:E) ratio was significantly increased in both periphery blood and bone marrow (Table 1).

### Detection of BACR-ABL1 fusion gene with the NGS

Bone marrow karyotype showed a phenotype of 46,XY,t (9;22) (q34;q11) [10/10] (Fig. 2). FISH analysis suggested a possible fusion between the *BCR* and *ABL1* genes.

**Table 1** Analysis of periphery blood smear and bone marrow aspiration

| Cell type | Blood smear | Bone marrow aspiration | |
|---|---|---|---|
| | Cell count (%) | Reference (Mean ± sem) | Cell count (%) |
| Myeloblast | 6.0 | 0.64 ± 0.33 | 5.4 |
| Promyelocyte | 4.0 | 1.57 ± 0.60 | 8.0 |
| Neutrophil | | | |
| N. myelocyte | 11.0 | 6.49 ± 2.04 | 18.2 |
| N. metamyelocyte | 8.5 | 7.90 ± 1.97 | 7.6 |
| N. band | 14.5 | 23.72 ± 3.50 | 14.6 |
| Neutrophil | 14.0 | 9.44 ± 2.92 | 13.8 |
| Eosinophil | 13.0 | 0.86 ± 0.61 | 11.0 |
| Basophil | 5.5 | 0.30 ± 0.05 | 1.8 |
| Lymphocyte | 16.0 | 22.78 ± 7.04 | 9.4 |
| Monocyte | 7.5 | 3.00 ± 0.88 | 4.2 |
| M:E ratio | 153:0 | 3.00 ± 1.00 | 215:1 |

However, fluorescent quantitative RT-PCR (qRT-PCR) failed to detect any previously characterized *BCR-ABL1* fusion transcripts p210 (e13-a2 and e14-a2), p190 (e1-a2), and p230 (e19-a2). To clarify whether a *BCR-ABL1* fusion occurred in this patient, we conducted whole genome sequencing (WGS) analysis on a next-generation sequencing (NGS) platform. We detected a *BCR-ABL1* fusion gene with novel breakpoints in the *BCR* intron 14 and the *ABL1* intron 2, respectively (Fig. 3a). Based on this finding, we predicted that the fusion junction in the novel *BCR-ABL1* fusion transcript was flanked by sequences from the *BCR* exon 14 (e14) and *ABL1* exon 3 (a3), which were used as templates for designing customized PCR primers. Through using these primers, we conducted RT-PCR followed by Sanger sequencing and identified the corresponding *BCR-ABL1* hybrid mRNA with an e14a3 junction (Fig. 3b). Through NGS, we also detected nonsynonymous single nucleotide variant (SNV) in several well-known leukemic genes, including FLT3 (c.A20G:p.D7G), KIT (c.A1621C:p.M541L), PAX5 (c.C878T:p.T293), and TP53 (c.C215G:p.P72R). However, it is not clear whether these mutations play any important roles in leukemogenesis due to either no or limited reports associated with each of these mutations in cancer.

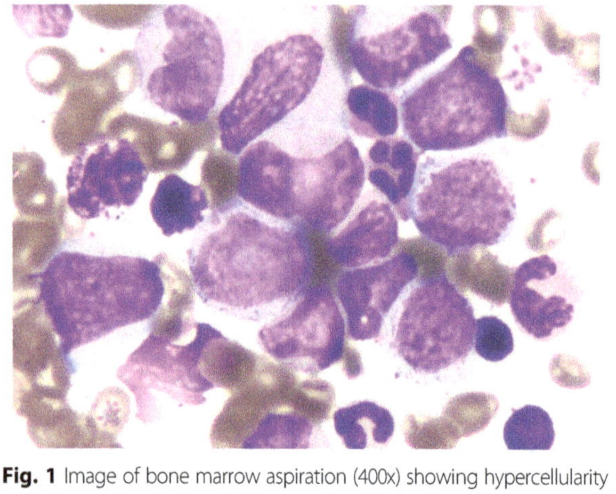

**Fig. 1** Image of bone marrow aspiration (400x) showing hypercellularity with elevated level of myeloblasts, eosinophils, and basophils

### Treatment

Diagnosed with CML, the patient was initially treated with hydroxyurea to improve blood count. Additional medicines, including antibiotics and anti-infection drugs, were also prescribed to relief fever, gum swelling and redness, and other complications. After detecting the novel *BCR-ABL1* fusion gene, imatinib was used at 400 mg/day as a targeted treatment. However, despite an improved blood count, the patient showed intolerant reactions, including raised fever, sore throat, right-side maxillofacial swelling, etc., after 40 days' treatment. The dosage of imatinib was then reduced to 300 mg/day. The full blood count was significantly improved with a WBC count at a relatively stable level (3 to 10 × $10^9$/L). The patient was then released with continued imatinib usage at 300 mg/day and with periodic follow-up examinations.

## Discussion

In this study, we reported that a novel *BCR-ABL1* fusion gene was identified by NGS technology, but not by a routinely-used, RT-qPCR-based method in a rare case of CML. Its mRNA transcript was subsequently detected using RT-qPCR with customized primers. Our result suggested that the NGS-based application can be employed as a diagnostic tool in those difficult cases with novel or complex genomic abnormalities.

CML, a malignant myeloproliferative disorder, originates from a hematopoietic stem cell that carries a Philadelphia chromosome, characterized by a reciprocal translocation between chromosomes 9 and 22, or t (9,22). This translocation generates a fusion gene with the juxtaposition of the *BCR* gene fragment at the 5′ end and the *ABL1* gene fragment at the 3′end [20]. An in-frame *BCR-ABL1* fusion gene is likely oncogenic, which can be transcribed into *BCR-ABL1* fusion mRNA and translated into BCR-ABL1 fusion protein. As discovered by genomic and cDNA sequencing in CML patients, the breakpoint in the *ABL1* gene is usually detected in a region between exon 1a and exon 2 [21]. In rare occasions, the breakpoints were detected in intron region downstream to the exon 2, resulting in a smaller fusion gene skipping exon 2 [22]. In the *BCR* gene, the breakpoints are most frequently detected in introns between exons 13 and 14 or exons 14 and 15 within a region recognized as the major breakpoint cluster region (M-*bcr*) covering exons 12–16 (e12-e16, or

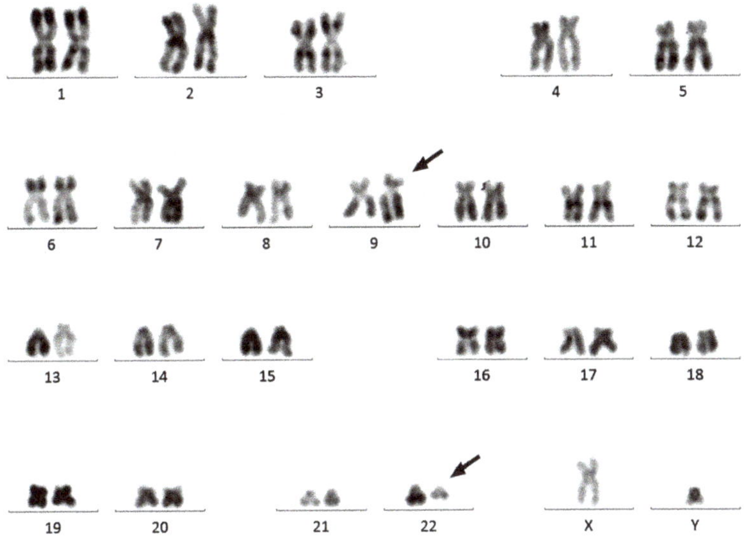


**Fig. 2** Cytogenetic analysis of bone marrow aspiration showing a karyotype 46,xy,t (9;22) (q34;q11). A gene translocation occurred between chromosomes 9 and 22 resulting Philadelphia chromosomes at the sites as indicated with *arrows*

historically known as b1-b5) [1]. The encoding proteins were termed based on their molecular weight as $p210^{BCR\text{-}ABL1}$ fusion proteins with junctions described as e13a2 or e14a2. In rare cases, the breakpoints were found in the minor bcr (m-bcr) between the two alternative exons e2′ and e2 [23] or μ-bcr between exons 19 and 20 [24–26]. Their encoding proteins were described as $p190^{BCR\text{-}ABL1}$ and $p230^{BCR\text{-}ABL1}$.

In this study, we reported a CML patient with constant low fever, swollen gums, bilaterally cervical lymphadenopathy, and splenomegaly. Interestingly, this patient showed otherwise normal physical and mental conditions. Upon blood and bone marrow tests, this patient was diagnosed as CML. Further cytogenetic analysis confirmed the existence of Philadelphia chromosome. However, routine fluorescent RT-qPCR screening cannot

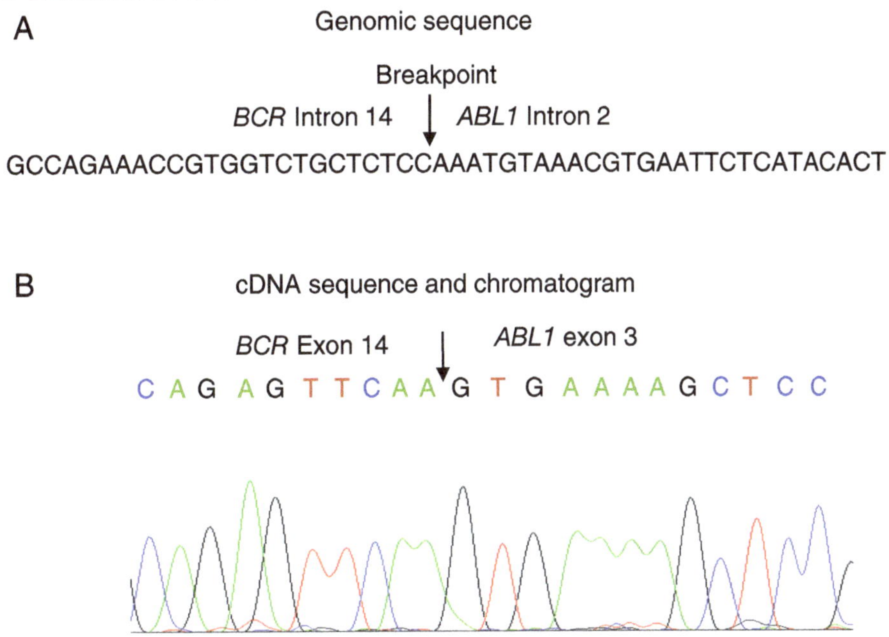


**Fig. 3** A novel BCR-ABL1 fusion gene and its transcript in a CML case. **a** Diagram showing the breaking point (or fusion junction) and flanking sequences from *BCR* Intron 14 and *ABL1* intron 2, which were identified using WGS in a NGS platform. **b** BCR-ABL1 cDNA sequence around the fusion junction and related chromatogram are shown. The junction is indicated with an *arrow*. The origins of cDNA sequences were also indicated

detect any form of *BCR-ABL1* fusion mRNAs that were previously characterized and detected in the majority of CML cases. To resolve the discrepancy, we performed WGS on an Illumina HiSeq X and identified a novel *BCR-ABL1* fusion gene. Although the breakpoint in the *BCR* gene is located in intron between exons 13 and 14 within the M-bcr region, the breakpoint in the *ABL1* is novel, located in intron 2, a region downstream to the exon 2. The resulting fusion gene is presumably transcribed into a smaller fusion mRNA with an e14a3 junction, skipping the entire exon 2 (174 nucleotides). This novel transcript was initially undetectable by routine RT-qPCR-based diagnostic screening as this type of fusion transcripts have only been reported in rare cases and have not been the subjects for detection using RT-PCR-based routine *BCR-ABL1* screening [22]. This rare fusion variant was only reported in 4 leukemia cases, including one case of CML [27] and three cases of acute lymphoblastic leukemia (ALL) [28–30], Unlike our study, none of these studies performed genomic sequencing to show the existence of this fusion gene on the genomic level. After NGS application, this novel fusion mRNA (cDNA) was eventually identified using RT-PCR with a pair of customized primers targeting the *BCR* exon 14 (e14) and *ABL1* exon 3 (a3), respectively, and followed by Sanger sequencing of PCR amplicons. Similar to our study, a recent publication has shown that an e14a3 transcript was detected by a customized PCR using primers targeting the *BCR* exon e13 and the *ABL1* exon a3, but not by the PCR using conventional primer sets [28]. Thus, if a *BCR-ABL1* negative result was obtained by conventional screening, care should be taken to avoid misdiagnosis, which may cause an adverse impact on therapeutic outcome. The correct diagnosis will allow physicians to make right decisions whether a targeted therapy (imatinib in this case) or other treatment plans should be used for better outcome achievement.

ABL1 protein is a nonreceptor tyrosine kinase containing a tyrosine kinase domain. The fusion with the *BCR* gene creates a fusion protein with an constitutively active ABL1 tyrosine kinases, which are believe to be causative in CML [31]. The majority of BCR-ABL1 proteins contain juxtaposed SH3-SH2 domains, which are located upstream to the tyrosine kinase domain and regulate kinase activity through their interactions with other proteins [32]. It has been shown that the interaction between BCR-ABL1 SH3 and RAD51 proline-rich regions caused RAD51 phosphorylation, resulting in secondary chromosomal aberrations that contribute to disease progression and relapse in CML [33]. In contrast, small protein apoptin, a tumor-selective killer [34], is a negative regulator of BCR-ABL1 kinase via its ability to interact with BCR-ABL1 SH3 domain [35]. Moreover, it has also been suggested that sensitivity to the ABL TKIs is altered by either SH3-SH2 mutations or the interaction between ABL1 SH3-SH2 and other proteins such as RIN1 [36, 37]. SH3 domain is encoded by ABL1 exons 2 and 3. In our case, the whole exon 2 sequence including 51 nucleotides used for encoding the part of the ABL1 SH3 domain, were excluded in this novel *BCR-ABL1* fusion gene. Thus, this fusion gene is predicted to encode a fusion protein with a compromised SH3 domain. It is not clear whether this SH3 domain truncation is associated with some of the less common clinical presentations and drug response including intolerance to the normal dose of imatinib. Further studies are warranted to clarify these questions.

Through NGS, we also detected nonsynonymous mutations in leukemic genes *TP53, FLT3, KIT,* and *PAX5,* which were co-existed with BCR-ABL1 fusion. This result suggested that this CML is highly heterogeneous. *TP53,* the most frequently mutated gene in cancer, has often been detected with mutation in acute myeloid leukemia (AML), ALL, and chronic lymphocytic leukemia (CLL), predicting poor prognosis [38–40]. Both *FLT3* and *KIT* mutations have been shown to be associated with poor prognosis in AML [41, 42], while mutation in the gene *PAX5* are considered as signature mutations in precursor B-ALL [43, 44]. Although all these genes are frequently mutated in leukemia, the particular *FLT3* and *PAX5* mutations identified in this CML patient have never been reported before in any type of cancer, while the *TP53* and *KIT* mutations were only described in prostate cancer and melanoma [45, 46]. It should be noted that these novel mutations would be less likely to be detected by routine PCR-based molecular screening due to their novelty. Meanwhile, it remains to be determine whether these mutations are recurrent and play any pathological role in CML.

## Conclusions

Through NGS application, we have identified a novel *BCR-ABL1* fusion (with an e14a3 junction) that is undetectable by routine qRT-PCR-based laboratory procedures in a rare case of CML. Due to the correct diagnosis, the physicians prescribed targeted therapy using imatinib to this patient, leading to a better treatment outcome. Our NGS result also suggested that this fusion gene encodes a protein containing a truncated SH3 domain, which may contribute to the unique clinical presentation and altered drug response in this patient. Moreover, novel nonsynonymous mutations in the *TP53, FLT3, KIT,* and *PAX5* genes, are co-existed with BCR-ABL1 fusion, indicating the high heterogeneity in this disease. Therefore, this study has demonstrated the value of NGS as a powerful diagnostic tool for identifying novel and complex genetic mutations.

## Abbreviations

CML, Chronic myeloid leukemia; FISH, Fluorescent In-Situ Hybridization; NGS, Next-generation sequencing; TKI, Tyrosine kinase inhibitor; WES, Whole exome sequencing; WGS, Whole genome sequencing

## Funding

This work was partly supported by National Natural Science Foundation of China (NSFC) grant 81470287.

## Authors' contributions

XL, JY and YS designed the study and wrote the manuscript. XW, JH, BL, YZ, ZG, BL, and RF performed the experiments and data analysis. All authors reviewed the manuscript. All authors read and approved the final manuscript.

## Competing interests

The authors declare that they have no competing interests.

## Author details

[1]School of Basic Medical Sciences, Zhengzhou University, Zhengzhou, Henan 450000, China. [2]Central Laboratory, the Affiliated Cancer Hospital of Zhengzhou University; Henan Cancer Hospital, Zhengzhou, Henan 450000, China. [3]Department of Hematology, the Affiliated Cancer Hospital of Zhengzhou University; Henan Cancer Hospital, Zhengzhou, Henan 450000, China.

## References

1. Melo JV. The diversity of BCR-ABL fusion proteins and their relationship to leukemia phenotype. Blood. 1996;88:2375–84.
2. Sorel N, Mayeur-Rousse C, Deverriere S, Roy L, Brottier-Mancini E, Guilhot F, et al. Comprehensive characterization of a novel intronic pseudo-exon inserted within an e14/a2 BCR-ABL rearrangement in a patient with chronic myeloid leukemia. J Mol Diagn. 2010;12(4):520–4.
3. van der Velden VHJ, Beverloo HB, Hoogeveen PG, Zwaan CM. A novel BCR-ABL fusion transcript (e18a2) in a child with chronic myeloid leukemia. Leukemia. 2007;21(4):833–5.
4. Callet-Bauchu E, Salles G, Gazzo S, Dalle S, Berger F, Hayette S. Identification of a novel e8/a4 BCR/ABL fusion transcript in a case of a transformed Sézary syndrome. Haematologica. 2007;92(9):1277–8.
5. Tchirkov A, Couderc JL, Périssel B, Goumy C, Regnier A, Uhrhammer N, et al. Major molecular response to imatinib in a patient with chronic myeloid leukemia expressing a novel form of e8a2 BCR-ABL transcript. Leukemia. 2006;20(1):167–8.
6. Demehri S, Paschka P, Schultheis B, Lange T, Koizumi T, Sugimoto T, et al. e8a2 BCR-ABL: More frequent than other atypical BCR-ABL variants? Leukemia. 2005;19(4):681–4.
7. Mdel Moreno P, Cortinas MN, Bonomi R, Cardeza A, Mdel Uriarte R. A novel BCR-ABL fusion transcript (e15a2) in 2 patients with atypical chronic myeloproliferative syndrome. Blood. 2001;97(11):3668–9.
8. Branford S, Rudzki Z, Hughes TP. A novel BCR-ABL transcript (e8a2) with the insertion of an inverted sequence of ABL intron 1b in a patient with Philadelphia-positive chronic myeloid leukaemia. Br J Haematol. 2000;109(3):635–7.
9. Hirota M, Hidaka E, Ueno I, Ishikawa M, Asano N, Yamauchi K, et al. Novel BCR-ABL transcript containing an intronic sequence insert in a patient with Philadelphia-positive acute lymphoblastic leukaemia. Br J Haematol. 2000;110(4):867–70.
10. Martinelli G, Terragna C, Amabile M, Montefusco V, Testoni N, Ottaviani E, et al. Alu and translisin recognition site sequences flanking translocation sites in a novel type of chimeric bcr-abl transcript suggest a possible general mechanism for bcr-abl breakpoints. Haematologica. 2000;85(1):40–6.
11. Leibundgut EO, Jotterand M, Rigamonti V, Parlier V, Muhlematter D, Tobler A, et al. A novel BCR-ABL transcript e2a2 in a chronic myelogenous leukaemia patient with a duplicated Ph-chromosome and monosomy 7. Br J Haematol. 1999;106(4):1041–4.
12. Byrne JL, Carter GI, Davies JM, Haynes AP, Russell NH, Cross NCP. A novel BCR-ABL fusion gene (e2/1a) in a patient with Philadelphia-positive chronic myelogenous leukaemia and an aggressive clinical course. Br J Haematol. 1998;103(3):791–4.
13. Frederick L, Beardell F, Viswanatha DS. Novel BCR-ABL1 fusion identified by targeted next-generation sequencing in a patient with an atypical myeloproliferative neoplasm. Hum Pathol. 2014;45(8):1784–9.
14. Roman J, Parziale A, Gottardi E, De Micheli D, Cilloni D, Tiribelli M, et al. Novel type of BCR-ABL transcript in a chronic myelogenous leukaemia patient relapsed after bone marrow transplantation. Br J Haematol. 2000;111(2):644–6.
15. Nakagawa H, Wardell CP, Furuta M, Taniguchi H, Fujimoto A. Cancer whole-genome sequencing: present and future. Oncogene. 2015;34(49):5943–50.
16. Bamshad MJ, Ng SB, Bigham AW, Tabor HK, Emond MJ, Nickerson DA, et al. Exome sequencing as a tool for Mendelian disease gene discovery. Nat Rev Genet. 2011;12(11):745–55.
17. Metzker ML. Sequencing technologies — the next generation. Nat Rev Genet. 2010;11(1):31–46.
18. McCutcheon JN, Giaccone G. Next-Generation Sequencing: Targeting Targeted Therapies. Clin Cancer Res. 2015;21(16):3584–5.
19. Guo Y, Ma J, Lyu X, Liu H, Wei B, Zhao J, et al. Non-small cell lung cancer with EML4-ALK translocation in Chinese male never-smokers is characterized with early-onset. BMC Cancer. 2014;14(1):834.
20. Apperley JF. Chronic myeloid leukaemia. Lancet. 2015;385(9976):1447–59.
21. Melo JV, Gordon DE, Cross NC, Goldman JM. The ABL-BCR fusion gene is expressed in chronic myeloid leukemia. Blood. 1993;81(1):158–65.
22. Melo JV. BCR-ABL gene variants. Baillieres Clin Haematol. 1997;10(2):203–22.
23. Chissoe SL, Bodenteich A, Wang YF, Wang YP, Burian D, Clifton SW, et al. Sequence and analysis of the human ABL gene, the BCR gene, and regions involved in the Philadelphia chromosomal translocation. Genomics. 1995; 27(1):67–82.
24. Pane F, Frigeri F, Sindona M, Luciano L, Ferrara F, Cimino R, et al. Neutrophilic-chronic myeloid leukemia: a distinct disease with a specific molecular marker (BCR/ABL with C3/A2 junction). Blood. 1996;88(7):2410–4.
25. Saglio G, Guerrasio A, Rosso C, Zaccaria A, Tassinari A, Serra A, et al. New type of Bcr/Abl junction in Philadelphia chromosome-positive chronic myelogenous leukemia. Blood. 1990;76(9):1819–24.
26. Wada H, Mizutani S, Nishimura J, Usuki Y, Kohsaki M, Komai M, et al. Establishment and molecular characterization of a novel leukemic cell line with Philadelphia chromosome expressing p230 BCR/ABL fusion protein. Cancer Res. 1995;55(14):3192–6.
27. Jinawath N, Norris-Kirby A, Smith BD, Gocke CD, Batista DA, Griffin CA, et al. A rare e14a3 (b3a3) BCR-ABL fusion transcript in chronic myeloid leukemia: diagnostic challenges in clinical laboratory practice. J Mol Diagn. 2009;11(4):359–63.
28. Kurita D, Hatta Y, Hojo A, Kura Y, Sawada U, Kanda Y, et al. Adult acute lymphoblastic leukemia with a rare b3a3 type BCR/ABL1 fusion transcript. Cancer Genet. 2016;209(4):161–5.
29. Kim J, Park TS, Lyu CJ, Song J, Lee KA, Kim SJ, et al. BCR/ABL rearrangement with b3a3 fusion transcript in a case of childhood acute lymphoblastic leukemia. Cancer Genet Cytogenet. 2009;189(2):132–7.
30. Inukai T, Sugita K, Suzuki T, Ijima K, Goi K, Tezuka T, et al. A novel 203 kD aberrant BCR-ABL product in a girl with Philadelphia chromosome positive acute lymphoblastic leukaemia. Br J Haematol. 1993;85(4):823–5.
31. Pinilla-Ibarz J, Sweet K, Emole J, Fradley M. Long-term BCR-ABL1 Tyrosine Kinase Inhibitor Therapy in Chronic Myeloid Leukemia. Anticancer Res. 2015;35(12):6355–64.
32. Colicelli J. ABL tyrosine kinases: evolution of function, regulation, and specificity. Sci Signal. 2010;3(139):re6.
33. Slupianek A, Dasgupta Y, Ren SY, Gurdek E, Donlin M, Nieborowska-Skorska M, et al. Targeting RAD51 phosphotyrosine-315 to prevent unfaithful recombination repair in BCR-ABL1 leukemia. Blood. 2011;118(4):1062–8.
34. Los M, Panigrahi S, Rashedi I, Mandal S, Stetefeld J, Essmann F, et al. Apoptin, a tumor-selective killer. Biochim Biophys Acta. 2009;1793(8):1335–42.

35. Jangamreddy JR, Panigrahi S, Lotfi K, Yadav M, Maddika S, Tripathi AK, et al. Mapping of apoptin-interaction with BCR-ABL1, and development of apoptin-based targeted therapy. Oncotarget. 2014;5(16):7198–211.
36. Sherbenou DW, Hantschel O, Kaupe I, Willis S, Bumm T, Turaga LP, et al. BCR-ABL SH3-SH2 domain mutations in chronic myeloid leukemia patients on imatinib. Blood. 2010;116(17):3278–85.
37. Thai M, Ting PY, McLaughlin J, Cheng D, Muschen M, Witte ON, et al. ABL fusion oncogene transformation and inhibitor sensitivity are mediated by the cellular regulator RIN1. Leukemia. 2011;25(2):290–300.
38. Hof J, Krentz S, van Schewick C, Korner G, Shalapour S, Rhein P, et al. Mutations and deletions of the TP53 gene predict nonresponse to treatment and poor outcome in first relapse of childhood acute lymphoblastic leukemia. J Clin Oncol. 2011;29(23):3185–93.
39. Zenz T, Eichhorst B, Busch R, Denzel T, Habe S, Winkler D, et al. TP53 mutation and survival in chronic lymphocytic leukemia. J Clin Oncol. 2010;28(29):4473–9.
40. Stirewalt DL, Kopecky KJ, Meshinchi S, Appelbaum FR, Slovak ML, Willman CL, et al. FLT3, RAS, and TP53 mutations in elderly patients with acute myeloid leukemia. Blood. 2001;97(11):3589–95.
41. Network TCGAR. Genomic and epigenomic landscapes of adult de novo acute myeloid leukemia. N Engl J Med. 2013;368(22):2059–74.
42. Kihara R, Nagata Y, Kiyoi H, Kato T, Yamamoto E, Suzuki K, et al. Comprehensive analysis of genetic alterations and their prognostic impacts in adult acute myeloid leukemia patients. Leukemia. 2014;28(8):1586–95.
43. Shah S, Schrader KA, Waanders E, Timms AE, Vijai J, Miething C, et al. A recurrent germline PAX5 mutation confers susceptibility to pre-B cell acute lymphoblastic leukemia. Nat Genet. 2013;45(10):1226–31.
44. Mullighan CG, Goorha S, Radtke I, Miller CB, Coustan-Smith E, Dalton JD, et al. Genome-wide analysis of genetic alterations in acute lymphoblastic leukaemia. Nature. 2007;446(7137):758–64.
45. Salgado CM, Basu D, Nikiforova M, Hamilton RL, Gehris R, Jakacki R, et al. Amplification of mutated NRAS leading to congenital melanoma in neurocutaneous melanocytosis. Melanoma Res. 2015;25(5):453–60.
46. Lo Iacono M, Buttigliero C, Monica V, Bollito E, Garrou D, Cappia S, et al. Retrospective study testing next generation sequencing of selected cancer-associated genes in resected prostate cancer. Oncotarget. 2016;7(12):14394–404.

12

# Mosaic UPD(7q)mat in a patient with silver Russell syndrome

Jiasun Su[1*], Jin Wang[1], Xin Fan[1], Chunyun Fu[1], ShuJie Zhang[1], Yue Zhang[1], Zailong Qin[1], Hongdou Li[1], Jingsi Luo[1], Chuan Li[1], Tingting Jiang[1] and Yiping Shen[1,2*]

**Abstract**

**Background:** Silver-Russell syndrome (SRS) is one of the imprinting disorders characterized by prenatal and postnatal growth restriction, relative macrocephaly, body asymmetry and characteristic facial features. ~ 10% of SRS cases are known to be associated with maternal uniparental disomy of chromosome 7 (UPD(7)mat). Mosaic maternal segmental UPD of 7q (UPD(7q)mat) is very rare, had only been described in one case before.

**Case presentation:** We reported a second case of mosaic segmental UPD involving 7q. The patient presented with dysmorphic features including thin and short stature, triangular face, moderate protruding forehead, relative macrocephaly, fifth toe clinodactyly and irregular teeth, meeting the clinical diagnosed criteria of SRS. This case indicated that ~ 80% of mosaic UPD(7q)mat lead to the manifestation of main phenotypes of Silver-Russell syndrome.

**Conclusions:** Our case support the notion that there are genes control postnatal growth on long arm of chromosome 7 and indicate that ~ 80% of UPD(7q)mat mosaicism level was contributed to the SRS phenotype.

**Keywords:** Silver-Russell syndrome, Maternal uniparental disomy, Mosaicism

## Background

The Silver-Russell syndrome (SRS; OMIM #180860) is one of the imprinting disorders characterized by prenatal and postnatal growth restriction, relative macrocephaly, body asymmetry and characteristic facial features. To date, more than 400 SRS cases have been reported since it was initially described by Silver et al. in 1953 [1] and Russell in 1954 [2]. The clinical and genetic heterogeneity of SRS make it difficult to define its clinical diagnostic criteria and genetic etiology. Several scoring systems for clinical diagnosis of SRS have been proposed [3–7]. Most recent proposal suggested that a patients can be considered to have likely SRS if at least four out of the following six criteria were met: (1) small for gestational age, birth length and/or weight ≤ −2SDS, (2) postnatal growth retardation (height ≤ −2SDS), (3) relative macrocephaly at birth, (4) body asymmetry, (5) feeding difficulties and/or body mass index (BMI) ≤ −2SDS in toddlers; (6) protruding forehead at the age of 1-3 years (Netchine-Harbison SRS Clinical Scoring System). About 10% of SRS case had maternal uniparental disomy of chromosome 7, so far about 60 SRS patients with matUPD(7) had been reported [8]. The imprinting genes on chromosome 7 are believed to be involved in the pathogenesis of the syndrome [9–13], the specific causal gene(s) are yet to be identified.

Five cases with segmental UPD(7q)mat in patients with SRS phenotype had been documented in literature since 2001. The only mosaic segmental UPD(7) that was reported by Reboul et al. in 2006 revealed a 7q21-qter mosaicism in a patient with SRS phenotype [14]. Identifying segmental UPD(7) in patients with SRS may help to narrow-down causal genes and regions.

Here, we reported a second case with mosaic segmental UPD(7q) mat, the patient presented with the main phenotypes of SRS [15]. We compared the clinical findings involving mosaic UPD(7q)mat documented in literature and the finding support the notion that imprinted genes on 7q contribute to the pathogenesis of SRS, even in a mosaic status.

* Correspondence: sujiasun@126.com; yiping.shen@childrens.harvard.edu
[1]Department of Genetic and Metabolic Central Laboratory, Guangxi Maternal and Child Health Hospital, Guangxi Birth Defects Prevention and Control Institute, No 59, Xiangzhu Road, Nanning, China
Full list of author information is available at the end of the article

## Case presentation

The patient was a six-year-old boy came to hospital due to severe developmental delay, short stature and mild dysmorphic features. He was a full term first child with two apparently healthy younger siblings. He was delivered via cesarean section without complication during pregnancy or delivery. His birth weight was 1.91 kg(< −3SD), indicating small for gestational age. His parents were non-consanguineous without family history of congenital anomalies. The paternal height was 162 cm, and the maternal height was 138 cm, the mother was not investigated for SRS and the height of the maternal family members were not applied. The patient was reported to have failure to thrive since birth. During his initial hospital visit at the age of 6, his height was 91.9 cm (~ − 6 SD), weight 9.5 kg(~ − 6SD) and head circumference 49 cm (~ − 1SD, thus a relative macrocephaly). The bone age was delayed. Mild dysmorphic features were noticed including triangular face, moderate protruding forehead, relative macrocephaly, fifth toe clinodactyly and irregular teeth (Fig. 1a). Although the obvious body asymmetry was not noticed in this patient, this patient can be clinical diagnosed as SRS based on the Netchine–Harbison clinical scoring system (the first four features are present in this patient) [16]. In addition, he had normal electroencephalogram and electromyography, the growth hormone (GH) stimulating peak was 5.08 μg/L and diagnosed as partial growth hormone deficiency. He was subsequently treated with recombinant human growth hormone at the doses of 1 IU/(kg/d). The treatment lasted 4 months and stopped due to no significant growth response. Cytogenetic and molecular analysis were performed.

## Method

### Chromosomal microarray (CMA) and cytogenetic analyses

DNA sample was extracted from peripheral blood lymphocytes by using Lab-Aid DNA kit (Zeesan Biotech Co, Ltd., China). Genomic wide single nucleotide polymorphism (SNP) array analysis was performed by Illumina HumanSNPcyto-12 v2.1 BeadChip array. And the SNP data were collected and analyzed by Illumina Genome Studio and KaryoStudio software, cytogenetic analysis was performed by conventional standard GTG-banding at 400–550 band resolution.

### Microsatellite analysis

Eight highly informative microsatellite markers (short tandem repeat, STR) spanning the whole of chromosome 7 (D7S2552, D7S506, D7S510, D7S517, D7S672, D7S2410, D7S2504, D7S523) were selected from Genethon Genetic Maps (http://www.bli.uzh.ch/BLI/Projects/genetics/maps/gthon.html) for parent-of-origin analysis. The forward PCR primers designed for each STR maker were modified at 5′ terminal base with carboxyfluorescein (FAM). All fluorescent PCR products were analyzed on ABI 3130 genetic analyzer and GeneMapper (Applied Biosystems), the size and loci of each STR marker was assigned manually by identifying the peak on the electropherogram.

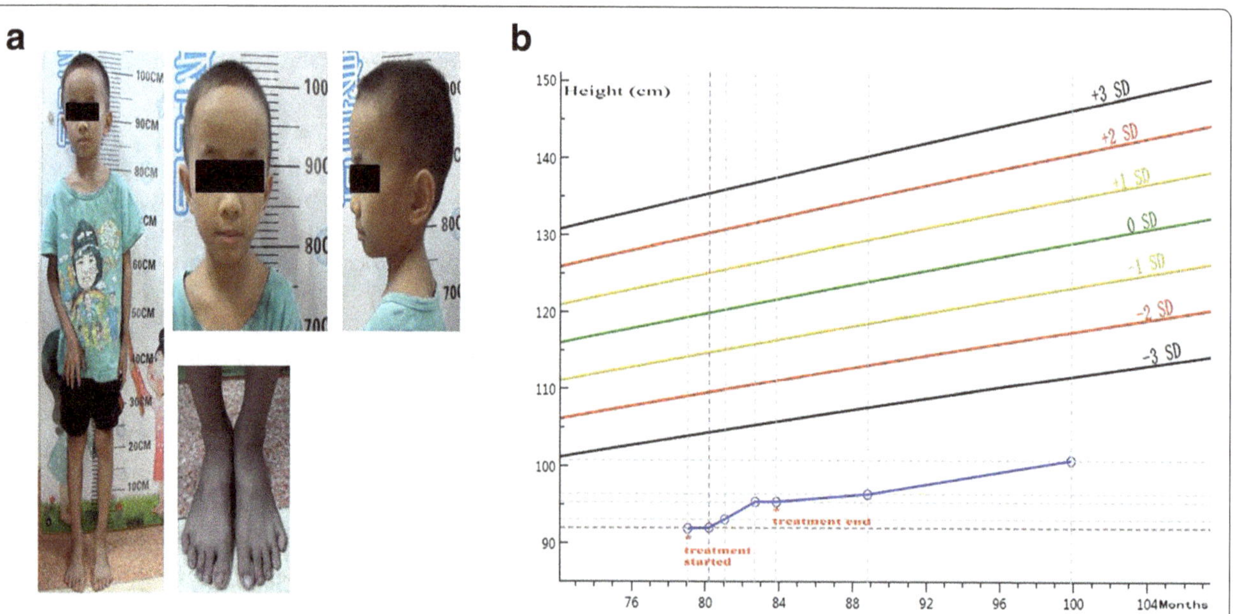


**Fig. 1** **a** Patient at age 8 years and 3 months. Dysmorphic features including thin and short stature, *triangular* face, moderate protruding forehead, relative macrocephaly, fifth toe clinodactyly and irregular teeth. **b** Growth curve of the patient: standard deviations (SD) were calculated based on the standardized growth charts for Chinese children and adolescents aged 0 to 18 [33], according to population-standard charts, the patient's growth improved but remained ~5.5 SD below the mean height for age

## Results

Uniparental disomy (UPD) of chromosome 7q was detected by CMA, spanned from the region of 7q11 to 7qter. The B allele frequency indicated that the UPD region was homozygous and mosaic (Fig. 2a), and the mosaicism level was estimated to be about 80% according to Conlin et al. [17]. G-band analysis presented normal karyotype. The STR makers analysis revealed that the UPD was maternal origin (Fig. 2b, c).

## Discussion

We reported a rare case of SRS due to mosaic segmental UPD(7q)mat. This is only the second such case ever reported [14] and the first case detected by SNP array. There are more than 60 UPD(7)mat cases documented in the literature since the first case of UPD(7)mat reported by Spence et al. [8, 18], we summarized the clinical features of typical SRS features and UPD(7)mat cases in Table 1. The body asymmetry phenotype was only ~ 39% prevalent among SRS cases. Relative macrocephaly (79.2%), SGA, BL and/or BW (61.6%), prominent forehead (61.6%), clinodactyly V digits (57.0%), feeding difficulties (46.5%), were the most common phenotype in the UPD(7)mat cases. Our patient presented with at least four common features, thus meet the clinical diagnosis of SRS (Netchine-Harbison SRS Clinical Scoring System, NH-CSS) [3].

Mosaic UPD(7)mat was a rare condition. Monk et al. did not find any evidence of somatic mosaicism in three UPD(7)mat probands in lymphocyte and fibroblasts using both Southern blot and FISH analyses [19], subsequently, five mosaic UPD(7) mat cases have been reported (Table 2). Karl Y et al. found the first case of trisomy 7 (T7)/upd(7) mosaicism by amniocentesis, and the fetus showed likely-SRS symptoms with SGA, low-set ears, prominent forehead, triangular face, obstructed micrognathia, clinodactyly of fifth finger bilaterally [20]. Miozzo et al. used haplotyping and cytogenetic-FISH studies characterized a newborn presented SRS phenotype with complete maternal isodisomy 7 (i7) and trisomy 7 mosaicism [21]. Complete maternal heterodisomy 7 and trisomy 7 mosaicism was also reported by Elisabeth et al. [22]. Patient with full UPD(7) mat abnormal cell lineage and normal cell lineage without trisomy 7 also present SRS phenotype [23]. Reboul et al. reported a patient had UPD (7) without the mosaic trisomy 7 [14]. A summary of

**a**

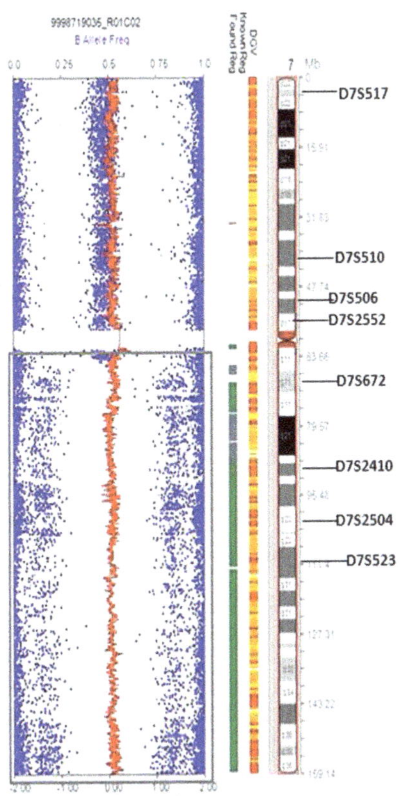


**b**

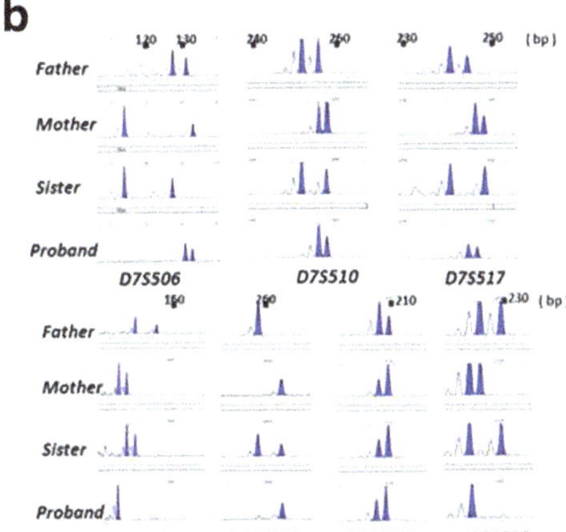


**c**

| Marks | Position | Father | Mother | C1 | Patient | Assessment |
|---|---|---|---|---|---|---|
| D7S2552 | 7p11.2 | 260/270 | 270/272 | 260/272 | -/- | Not informative |
| D7S506 | 7p12.1 | 127/130 | 114/133 | 114/127 | 130/133 | biparental |
| D7S510 | 7p14.1 | 252/256 | 256/258 | 252/258 | 256/258 | biparental |
| D7S517 | 7p22.2 | 241/244 | 246/248 | 241/248 | 244/246 | biparental |
| D7S672 | 7q11.22 | 142/152 | 134/139 | 139/141 | 134/134 | Maternal |
| D7S2410 | 7q21.13 | 257/257 | 264/264 | 257/264 | 264/264 | Maternal |
| D7S2504 | 7q22.1 | 208/210 | 208/210 | 208/210 | 208/210 | Not informative |
| D7S523 | 7q31.1 | 226/230 | 225/226 | 225/230 | 225/225 | Maternal |

**Fig. 2 a** The scatterplot representation of SNP microarray revealed the mosaic UPD region from 7q11 to 7qter. **b** Electropherograms of the D7S2552, D7S506, D7S510, D7S517, D7S672, D7S2410, D7S2503, D7S523 microsatellites in the proband (*bottom panel*), father (*top panel*) and mother (second panel). **c** The results of microsatellite analysis, the Arabic numbers denote the PCR product sizes in bp, D7S672, D7S2410, D7S523 loci revealed the UPD region detected by array was maternal origin

**Table 1** Phenotypic comparison of typical SRS cases and SRS due to UPD(7) mat

| Clinical findings | SRS[a] (*NH-CSS*) | UPD(7) mat cases[b] | mosaic UPD(7) mat cases[c] $n = 5$ | Our patient |
|---|---|---|---|---|
| Relative macrocephaly | + | 61/77(79.2%) | 3 | + |
| SGA, BL and/or BW ≤ −2SD | + | 53/86(61.6%) | 5 | + |
| Asymmetry | + | 30/77(39.0%) | 1 | – |
| Feeding difficulties | + | 40/86(46.5%) | 2 | – |
| Retarded bone age | + | 24/77(31.2%) | 1 | + |
| Clinodactyly V digits | 75% | 49/86(57.0%) | 3 | + |
| Triangular face | 94% | 24/86(28.0%) | 3 | + |
| prominent forehead | + | 53/86(61.6%) | 3 | + |
| Teeth anomalies | 37% | 14/77(18.2%) | 1 | + |
| Low set ears | 49% | 16/68(23.5%) | 2 | – |
| small chin | 62% | 10/86(11.6%) | 1 | + |

Clinical findings: +, present; –, absent, *SGA* small for gestational age, *BL* birth length, *BW* birth weight
*NH-CSS* netchine-harbison SRS clinical scoring system
[a]data from Wakeling et al. [16], [b]data from Kotzot, D. [34], Hannula et al. [35] and Fuke et al. [36], [c]cases from Miozzo et al. [21], Bilimoria et al. [20], Flori et al. [22], Reboul et al. [14], and Tomoko et al. [23]

the clinical features of the five previously reported patients with mosaic UPD(7)mat and our present case is listed in Table 2. Collectively, these cases indicated that SRS phenotype could raise from mosaic UPD(7)mat status.

Five segmental UPD(7q) mat cases associated with SRS phenotypes had been documented in literature since 2001 [14, 24–26] (Table 3). The involved region would span the whole 7q and the smallest region was ~ 31 Mb to 7qter (Fig. 3). Clinical features of segmental UPD(7q)mat were compared in Table 3. The most common were relative macrocephaly and triangular face (5/5). Notably, psychomotor delay was present in the case reported by Eggermann et al. [25] and Begemann et al. [26], but not in the rest of cases. Additionaly, The relevance of 7p for the SRS phenotype currently known are maternal duplication of 7p12.1 (including gene *GRB10*) [27, 28], These findings are consistent with the notion that the imprinted gene(s) on chromosome 7q are the causes of SRS phenotype [9].

The only previously reported a mosaic segment UPD(7q)mat from 7q21-qter mosaicism by Reboul et al. in a patient presented with SGA, relative macrocephaly, triangular face, severe growth retardation [14]. Our patient had only slightly larger size and presented with very similar phenotypes. The mosaicism level of Reboul's case was not evaluated.

**Table 2** Clinical features of mosaic UPD(7) mat cases

| | Miozzo et al. | Bilimoria et al. | Elisabeth et al. | Reboul et al. | Tomoko et al. | Our patient |
|---|---|---|---|---|---|---|
| *Mosaicism UPD type* | Mixture of i7 andT7 | Mixture of i7 and T7 | Mixture of het 7 and T7 | Mosaic segmental UPD7(q21-qter) | Mixture of i7 and N7 | Mosaic UPD7 (q11-qter) |
| *Evaluation analysis* | Microsatellite Metaphase FISH karyotyping | Microsatellite, karyotyping | Microsatellite, FISH | microsatellite analysis | microsatellite karyotype methylation | SNP array microsatellite |
| *tissuses* | Peripheral blood placental cotyledons | AF: ~ 27%[a] | AF: ~ 44% Intestine: 15% Skin: metaphases (5.5%) = nuclei (4%) | Peripheral blood | Peripheral blood: 92% Salivary:91% | Peripheral blood: ~ 80% |
| *Major Clinical findings* | IUGR, low birth weight, PNGR, relative macrocephaly, triangular face, prominent forehead, asymmetry | SGA, low-set ears, prominent forehead, small chin, triangular face, micrognathia, reversed epicanthal folds, clinodactyly of fifth finger bilaterally | Prominent large forehead, low osterior-rotated ears, small and retruded chin, bilateral clinodactyly of fifth fingers, VSD, PNGR, relative macrocephaly, feeding difficulties, triangular-shaped face, BAD | Growth failure, SGA, low birth weight, not show any craniofacial dysmorphic features. | Low birth weight/ length, VSD, hydronephrosis, Feeding difficulty, speech delay, short stature, relative macrocephaly, abnormal teeth, 5th finger clinodactyly | Short stature triangular face, moderate protruding forehead, relative macrocephaly, fifth toe buckling and irregularly teeth. |

*AF* amniotic fluid, *IUGR* intrauterine growth retardation, *PNGR* post-natal growth retardation, *SGA* small for gestational age, *VSD* ventricular septal defect, *BAD* bone age delayed
[a]the percentage in table stand for the mosaicism level

**Table 3** The clinical features of segment UPD(7q) mat

| | Hannula et al. | Reboul et al. | Eggermann et al. | Eggermann et al. | Begemann et al. | Total | Our patient |
|---|---|---|---|---|---|---|---|
| UPD region | D7S686 to qter | D7S2429 to qter | D7S663 to qter | D7S2429 to qter | chr7: 127,240,160-159,138,663 | *N* = 6 | chr7: 65,350,058-159,138,663 mos |
| Evaluation analysis | Microsatellite | Microsatellite | Microsatellite | Microsatellite | microsatellite | | Array, microsatellite |
| gender | F | M | F | M | F | 3F/2M | male |
| SGA | + | + | + | + | + | 5/5 | N |
| gestational age(weeks) | 37.5 | 27 | 3 weeks before term | 3 weeks before term | 39 | | term |
| birth weight(g) | 1510(−4.3SD) | 600 (−3.5 SD) | 2800 (−0.45SD) | 2180 (−2.28 SD) | 2410 (−2.74 SD) | | 1910 |
| length(cm) | 40 (−4.9SD) | N | 46 (−1.16 SD) | 45 (−1.97 SD) | 44 (−3.7 SD) | | N |
| head circumference | 47 (0.2SD) | N | N | 32 (−1.34 SD) | 32 (− 2.77 SD) | | N |
| age at evaluation(years) | 1.35 | 33 months | 5.3 | 1 4/12 | 3 2/12 | | 6 7/12 |
| weight(kg) | 6.95 | 9.4 (−3.5 SD) | N | 6.7 (−4.12 SD) | 10.5 (BMI: 14.36) | | 9.5 (~ − 6SD) |
| height (cm) | 71.5 (−2.9SD) | 82 (−3.5 SD) | 99.5 (−2.86SD) | 73 (−3.60 SD) | 85.5 (SD −3.09) | | 91.9 (~ − 6 SD) |
| feeding difficulties | − | − | + | − | + | 2/5 | − |
| relative macrocephaly | + | + | + | + | + | 5/5 | + |
| triangular face | + | + | + | + | + | 5/5 | + |
| protruding forehead | + | − | + | − | + | 3/5 | + |
| asymmetry | + | − | − | − | − | 1/5 | − |
| clinodactyly of the fifth fingers fingers/toes | + | − | − | + | + | 3/5 | fifth toe buckling |
| irregularly teeth | + | − | − | − | − | 1/5 | + |
| downturned mouth corners | + | − | − | + | − | 2/5 | − |
| ear anomalies | − | − | − | + | large prominent ears | 2/5 | − |
| development delay | − | − | − | + | + | 2/5 | − |
| other dysmorphic features | slender in appearance | − | − | single cafe'-au-lait spot | broad nasal bridge, ridge and tip, broad lips, retrognathia, epicanthal folds | | slender in appearance |

***F* female, *M* male, *N* not apply**

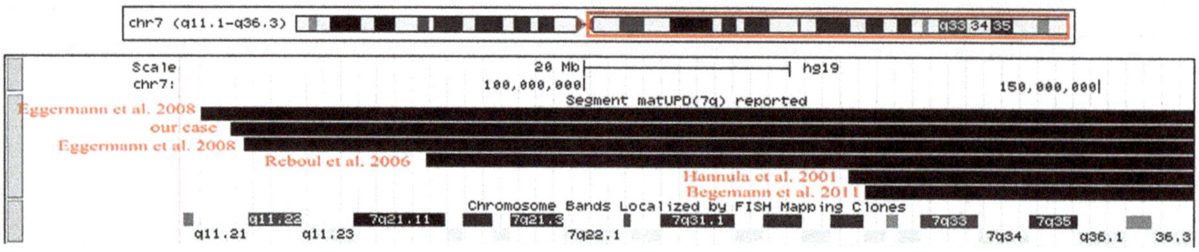


**Fig. 3** Schematic representation referred to segment mat UPD(7q) cases reported (UCSC genome browser custom track, hg19)

We detected and confirmed the mosaicism by both microsatellite and SNP array, the formulation to calculated the mosaic level proposed by Bliek et al. [29] by STR maker may be not accurate [30]. The pattern of B allele by SNP array offered an alternative and probable more accurate method for mosaic level assessment. Correlation between the level of mosaicism and SRS phenotype should be performed when more such cases are detected.

Complex and segmental UPD could resulting from either meiotic, mitotic, or meiotic and subsequent mitotic abnormal recombinations. Interestingly, apart from full upid(7)mat mosaicism which was likely result from mitotic non-disjunction and subsequent trisomy rescue, our case present the existence of normal cell line and UPD(7q11-qter) cell line, indicate the mosaicism may arise from somatic recombination [31, 32], further study would need to prove this hypothesis. Meanwhile, mosaicism could be tissue specific, but no more research for other tissue of our patient was performed because the father did not gave the consent.

## Conclusions

In summary, we described a second case with rare segmental maternal UPD(7q11-qter) mosaicism. This was the first report of UPD(7q11-qter) mosaicism detected by SNP array. Our case support the notion that there are genes control postnatal growth on long arm of chromosome 7 and indicate that ~ 80% of 7q11-qter mosaicism level was contributed to the SRS phenotype.

### Abbreviations

AF: Amniotic fluid; BL: Birth length; BW: Birth weight; CMA: Chromosome microarray analysis; IUGR: Intrauterine growth retardation; matUPD(7): Maternal uniparental disomy of chromosome 7; PNGR: Post-natal growth retardation; SD: Standard deviation; SGA: Small for gestational age; SNP: Single nucleotide polymorphisms; SRS: Silver-russell syndrome; UPD: Uniparental disomy

### Acknowledgments

We thank the family for their support and all authors work in this study.

### Funding

This work is supported by the project of science and technology of Guangxi Zhuang Autonomous Region (gui-ke-gong 14,124,004-1-8).

### Authors' contributions

Wrote the manuscript: JSS, YPS. Conceived and designed the experiments: XF, YPS. Performed the experiments: JSS, CYF and SJZ. XF, JSL, JW, TTJ were involved in SNP array analysis. CL and DHL helped to revise the manuscript. All authors read and approved the final manuscript.

### Competing interests

The authors declare that they have no competing interests.

### Author details

[1]Department of Genetic and Metabolic Central Laboratory, Guangxi Maternal and Child Health Hospital, Guangxi Birth Defects Prevention and Control Institute, No 59, Xiangzhu Road, Nanning, China. [2]Department of Laboratory Medicine, Boston Children's Hospital, Harvard Medical School, 300 Longwood Avenue, Boston, MA 02115, USA.

### Reference

1. Silver HK, et al. Syndrome of congenital hemihypertrophy, shortness of stature, and elevated urinary gonadotropins. Pediatrics. 1953;12(4):368–76.
2. Russell A. A syndrome of intra-uterine dwarfism recognizable at birth with cranio-facial dysostosis, disproportionately short arms, and other anomalies (5 examples). Proc R Soc Med. 1954;47(12):1040–4.
3. Azzi S, et al. A prospective study validating a clinical scoring system and demonstrating phenotypical-genotypical correlations in silver-Russell syndrome. J Med Genet. 2015;52(7):446–53.
4. Bartholdi D, et al. Epigenetic mutations of the imprinted IGF2-H19 domain in silver-Russell syndrome (SRS): results from a large cohort of patients with SRS and SRS-like phenotypes. J Med Genet. 2009;46(3):192–7.
5. Netchine I, et al. 11p15 imprinting center region 1 loss of methylation is a common and specific cause of typical Russell-silver syndrome: clinical scoring system and epigenetic-phenotypic correlations. J Clin Endocrinol Metab. 2007;92(8):3148–54.
6. Price SM, et al. The spectrum of silver-Russell syndrome: a clinical and molecular genetic study and new diagnostic criteria. J Med Genet. 1999;36(11):837–42.
7. Eggermann T, et al. Broad clinical spectrum in silver-Russell syndrome and consequences for genetic testing in growth retardation. Pediatrics. 2009;123(5):e929–31.
8. Spence JE, et al. Uniparental disomy as a mechanism for human genetic disease. Am J Hum Genet. 1988;42(2):217–26.
9. Preece MA, et al. An analysis of the distribution of hetero- and isodisomic regions of chromosome 7 in five mUPD7 silver-Russell syndrome probands. J Med Genet. 1999;36(6):457–60.
10. Eggerding FA, et al. Uniparental isodisomy for paternal 7p and maternal 7q in a child with growth retardation. Am J Hum Genet. 1994;55(2):253–65.
11. Riesewijk AM, et al. Monoallelic expression of human PEG1/MEST is paralleled by parent-specific methylation in fetuses. Genomics. 1997;42(2):236–44.
12. Blagitko N, et al. gamma2-COP, a novel imprinted gene on chromosome 7q32, defines a new imprinting cluster in the human genome. Hum Mol Genet. 1999;8(13):2387–96.

13. Yoshihashi H, et al. Imprinting of human GRB10 and its mutations in two patients with Russell-silver syndrome. Am J Hum Genet. 2000;67(2):476–82.
14. Reboul MP, et al. Mosaic maternal uniparental isodisomy for chromosome 7q21-qter. Clin Genet. 2006;70(3):207–13.
15. Ishida M. New developments in silver-Russell syndrome and implications for clinical practice. Epigenomics. 2016;8(4):563–80.
16. Wakeling EL, et al. Diagnosis and management of silver-Russell syndrome: first international consensus statement. Nat Rev Endocrinol. 2017;13(2):105–24.
17. Conlin LK, et al. Mechanisms of mosaicism, chimerism and uniparental disomy identified by single nucleotide polymorphism array analysis. Hum Mol Genet. 2010;19(7):1263–75.
18. Liehr T. Cases with uniparental disomy. 2017. http://upd-tl.com/upd.html. Accessed 10/10/2017.
19. Monk D, et al. Chromosome 7p disruptions in silver Russell syndrome: delineating an imprinted candidate gene region. Hum Genet. 2002;111(4-5):376–87.
20. Bilimoria KY, Rothenberg JM. Prenatal diagnosis of a trisomy 7/maternal uniparental heterodisomy 7 mosaic fetus. Am J Med Genet A. 2003;118A(1):60–3.
21. Miozzo M, et al. Post-zygotic origin of complete maternal chromosome 7 isodisomy and consequent loss of placental PEG1/MEST expression. Placenta. 2001;22(10):813–21.
22. Flori E, et al. Trisomy 7 mosaicism, maternal uniparental heterodisomy 7 and Hirschsprung's disease in a child with silver-Russell syndrome. Eur J Hum Genet. 2005;13(9):1013–8.
23. Fuke-Sato T, et al. Mosaic upd(7)mat in a patient with silver-Russell syndrome. Am J Med Genet A. 2012;158A(2):465–8.
24. Hannula K, et al. A narrow segment of maternal uniparental disomy of chromosome 7q31-qter in silver-Russell syndrome delimits a candidate gene region. Am J Hum Genet. 2001;68(1):247–53.
25. Eggermann T, et al. Segmental maternal UPD(7q) in silver-Russell syndrome Clin Genet. 2008;74(5):486–9.
26. Begemann M, et al. Segmental maternal uniparental disomy 7q associated with DLK1/GTL2 (14q32) hypomethylation. Am J Med Genet A. 2012; 158A(2):423–8.
27. Monk D, et al. Duplication of 7p11.2-p13, including GRB10, in silver-Russell syndrome. Am J Hum Genet. 2000;66(1):36–46.
28. Joyce CA, et al. Duplication of 7p12.1-p13, including GRB10 and IGFBP1, in a mother and daughter with features of silver-Russell syndrome. Hum Genet. 1999;105(3):273–80.
29. Bliek J, et al. Increased tumour risk for BWS patients correlates with aberrant H19 and not KCNQ1OT1 methylation: occurrence of KCNQ1OT1 hypomethylation in familial cases of BWS. Hum Mol Genet. 2001;10(5):467–76.
30. Russo S, et al. A fluorescent method for detecting low-grade 11patUPD mosaicism in Beckwith-Wiedemann syndrome. Mol Cell Probes. 2003;17(6):295–9.
31. Kotzot D. Complex and segmental uniparental disomy (UPD): review and lessons from rare chromosomal complements. J Med Genet. 2001;38(8):497–507
32. Chantot-Bastaraud S, et al. Formation of upd(7)mat by trisomic rescue: SNP array typing provides new insights in chromosomal nondisjunction. Mol Cytogenet. 2017;10:28.
33. Li H, et al. Height and weight standardized growth charts for Chinese children and adolescents aged 0 to 18 years. Zhonghua Er Ke Za Zhi. 2009; 47(7):487–92.
34 Kotzot D. Maternal uniparental disomy 7 and silver-Russell syndrome - clinical update and comparison with other subgroups. Eur J Med Genet. 2008;51(5):444–51.
35 Hannula K, et al. Do patients with maternal uniparental disomy for chromosome 7 have a distinct mild silver-Russell phenotype? J Med Genet. 2001;38(4):273–8.
36 Fuke T, et al. Molecular and clinical studies in 138 Japanese patients with silver-Russell syndrome. PLoS One. 2013;8(3):e60105.

# 13

# Prenatal diagnosis of 1p34.3 interstitial microdeletion by aCGH in a fetus with jaw bone abnormalities

Themistoklis Dagklis[3,4], Elena Papageorgiou[1,2], Elisavet Siomou[1,2], Vassilis Paspaliaris[1,2], Christina Zerva[4], Panagiotis Chatzis[5], Loretta Thomaidis[6], Emmanouil Manolakos[1,2,6,7*] and Ioannis Papoulidis[1]

**Abstract**

**Background:** Interstitial microdeletions in 1p are extremely rare, as very few cases have been reported postnatally and only one prenatally, yet. There is a variability of phenotypic findings such as hypotonia, facial dysmorphisms, mild microcephaly, with being most common developmental delay.

**Case presentation:** The present case involved a female fetus with an interstitial deletion on 1p, presenting with micrognathia in the 2nd trimester routine ultrasound examination. Array-based comparative genomic hybridization (a-CGH) revealed a 2,7 Mb deletion located on 1p34.3 which could not be detected by standard karyotyping.

**Conclusions:** This is the first prenatal case of an interstitial deletion in 1p34.3 with facial dysmorphism detected by a-CGH. Due to the use of a-CGH techniques submicroscopic imbalances could be detected, and a refined genotype-phenotype correlation could be achieved.

**Keywords:** Array-based Comparative Genomic Hybridization array (a-CGH), Chromosome 1, Genotype-phenotype correlation, Microdeletions, Prenatal diagnosis

## Background

Array-based comparative genomic hybridization (array CGH) is a powerful method that allows the detection of submicroscopic alterations in human genome and thus identifies underlying genetic causes that may contribute to various phenotypic abnormalities. On the short arm of chromosome 1, a subtelomeric microdeletion on 1p36 has been well established [1], but interstitial microdeletions in chromosome 1p have rarely been reported. Likewise, some efforts have been made to correlate submicroscopic deletions in 1p34 with a phenotype and such deletions have been associated with dysmorphic features and severe developmental delay [2, 3].

Furthermore, specific genes of this chromosomal region have been associated with distinct phenotypic malformations. More precisely, *GLUT1* deficiency may cause a specific syndrome which correlates with hyperactivity and developmental delay [3, 4], *RIMS3* is considered to be a novel candidate for autism [5], *GRIK3* has also been associated with developmental delay [6], and *AGO1/AGO3* may be responsible for neurocognitive deficits [7]. Furthermore, the chromosomal region 1p34 has been characterized as a tumor suppressor gene locus suggesting a role in cancer development [8].

Until today, there is only 1 case reported in the literature with an interstitial deletion of 1p that was diagnosed prenatally. The deletion spanned the region 1p36.11 to 1p34.3 and was detected by banding cytogenetic method and fluorescence in situ hybridization (FISH) [9]. Here, we report a 2.7 Mb *de novo* interstitial deletion within chromosomal subband 1p34.3, which was diagnosed prenatally in a fetus with micrognathia.

## Case presentation

At 22 weeks of gestation a 34-year-old pregnant female was referred to our lab for prenatal genetic

* Correspondence: manolakos@atg-labs.gr
[1]Access To Genome - ATG P.C, Clinical Laboratory Genetics, 33A Ethn. Antistaseos str, 55134 Thessaloniki, Greece
[2]Access To Genome - ATG P.C, Clinical Laboratory Genetics, 8 Sisini str, 11528 Athens, Greece
Full list of author information is available at the end of the article

**Table 1** Autopsy observations of the embryo and the placenta

| *Embryo* | *Placenta* |
|---|---|
| • Cleft palate<br>• Craniofacial malformations (severe posterior micrognathia, microtia)<br>• Narrow trunk with 11 pairs of thoracic and 1 pair of nuchal sides<br>• Abnormal position of fingers<br>• Talipes varus<br>• Knee flexion<br>• Dilatation of fourth ventricle<br>• Malformation of mitral valve | • Underweight placenta with increased fetus-placenta ratio<br>• Mitral decidual arteriopathy<br>• Low-grade acute chorioamniotis maternally derived, without any inflammatory reaction observed in the fetus |

testing after amniocentesis due to the presence of micrognathia detected at the routine 2nd trimester ultrasound examination. The prospective parents were healthy and of Greek origin. This was their first pregnancy and they had no previous medical history. The molecular cytogenetic analysis (see below) revealed a deletion in 1p. Genetic counseling was offered to the couple. At the parents' request the pregnancy was terminated at 22 weeks of gestation. Subsequently, the female fetus was sent for an autopsy.

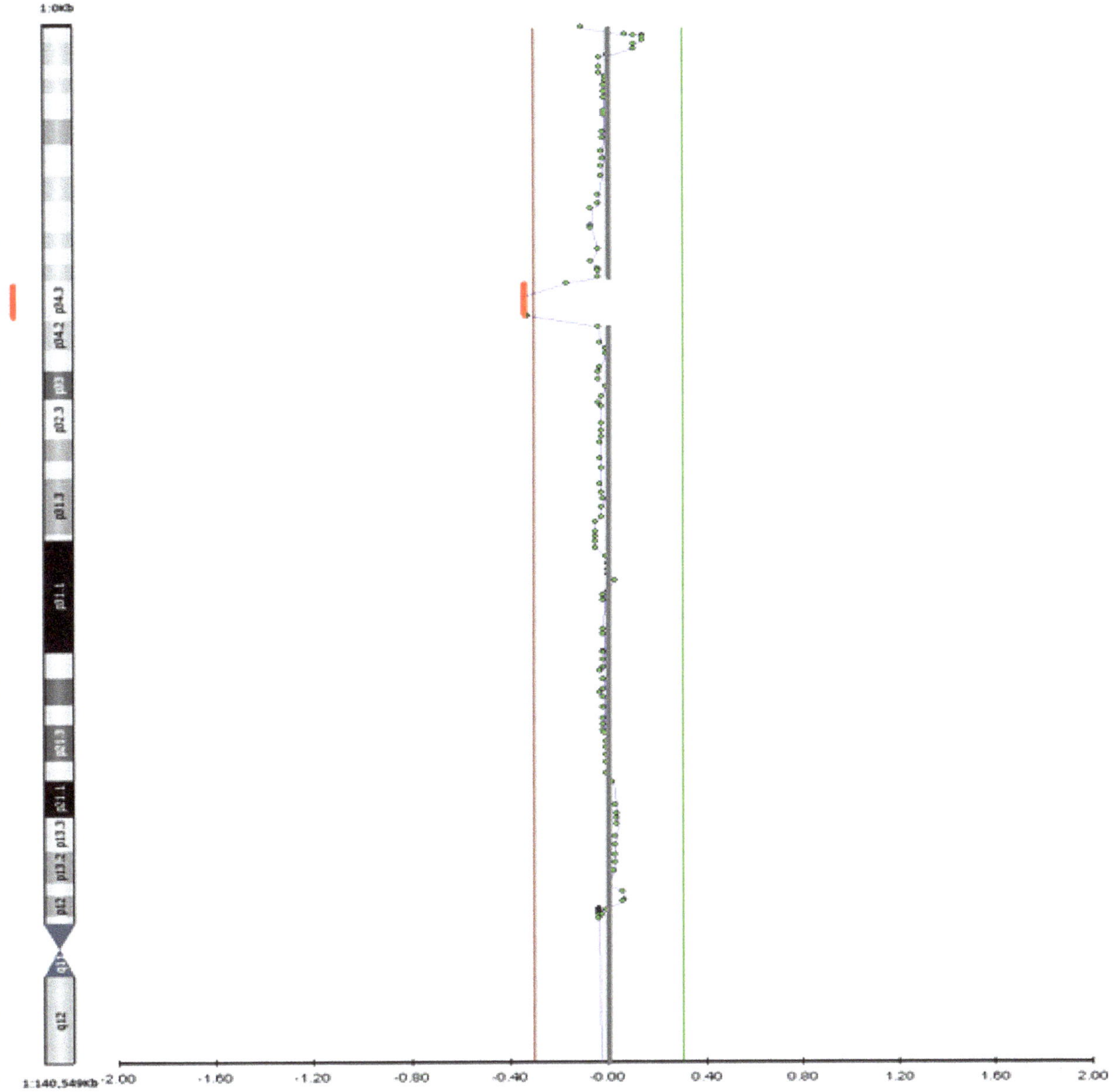


**Fig. 1** Array-CGH analysis illustrating in depth the *de novo* interstitial microdeletion of approximately 2,7 Mb in size on the short arm of chromosome 1 at chromosomal band 1p34.3 (location: 36,901,642 – 39,606,756 using build GRCh37 (hg19))

### Fetal autopsy

The fetus was of normal growth according to the weeks of gestation (~21/40) weighing 438 g without essential autolytic changes of intrauterine death. The autopsy's observations are shown in Table 1.

The mitral decidual arteriopathy observed in the placenta indicated pathological implantation, which possibly caused uteroplacental insufficiency and relevant gestational complications uteroplacental ischemia. In the present case, however it is possible that the decidual arteriopathy and the underweight placenta just reflect the pathological implantation and the abnormal placentation of a genetically pathological fetus.

### Molecular cytogenetic analysis

Molecular karyotype analysis by array CGH using "Illumina Cytochip Focus Constitutional array with BAC technology" was performed on DNA isolated from uncultured amniocytes according to the manufacturer's protocol. The Illumina Cytochip Focus Constitutional array is a commercially available whole-genome BAC array with a median resolution of 0.5–1 Mb. (Cytochip Focus Constitutional, Illumina).

The parent's blood derived DNA samples were prepared from peripheral blood leukocytes (Promega, Madison, WI, USA). Array data was analyzed using Bluefuse software analysis (BlueGnome Ltd., UK) using GRCh37/hg19 UCSC assembly and compared to known duplication listed in public available databases [Database of Genomic Variants (DGV, http://projects.tcag.ca/variation/webcite), ENSEMBL (http://www.ensembl.orgwebcite), and DECIPHER (http://decipher.sanger.ac.ukwebcite) Accessed at 25/01/2015].

A female profile was revealed with a 2,7 Mb deletion at chromosome 1p34.3 extending from position 36,901,642 to 39,606,756 (GRCh37/hg19 Feb.2009) (Fig. 1). No other copy number variant was detected at the referred sample. Using the UCSC Genome Browser and the OMIM database we observed that the deleted region contains 27 OMIM genes, listed in Table 2. Parental blood testing with a-CGH method revealed that the deletion occured *de novo.*

**Table 2** OMIM genes included in the deleted region

| Gene symbol | OMIM number |
|---|---|
| *OSCP1* | 608854 |
| *MRPS15* | 611979 |
| *CSF3R* | 138971 |
| *GRIK3* | 138243 |
| *ZC3H12A* | 610562 |
| *MEAF6* | 611001 |
| *SNIP1* | 608241 |
| *DNALI1* | 602135 |
| *GNL2* | 609365 |
| *RSPO1* | 609595 |
| *C1orf109* | 614799 |
| *CDCA8* | 609977 |
| *EPHA10* | 611123 |
| *YRDC* | 612276 |
| *MTF1* | 600172 |
| *INPP5B* | 147264 |
| *SF3A3* | 605596 |
| *FHL3* | 602790 |
| *UTP11L* | 609440 |
| *POU3F1* | 602479 |
| *RRAGC* | 608267 |
| *MYCBP* | 606535 |
| *GJA9* | 611923 |
| *RHBDL2* | 608962 |
| *AKIRIN1* | 615164 |
| *NDUFS5* | 603847 |
| *MACF1* | 608271 |

## Discussion

We report a prenatal case, which involves an interstitial microdeletion within chromosome 1p34.3. Most of the cases that have been reported with similar deletions are postnatal and only 1 is a prenatal report [9]. There is no specific phenotype or known syndrome that has been associated to this kind of deletion. To our knowledge there are only about 8 comparable patients, and in most cases the detected rearrangement was de novo as in our case. These patients showed a variability of phenotypic findings with developmental delay to be apparently present in almost all of them (Table 3).

Takenounci et al. [6] reported about a young girl, showing severe developmental delay, mild retrognathia and slightly downslanting papebral fissures. The deleted chromosomal regions in this proband and in the present case encompass the *GRIK3* gene which was suggested to be responsible for neurodevelopmental manifestations by Takenounci et al. [6].

Another gene that might contribute to craniofacial malformation and it is haploinsufficient in this case is *SNIP1*. Puffenberger et al. [10] identified a homozygous 1097A-G transition in the *SNIP1* gene in 3 Amish patients with severe craniofacial dysmorphism. Western blot analysis showed decreased levels of the mutant homologous murine protein, suggesting that it is unstable. Puffenberger et al. [10] postulated that decreased abundance of SNIP1 likely affects c-Myc activity, TGF-beta, and NF-kappa-B signaling, as

**Table 3** Overview of patients with 1p34.3 deletion. NM: Not Mentioned

| | Tokita et al. [7] proband 1 | Tokita et al. [7] proband 2 | Tokita et al. [7] proband 3 | Tokita et al. [7] proband 4 | Tokita et al. [7] proband 5 | Martinez et al. [2] proband 1 | Martinez et al. [2] proband 2 | Takenouchi et al. [6] |
|---|---|---|---|---|---|---|---|---|
| Gender | F | F | F | M | M | M | F | F |
| Delivery age (weeks) | 38 | 37 | 42 | 41 | 38 | NM | NM | 37 |
| Pregnancy and delivery | Uncomplicated | Uncomplicated | Uncomplicated | IUGR, neonatal sepsis | IUGR, perinatal asphyxia | NM | NM | Uncomplicated |
| Feeding difficulties | No | Yes | Yes | Yes | Yes | No | No | Yes |
| Age | 3y 9 m | 10y 6 m | 18y | 17 m | 13y | 13y | 8y | 8y |
| Height (percentile) | 24th | 25th | 50th | <1st | 90th-97th | 50th | 50th | NM |
| Weight (percentile) | 15th | 2nd | 5th | 1st | >97th | 50th | 50th | NM |
| OFC (percentile) | 3rd-10th | 25th | <<3rd | <1st | 2nd-10th | 50th | 50th | NM |
| Developmental delay | Yes | Yes | Yes | Yes | Yes | No | No | Yes |
| Facial deformities | Yes | Yes | Yes | Yes | Yes | Yes | No | No |
| Hypotonia | Yes | Yes | Yes | Yes | Yes | No | No | No |

SNIP1 protein interacts with these pathways [11–13], and this effect may cause abnormal brain and skull development.

Recent data from Tokita et al. [7] describe five children with microdeletions on 1p34.3 that showed, apart from hypotonia and developmental delay, craniofacial dysmorphisms such as retrognathia and small ears, as well feet and fingers malformations. The deletion that we report here overlaps with 4 deleted chromosomal loci, except a region between 38,622,840–39,141,084 (Fig. 2). In this region there is the 5' end of *MACF1* gene (chr1:39,084,166–39,487,137). MACF1 protein was found to be greatly up-regulated upon differentiation of myoblasts into myotubes [14], while Kodama et al. [15] showed that mouse *MACF1* (or *Acf7*) is an essential integrator of microtubule-actin dynamics. In the absence of MACF1 the consequences were long, less stable microtubules with skewed cytoplasmic trajectories and altered dynamic instability [15]. Taking these into account it might be explained the fact that the present case exhibited dilatation of fourth ventricle and malformation of mitral valve, while none of the cases of Table 3 presented any heart defect.

The fetal autopsy also showed pathological implantation of the fetus, and a possible explanation is that the placenta exhibited abnormal extracellular matrix. Ephrins are membrane-bound proteins that interact with Eph receptors, and have a crucial role in many developmental processes like guidance of neuron axon growth cones, cell migration and formation of tissue boundaries [16]. In the present case, 1 Eph receptor, *EPHA10*, is haploinsufficient, and is possibly 1 of the causes of improper implantation of the fetus, due to abnormal interaction of placental and uterus tissue boundaries.

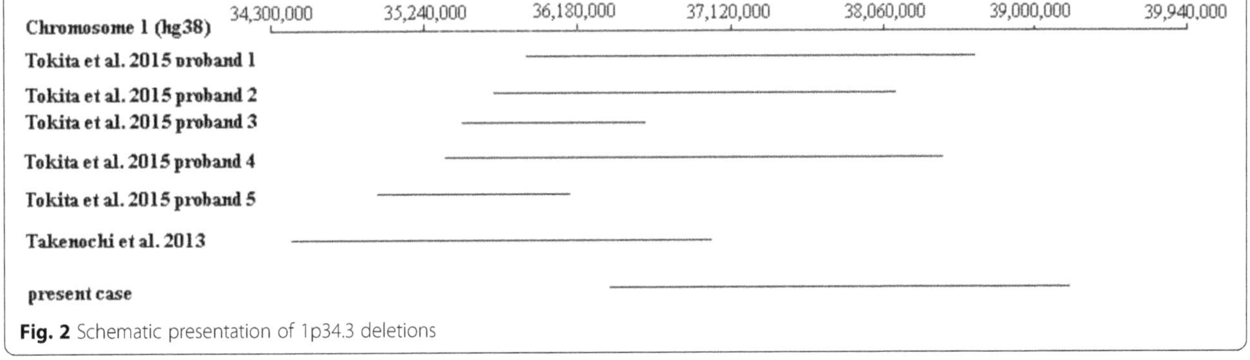


**Fig. 2** Schematic presentation of 1p34.3 deletions

## Conclusion

Array-based comparative genomic hybridization has been placed in the routine prenatal genetic testing and novel microscopic imbalances through the genome come to light. The comparison with similar findings in other patients is still not possible in most of the cases, but collecting data from such cases is crucial for genetic counselors to interpret prenatal cases, and achieve more accurate reports about clinical manifestations.

### Abbreviations

aCGH: Array comparative genomic hybridization; OFC: Orbito-frontal cortex

### Acknowledgments

The authors would like to thank the prospective parents for their collaboration.

### Funding

The whole study was funded by the private company Access to Genome, Clinical Laboratory Genetics, 33A Ethn. Antistaseos str, 55134 Thessaloniki, Greece.

### Authors' contribution

EP and CS wrote the manuscript; TD, CZ, PC, and LT coordinated the clinical analysis of the patient; ES and VP performed the cytogenetic analysis; IP signed out the molecular cytogenetic results; TD, EM, IP coordinated the study; All authors have read and approved the manuscript.

### Competing interests

The authors declare that they have no competing interests.

### Author details

[1]Access To Genome - ATG P.C, Clinical Laboratory Genetics, 33A Ethn. Antistaseos str, 55134 Thessaloniki, Greece. [2]Access To Genome - ATG P.C, Clinical Laboratory Genetics, 8 Sisini str, 11528 Athens, Greece. [3]3rd Department of Obstetrics and Gynecology, Aristotle University of Thessaloniki, Hippokration Hospital, Thessaloniki, Greece. [4]Embryomitriki, Prenatal Diagnostic Center, Thessaloniki, Greece. [5]2nd Department of Obstetrics and Gynecology, Aristotle University of Thessaloniki, Hippokration Hospital, Thessaloniki, Greece. [6]Developmental assessment unit, 2nd department of pediatrics, P. & A. Kyriakou children's hospital, School of medicine, National and Kapodistrian University of Athens, Athens, Greece. [7]Department of Medical Genetics, University of Cagliari, Binaghi Hospital, Cagliari, Italy.

### References

1. Shimada S, Shimojima K, Okamoto N, Sangu N, Hirasawa K, Matsuo M, Ikeuchi M, Shimakawa S, Shimizu K, Mizuno S, Kubota M, Adachi M, Saito Y, Tomiwa K, Haginoya K, Numabe H, Kako Y, Hayashi A, Sakamoto H, Hiraki Y, Minami K, Takemoto K, Watanabe K, Miura K, Chiyonobu T, Kumada T, Imai K, Maegaki Y, Nagata S, Kosaki K, Izumi T, Nagai T, Yamamoto T. Microarray analysis of 50 patients reveals the critical chromosomal regions responsible for 1p36 deletion syndrome-related complications. Brain Dev. 2015;37:515–26.
2. Martinez JE, Tuck-Muller CM, Gasparrini W, Li S, Wertelecki W. 1p microdeletion in sibs with minimal phenotypic manifestations. Am J Med Genet. 1999;15:107–9.
3. Vermeer S, Koolen DA, Visser G, Brackel HJ, van der Burgt I, de Leeuw N, Willemsen MA, Sistermans EA, Pfundt R, de Vries BB. A novel microdeletion in 1(p34.2p34.3), involving the SLC2A1 (GLUT1) gene, and severe delayed development. Dev Med Child Neurol. 2007;49:380–4.
4. Aktas D, Utine EG, Mrasek K, Weise A, von Eggeling F, Yalaz K, Posorski N, Akarsu N, Alikasifoglu M, Liehr T, Tuncbilek E. Derivative chromosome 1 and GLUT1 deficiency syndrome in a sibling pair. Mol Cytogenet. 2010;3(1):10. doi:10.1186/1755-8166-3-10.
5. Kumar RA, Sudi J, Babatz TD, Brune CW, Oswald D, Yen M, Nowak NJ, Cook EH, Christian SL, Dobyns WB. A de novo 1p34.2 microdeletion identifies the synaptic vesicle gene RIMS3 as a novel candidate for autism. J Med Genet. 2010;47:81–90.
6. Takenouchi T, Hashida N, Torii C, Kosaki R, Takahashi T, Kosaki K. 1p34.3 deletion involving GRIK3: Further clinical implication of GRIK family glutamate receptors in the pathogenesis of developmental delay. Am J Med Genet A. 2014;164A:456–60.
7. Tokita MJ, Chow PM, Mirzaa G, Dikow N, Maas B, Isidor B, Le Caignec C, Penney LS, Mazzotta G, Bernardini L, Filippi T, Battaglia A, Donti E, Earl D, Prontera P. Five children with deletions of 1p34.3 encompassing AGO1 and AGO3. Eur J Hum Genet. 2015;23:761–5.
8. Sulman EP, White PS, Brodeur GM. Genomic annotation of the meningioma tumor suppressor locus on chromosome 1p34. Oncogene. 2004;23:1014–20.
9. Yang H, Lee CL, Young DC, Shortliffe M, Yu W, Wright JR. A rare case of interstitial del(1)(p34.3p36.11) diagnosed prenatally. Fetal Pediatr Pathol. 2004;23:251–5.
10. Puffenberger EG, Jinks RN, Sougnez C, Cibulskis K, Willert RA, Achilly NP, Cassidy RP, Fiorentini CJ, Heiken KF, Lawrence JJ, Mahoney MH, Miller CJ, et al. Genetic mapping and exome sequencing identify variants associated with five novel diseases. PLoS ONE. 2012;7(1):e28936.
11. Fujii M, Lyakh LA, Bracken CP, Fukuoka J, Hayakawa M, Tsukiyama T, Soll SJ, Harris M, Rocha S, Roche KC, Tominaga S, Jen J, Perkins ND, Lechleider RJ, Roberts AB. SNIP1 is a candidate modifier of the transcriptional activity of c-Myc on E box-dependent target genes. Molec Cell. 2006;24:771–83.
12. Kim RH, Flanders KC, Reffey SB, Anderson LA, Duckett CS, Perkins ND, Roberts AB. SNIP1 inhibits NF-kappa-B signaling by competing for its binding to the C/H1 domain of CBP/p300 transcriptional co-activators. J Biol Chem. 2001;276:46297–304.
13. Kim RH, Wang D, Tsang M, Martin J, Huff C, de Caestecker MP, Parks WT, Meng X, Lechleider RJ, Wang T, Roberts AB. A novel Smad nuclear interacting protein, SNIP1, suppresses p300-dependent TGF-beta signal transduction. Genes Dev. 2000;14:1605–16.
14. Sun Y, Zhang J, Kraeft SK, Auclair D, Chang MS, Liu Y, Sutherland R, Salgia R, Griffin JD, Ferland LH, Chen LB. Molecular cloning and characterization of human trabeculin-alpha, a giant protein defining a new family of actin-binding proteins. J Biol Chem. 1999;274:33522–30.
15. Kodama A, Karakesisoglou I, Wong E, Vaezi A, Fuchs E. ACF7: an essential integrator of microtubule dynamics. Cell. 2003;115:343–54.
16. Davy A, Soriano P. Ephrin signaling in vivo: look both ways. Dev Dyn. 2005; 232:1–10.

# 14

# Partial monosomy14q involving *FOXG1* and *NOVA1* in an infant with microcephaly, seizures and severe developmental delay

H. Fryssira[1], E. Tsoutsou[1], S. Psoni[1], S. Amenta[2], T. Liehr[6], E. Anastasakis[7], Ch Skentou[5], A. Ntouflia[3], I. Papoulidis[3], E. Manolakos[3,8*] and N. Chaliasos[4]

**Abstract**

**Background:** *FOXG1* gene mutations have been associated with the congenital variant of Rett syndrome (RTT) since the initial description of two patients in 2008. The on-going accumulation of clinical data suggests that the FOXG1-variant of RTT forms a distinguishable phenotype, consisting mainly of postnatal microcephaly, seizures, hypotonia, developmental delay and corpus callosum agenesis.

**Case presentation:** We report a 6-month-old female infant, born at 38 weeks of gestation after in vitro fertilization, who presented with feeding difficulties, irritability and developmental delay from the first months of life. Microcephaly with bitemporal narrowing, dyspraxia, poor eye contact and strabismus were also noted. At 10 months, the proband exhibited focal seizures and required valproic acid treatment. Array-Comparative Genomic Hybridization revealed a 4.09 Mb deletion in 14q12 region, encompassing the *FOXG1* and *NOVA1* genes. The proband presented similar feature with patients with 14q12 deletions except for dysgenesis of corpus callosum. Disruption of the *NOVA1* gene which promotes the motor neurons apoptosis has not yet been linked to any human phenotypes and it is uncertain if it affects our patient's phenotype.

**Conclusions:** Since our patient is the first reported case with deletion of both genes (*FOXG1-NOVA1*), thorough clinical follow up would further delineate the Congenital Rett-Variant phenotypes.

**Keywords:** FOXG1 syndrome, Rett syndrome, *NOVA1*, Array-CGH, Postnatal microcephaly, Seizures

## Background

Since 2008, when mutations in the *FOXG1* gene were initially described in two patients with Rett-like symptoms, more than 90 patients have been reported to have mutations involving the *FOXG1* gene [1–6]. Rett syndrome is typically an X-linked neurodegenerative condition [6] that was initially described by Andreas Rett in 1966. Common clinical features of Rett syndrome include postnatal microcephaly, autism, seizures, breathing abnormalities, growth retardation and gait apraxia [7, 8]. The majority of patients with typical Rett syndrome carry mutations in the gene encoding Methyl-CpG-binding protein 2 (*MECP2*) located at Xq28. Variant forms of Rett syndrome have been revised in 2010 by Neul et al [7]. He classified them in to three main variant categories: 1. Preserved speech, 2. early seizures and, 3. the congenital variant. Mutations in the cyclin-dependent kinase-like 5 (*CDKL5*) gene located in Xp22 are found in most cases of early-onset seizure variants, while the congenital variant of the syndrome has recently been found to be associated with heterozygous mutations or deletions in the forkhead box protein G1 (*FOXG1*) gene, located in the 14q12 chromosomal region [7, 9–11]. In this study, we report a new case of atypical Rett Syndrome with a 14q12 deletion, 4.09 Mb in size, encompassing only two genes, the *FOXG1* and the *NOVA1* and we discuss the role of the *NOVA1* haploinsufficiency.

* Correspondence: manolakos@atg-labs.gr
[3]"Access to Genome" Clinical Laboratory Genetics, Athens Thessaloniki, Greece
[8]Department of Medical Genetics, Binaghi Hospital, University of Cagliari, Cagliari, Italy
Full list of author information is available at the end of the article

## Case presentation

Our patient was a 6-month- old female infant and the only child of non-consanguineous parents. She was born by caesarean section at 38 weeks of gestation. Her birth weight was 2.990 gr ($25^{th}$ -$50^{th}$ centile), her length was 49 cm ($25^{th}$ -$50^{th}$ centile) and her head circumference was 33 cm (10–25th centile).

It should be noted that the embryo was the product of in vitro fertilization (IVF) by intracytoplasmic sperm injection (ICSI) due to the husband's low sperm count. The mother underwent treatment with Follitropin Beta (Puregon), human Chorionic Gonadotropin, hCG (Pregnyl), and Cetrorelix Acetate (Cetrotide).

The patient as a neonate was hypotonic. She was referred for clinical evaluation at the age of 6 months due to irritability and feeding difficulties. The examinations revealed peripheral hypertonia, psychomotor retardation (limited facial expression—no smile, poor eye contact), borderline microcephaly (head circumference of 39 cm, at $3^{rd}$ centile) (Fig. 1a), periodical stereotypic movements and minor dysmorphic features such as a small forehead with bitemporal narrowing, strabismus, broad base to nose and long philtrum. Her weight was 6.18 kg (25th centile) and her height was 62 cm (25th centile).

Due to gastroesophageal reflux she was treated with ranitidine.

Haematological, biochemical, metabolic, thyroid, ammonia and blood gasses were all normal. The ultrasounds of the heart and abdomen were also normal.

At 10 months the proband exhibited focal seizures and required valproic acid treatment. Sleep deprived EEG examination revealed slower focal activity for her age and sleep spindles which are indicative signs of focal cerebral dysfunction. Brain magnetic resonance imaging (MRI) showed no serious findings except for a septum pellucidum cyst and brain asymmetry—the left hemisphere was larger than the right one.

At the age of 12 months, the head circumference was 40.7 cm (<< $3^{rd}$ centile) (Fig. 1a) while the height and

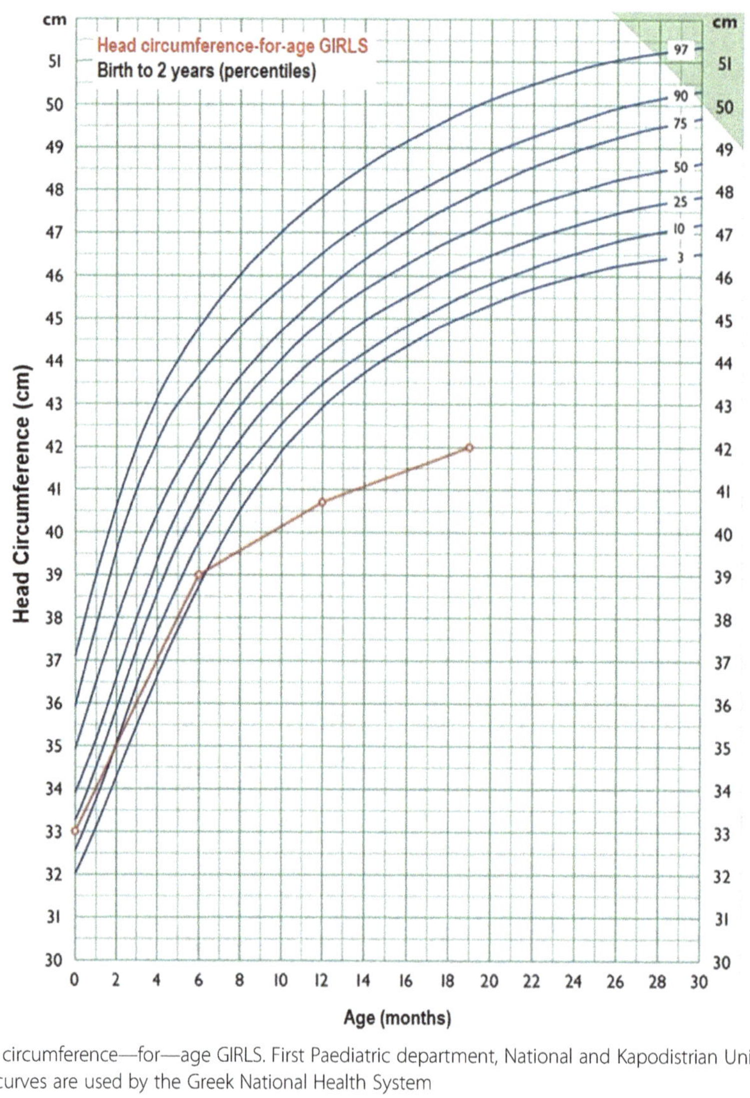


**Fig. 1** Growth curve "Head circumference—for—age GIRLS. First Paediatric department, National and Kapodistrian University of Athens. Professor G.Chroussos. The standard curves are used by the Greek National Health System

weight remained between 10th and 25th centile. Severe neurodevelopmental delay was obvious.

Re-examination at the age of 19- months and 2-years, revealed head circumference of 42 cm (<< 3rd centile) (Fig. 1a), height of 75.5 cm (slightly below the 3rd centile) and weight of 9 Kg (slightly below the 3rd centile). The proband exhibited severe psychomotor retardation as she could neither sit independently nor speak at all.

### Chromosome and array-based analysis

Metaphase chromosomes were obtained from phytohemagglutinin (PHA)-stimulated peripheral blood lymphocytes and high resolution (550–650 bands) thymidine treatment G-banding karyotype analysis was performed, using standard procedures. Twenty metaphase spreads were analysed, and the result was a normal female karyotype (46, XX). The molecular analysis of the *MECP2* gene was normal also.

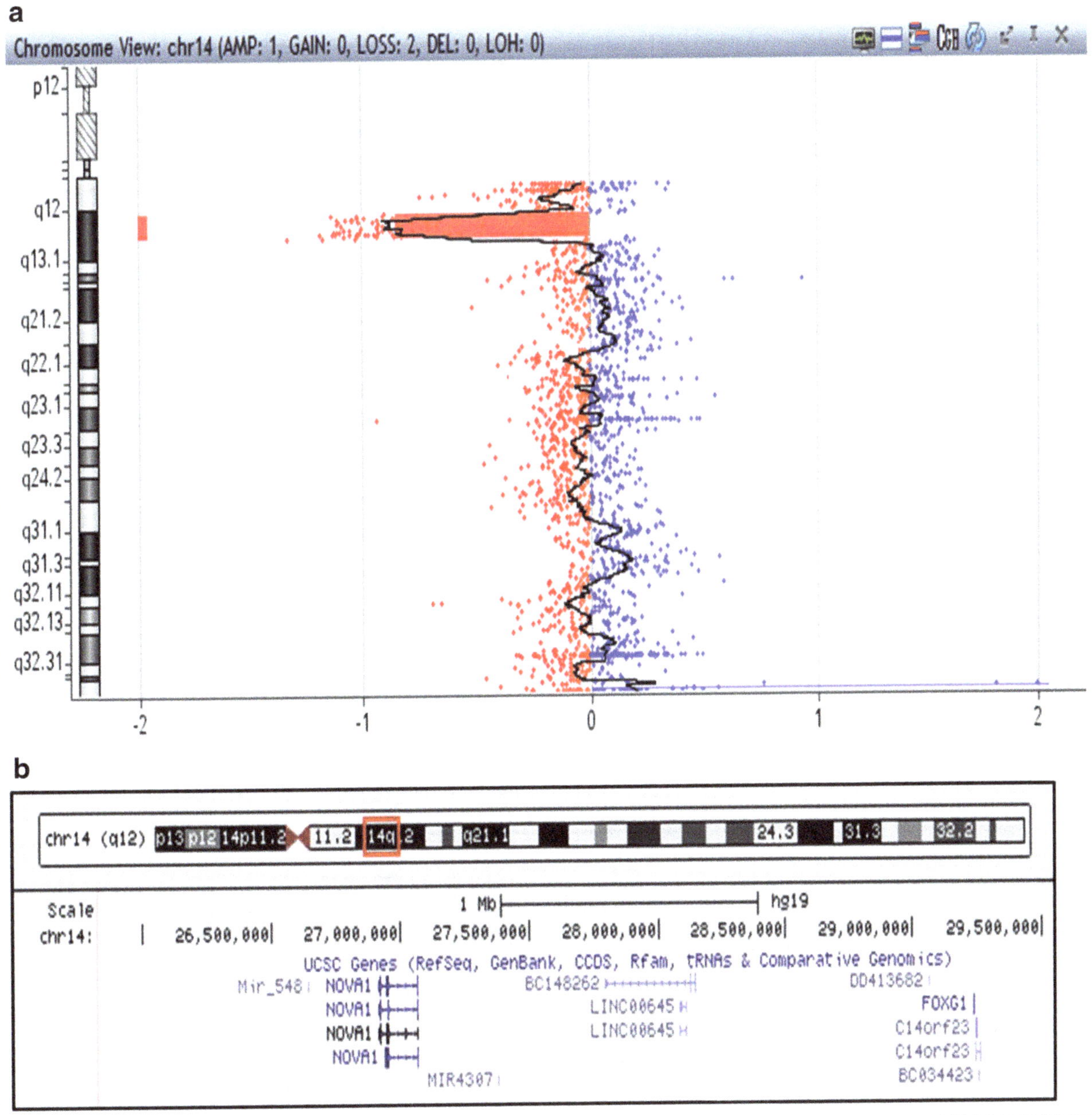


**Fig. 2** Array-CGH analysis detected a 4.09 Mb loss of the copy numbers in the spanning region 14q12. **b** Chromosome 14, region 25,843,560-29,938,629. Represents the 4,095,070 bp deletion described in our case report. The region includes both *FOXG1* and *NOVA1* genes. Figure adapted from http://genome.ucsc.edu/ Accessed at 18/10/2015

Further investigation with array-Comparative Genomic Hybridization was performed by hybridizing the sample against a male human reference commercial DNA sample (Promega biotech) using an array-CGH platform that includes 60,000 oligonucleotides distributed across the entire genome (Agilent Technologies). The statistical test used as parameter to estimate the number of copies was ADAM-2 (provided by the DNA analytics software, Agilent Techn.) with a window of 0.5 Mb, A = 6. Only those copy number changes that affect at least 5 consecutive probes with identically oriented change were considered as Copy Number Variations (CNV). For the majority of the genome, the average genomic power of resolution of this analysis was 200 kilobases. Array-CGH analysis detected a 4.09 Mb loss in the 14q12 region (Fig. 2a). The deleted segment was mapped at chr14:25,843,560-29,938,629 region. The genomic coordinates are listed according to genomic build GRCh37/hg19, and includes *FOXG1* and *NOVA1* genes (Fig. 2b).

The result of array-CGH was confirmed with FISH. Ten metaphases were analysed from phytohemagglutinin (PHA)-stimulated peripheral blood lymphocytes of the patient with RP11-120I18 in 14q12 and wcp 14 probes. The rearrangement was molecular cytogenetically unbalanced (data not shown), therefore the karyotype is: 46,XX, del[12](q12q12).ish14q12(RP11-120I18-). arr[hg19]14q12 (25,843,560-29,938,629)x1. Blood samples from both parents were examined with FISH in order to exclude any chromosome rearrangement like inversion. Ten metaphases were analysed from each subject with RP11-332 N6 in 14q11.2, RP11-120I18 in 14q12 and wcp 14 probes, and no rearrangement was detected (data not shown).

## Discussion

Recently, the *FOXG1* congenital variant of Rett syndrome has been described as a clinically identifiable phenotype, called the "*FOXG1* syndrome" [13]. This is an epileptic-dyskinetic developmental encephalopathy with features of classic Rett syndrome, but earlier onset from the first months of life. The main phenotype comprises postnatal microcephaly, severe developmental delay and lack of speech, hypotonia, dyskinesia and corpus callosum hypoplasia. Other symptoms include strabismus, feeding difficulties, bruxism and seizures [8, 12–16].

In the present study, a novel *FOXG1* and a *NOVA1* deletion is described. According to the diagnostic criteria for typical and atypical Rett syndrome [7], our patient possesses only some of the diagnostic criteria for the atypical Rett syndrome. She has slight facial dysmorphism, feeding difficulties, severe psychomotor retardation, postnatal microcephaly, seizures and focal cerebral dysfunction, strabismus and hypertonia. A deletion of 4.09 Mb on chromosome 14q12 including the *FOXG1* and *NOVA1* genes was identified by array-CGH technique. The clinical phenotypes vary between the reported cases that have mutations or deletions involving the *FOXG1* gene and other genes (Table 1, Fig. 3). Our case differs as only two genes, *FOXG1* and *NOVA1*, are involved. These genes were found to be highly expressed in the human brain throughout ontogeny, and double strand breaks in 14q12 region are implicated in the neurodegenerative disease: ataxia telangiectasia [17].

Different clinical features have also been described in patients with *FOXG1* point mutations. The severity or lack of the symptoms among cases could depend

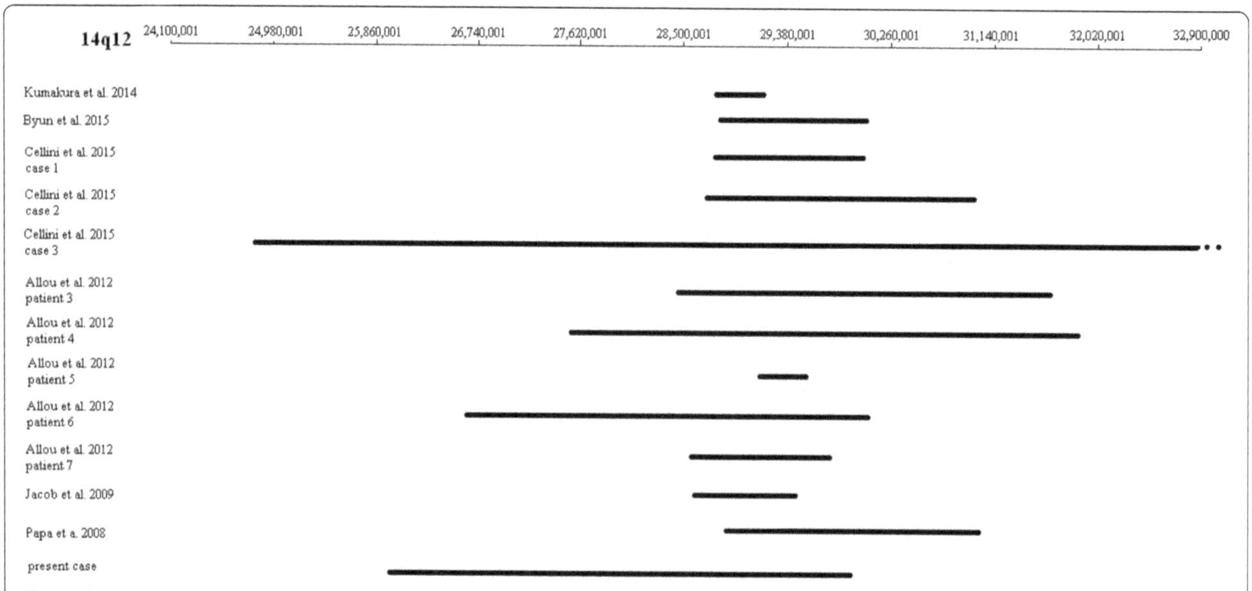


**Fig. 3** Ideogram of the deletions described in Table 1. The upper thin line indicates the 14q12 region (hg38), and the bold lines indicate the region which is deleted in each case. Cellini et al. 2015 case 3 has a deletion beyond 14q12 and is drawn with a discontinued line

**Table 1** Clinical presentation of patients with FOXG1 mutations and 14q12 deletions

| | *Kumakura* et al. *2014* | *Byun* et al. *2015* | *Patients (n = 8) Cellini* et al. *2015* | | | | | *Patients (n = 7) Allou* et al. *2012* | *Patients (n = 2) Philippe* et al. *2011* | *Jacob* et al. *2009* | *Yeung* et al. *2009* | *Patients (n = 2) Ariani* et al. *2008* | *Papa* et al. *2008* | *Present case* |
|---|---|---|---|---|---|---|---|---|---|---|---|---|---|---|
| | | | *1* | *2* | *3* | *4* | *4 cases with point mutations in FOXG1* | | | | | | | |
| Age (Y,M) | 8.0 | 8.0 | 9.0 | 3.6 | 2.0 | 10.0 | 2.6–17.0 | N/A | 22.0 and 10.0 | 3.0 | 9.0 | 22.0 and 7.0 | 7.0 | 0.6 |
| Sex | M | F | F | M | F | F | 3 F, 1 M | 4 F, 3 M | F | F | F | F | F | F |
| FOXG1 mutation on 14q12 CNV (Mb) | 0.54 Mb Del | 2.5 Mb Del | 2.5 Mb Del | 2.8 Mb Del | 9.1 Mb Del | 7.3 Mb Dup (de novo) | p.Gln100Serfs*92, p.Q46X, p.Glu154Glyfs*301, p.Gln86Argfs*106 (de novo) | 0.4–4.1 Mb | p.Trp308X and p.Tyr400X | 2.594 Mb Del | 4.45 Mb Dup | p.W255X and p.S323fsX325 | 3 Mb Del | 4,09 Del |
| Genes involved in mutation or point mutations | *FOXG1, C14orf23 (de novo)* | *FOXG1, C14orf23, PRKD1* (de novo) | *FOXG1, C14orf23, PRKD1* | *FOXG1, C14orf23, PRKD1, SCFD1, G2E3, COCH, STRN3* (de novo) | *STXBP6, NOVA1, FOXG1, C14orf23, PRKD1, SCFD1, G2E3, COCH, STRN3, AP4S1, HECTD1, DTD2, NUBPL, ARHGAP5, AKAP, NPAS3* (de novo) | *FOXG1 and 50 additional genes (de novo)* | *FOXG1* | *Deletions in 5 cases, 3 of them distal to FOXG1 and 2 cases of point mutations involving FOXG1* | *FOXG1* | *FOXG1, C14orf23* | *FOXG1, NOVA1, c14orf23, PRKD1, G2E3, SDFD, COCH* | *FOXG1* | *FOXG1, PRKD1, SCFD1, G2E3, COCH, STRN3* | *FOXG1, NOVA1* |
| Postnatal microcephaly | yes | yes | yes | yes | yes | no | yes | yes | yes | yes | no | yes | yes | yes |
| Psychomotor retardation | yes | yes | yes | yes | yes | yes | yes | yes | yes | yes | yes | yes | yes | yes |
| Hypotonia | yes | no | yes | yes | yes | yes | 2/4 cases hypotonic | All except 1 case | 1/2 cases | yes | yes | yes | yes | Hypertonia |
| Diskinesia | yes | yes | yes | yes | yes | yes | 3/4 cases diskinetic | 3/7 cases | yes | yes | yes | yes | yes | yes |
| Speech | no | no | no | no | no | no | no | no | no | no | no | no | no | no |
| Hand stereotypies | no | other sterotypies | yes | no | yes | yes | yes | 4/7 cases | yes | yes | hand flapping only | yes | yes | yes |
| Corpus callosum hypogenesis | yes | no | yes | yes | yes | no | 3/4 cases with hypoplasia | brain abnormalities in all cases | 1/2 cases | no, brachycephaly observed | no | yes | no | no |
| Seizures | yes | yes | yes | yes | yes | yes | yes | 5/7 cases | 1/2 cases | yes | yes | yes | yes | yes |
| Developmental delay | yes | yes | yes | yes | yes | yes | yes | 5/7 cases | 1/2 cases | yes | yes | yes | yes | yes |

***F*** **female, *M* male, *Y* years, *M* months, *Del* deletion, *Dup* duplication**

additionally on genetic and/or environmental factors [13]. Jacob F. et al. in 2009 [9] reported a case of a 2.594 Mb deletion involving the *FOXG1* and *C23orf14* (Table 1). As in our case, patient had a normal corpus callosum but showed all the typical characteristics found in patients with *FOXG1* alterations. Table 1 indicates that almost all cases suffer from microcephaly, dyskinesia, lack of speech, seizures and developmental delay. On the other hand, hypotonia and corpus callosum hypoplasia are not apparent in every case. Progressive hypertonia was obvious in our patient and in at least 10 other reported cases with *FOXG1* point mutations [8].

Forkhead BOX G1 *(FOXG1)* gene (OMIM*164874) encodes a developmental transcription factor with repressor activity, important for the development of the ventral telencephalon in the embryonic forebrain and crucial for the regulation of neurogenesis and neurite outgrowth. It is also expressed in neurogenetic regions of the postnatal brain [15]. Postnatal microcephaly is another common feature of FOXG1 syndrome. In cases with a duplication of the *FOXG1* gene, microcephaly is not found (Table 1), indicating that the phenotype is dependent on *FOXG1* dosage. Furthermore, other reported cases with deletions close but not disturbing the *FOXG1* gene have a similar phenotype as patients with "FOXG1 syndrome", suggesting that a position effect causing altered expression of *FOXG1* gene may be the cause. The protein Kinase D1 (*PRKD1)* gene (OMIM*605435), located close to *FOXG1* gene has been reported to be implicated in transcription and expression of *FOXG1* gene [14].

Neuro-Oncological Ventral Antigen 1 (*NOVA1)* gene (OMIM*602157) encodes a neuron-specific RNA-binding protein that is inhibited by paraneoplastic antibodies [18]. Recently, Storchel H et al., 2015 [19] found that NOVA1 protein converges on Ago proteins and controls miRNA-induced silencing complex (miRISC), possibly resulting on the regulation of neuronal development and synaptic plasticity. Despite the significant role of the *NOVA1* gene, it has not been linked to any human phenotype yet. In the case of our patient with FOXG1 syndrome, we are unable to estimate the impact of the *NOVA1* haploinsufficiency. *NOVA1* haploinsufficiency may act synergistically with the *FOXG1* gene or it may cause no difference in the final clinical outcome. Also, we cannot define whether the IVF by ICSI plays a role in the microdeletion of chromosome 14q12 region. Further research should investigate if ICSI could be associated with haploinsufficiency as was the case in our patient.

In conclusion, we present a female patient with clinical features compatible with the congenital variant of Rett syndrome.

## Conclusion

Since our patient is the only one with a deletion encompassing only *FOXG1* and *NOVA1* genes, in the future the thorough clinical follow-up of her neurological status will help for further delineation of the role of these genes.

#### Abbreviations

CGH, comparative genomic hybridization; EEG, electroencephalogram; ICSI, intracytoplasmic sperm injection; IVF, in vitro fertilization; MRI, magnetic resonance imaging; PHA, phytohemagglutinin; RTT, Rett syndrome

#### Acknowledgments

The authors would like to thank the members of the family of the patient for their collaboration.

#### Funding

The whole study was funded by the private company Access to Genome, Clinical Laboratory Genetics, 33A Ethn. Antistaseos str, 55134 Thessaloniki, Greece.

#### Authors' contributions

AN and CS wrote the manuscript; HF, ET, SP and SA coordinated the clinical analysis of the patient; EM performed the cytogenetic analysis; IP signed out the molecular cytogenetic results; EM, IP and NC coordinated the study; All authors have read and approved the manuscript.

#### Competing interests

The authors declare that they have no competing interests.

#### Author details

[1]Medical genetics, School of Medicine, National and Kapodistrian University of Athens, "Aghia Sophia" Children's Hospital, Athens, Greece. [2]"Mitera" Maternity Hospital, Athens, Greece. [3]"Access to Genome" Clinical Laboratory Genetics, Athens Thessaloniki, Greece. [4]Child Health Department, University Hospital of Ioannina (UHI), Ioannina, Greece. [5]"Mitera kai emvrio" Medical centre, Larisa, Greece. [6]Institute of Human Genetics, Jena University Hospital, Friedrich Schiller University, Jena, Germany. [7]Hellenic Navy Hospital, Deinokratous 70, Athens 11521, Greece. [8]Department of Medical Genetics, Binaghi Hospital, University of Cagliari, Cagliari, Italy.

#### References

1. Ariani F, Hayek G, Rondinella D, et al. FOXG1 is responsible for the congenital variant of Rett syndrome. Am J Hum Genet. 2008;83:89–93.
2. Takagi M, Sasaki G, Mitsui T, Honda M, Tanaka Y, Hasegawa T. A 2.0 Mb microdeletion in proximal chromosome 14q12, involving regulatory elements of FOXG1, with the coding region of FOXG1 being unaffected, results in severe developmental delay, microcephaly, and hypoplasia of the corpus callosum. Eur J Med Genet. 2013;56(9):526–8.
3. Perche O, Haddad G, Menuet A, Callier P, Marcos M, Briault S, Laudier B. Dysregulation of FOXG1 pathway in a 14q12 microdeletion case. Am J Med Genet. 2013;161A(12):3072–7.
4. Ellaway CJ, Ho G, Bettella E, Knapman A, Collins F, Hackett A, McKenzie F, Darmanian A, Peters GB, Fagan K, Christodoulou J. 14q12 microdeletions excluding FOXG1 give rise to a congenital variant Rett syndrome-like phenotype. Eur J Hum Genet. 2013;21(5):522–7.
5. Stenson PD, Mort M, Ball EV, Shaw K, Phillips A, Cooper DN. The Human Gene Mutation Database: building a comprehensive mutation repository for

clinical and molecular genetics, diagnositic testing and personalized genomic medicine. Hum Genet. 2014;133:1–9.

6. Kumakura A, Takahashi S, Okajima K, Hata D. A haploinsufficiency of *FOXG1* identified in a boy with congenital variant of Rett syndrome. Brain Dev. 2014;36(8):725–9.
7. Neul JL, Kaufmann WE, Glaze DG, et al. Rett Syndrome: revised diagnostic criteria and nomenclature. Ann Neurol. 2010;68:944–50.
8. Byun CK, Lee JS, Lim BC, Kim KJ, Hwang YS and Chae J. FOXG1 Mutation is a Low-Incidence Genetic Cause in Atypical Rett Syndrome. Child Neurology Open. 2015;8:1-5
9. Jacob F, Ramaswamy V, Andersen J, Bolduc F. Atypical Rett syndrome with selective FOXG1 deletion detected by comparative genomic hybridization: case report and review of literature. Eur J Hum Genet. 2009;17:1577–81.
10. Papa FT, Mencarelli MA, Caselli R, et al. A 3 Mb Deletion in 14q12 Causes Severe Mental Retardation, Mild Facial Dysmorphisms and Rett-like Features. Am J Med Genet. 2008;146:1994–8.
11. Pantaleón FG, Juvier RT. Molecular basis of Rett syndrome: A current look. Rev Chil Pediatr. 2015;86:142–51.
12. Allou L, Lambert L, Amsallem D, Bieth E, Edery P, Destree A, et al. 14q12 and severe Rett-like phenotypes: new clinical insights and physical mapping of FOXG1-regulatory elements. Eur J Hum Genet. 2012;20:1216–23.
13. Kortüm F, Das S, Flindt M, Morris-Rosendahl DJ, Stefanova I, Goldstein A, et al. The core FOXG1 syndrome phenotype consists of postnatal microcephaly, severe mental retardation, absent language, dyskinesia, and corpus callosum hypogenesis. J Med Genet. 2011;48:396–406.
14. Pratt DW, Warner JV, Williams MG. Genotyping FOXG1 mutations in patients with clinical evidence of the FOXG1 syndrome. Mol Syndromol. 2013;3(6): 284–7.
15. Florian C, Bahi-Buisson N, Bienvenu T. FOXG1-related disorders: from clinical description to molecular genetics. Mol Syndromol. 2012;2:153–63.
16. Cellini E, Vignoli A, Pisano T, et al. The hyperkinetic movement disorder of FOXG1-related epileptic-dyskinetic encephalopathy. Dev Med Child Neurol. 2016;58:93–7.
17. Iourov IY, Vorsanova SG, Liehr T, Kolotii AD, Yurov YB. Increased chromosome instability dramatically disrupts neural genome integrity and mediates cerebellar degeneration in the ataxia-telangiectasia brain. Hum Mol Genet. 2009;18:2656–69.
18. Buckanovich RJ, Yang YY, Darnell RB. The onconeural antigen Nova-1 is a neuron-specific RNA-binding protein, the activity of which is inhibited by paraneoplastic antibodies. J Neurosci. 1996;16:1114–22.
19. Störchel PH, Thümmler J, Siegel G, Aksoy-Aksel A, Zampa F, Sumer S, et al. A large-scale functional screen identifies Nova1 and Ncoa3 as regulators of neuronal miRNA function. EMBO J. 2015;34:2237–54.

# 15

# A high complex karyotype involving eleven chromosomes including three novel chromosomal aberrations and monoallelic loss of *TP53* in case of follicular lymphoma transformed into B-cell lymphoblastic leukemia

Abdulsamad Wafa[1], Faten Moassass[1], Thomas Liehr[2], Samarth Bhatt[2], Abdulmunim Aljapawe[3] and Walid Al Achkar[1*]

**Abstract**

**Background:** Follicular lymphoma (FL) is one of the most common B-cell non-Hodgkin's lymphoma (NHL). A subset of FL cases transform into more aggressive malignancies, most often to diffuse large B-cell lymphoma (DLBCL); in addition, lymphoblastic lymphoma and acute lymphoblastic leukemia (ALL) have also been rarely reported. The most common cytogenetic abnormalities associated with FL are translocation t(14;18)(q32;q21) with *BCL2* rearrangements, present in 80–90% of all FL. However, that translocation alone is insufficient to cause FL and additional genomic events specifically leading to this kind of disease are still to be determined. The most frequently reported secondary changes are gains of chromosomes 7p or 7q, Xp, 12q and 18q, as well as losses on 6q and mutations within *BCL2* and/or *BCL6* genes. The presence of additional genomic aberrations, in particular 17p and 6q deletions is more frequent in grade 2 and 3 FL patients and correlated with shorter survival and a higher rate of transformation into DLBCL.

**Case presentation:** We describe here, an adult FL grade 2 patient that had transformed to B-ALL at diagnosis. Banding cytogenetics, refined by multi-color fluorescence in situ hybridization including array-proven multicolor banding revealed a unique complex karyotype involving eleven chromosomes, translocation t(X;20)(p21.3;q11.2), translocation t(3;20)(q26.2;q12), and a dicentric dic(17;18). Interestingly, the dicentric chromosome led to monosomy of the tumor suppressor gene TP53. The case had an immunophenotype consistent with follicular center cell lymphoma according to the World Health Organization (WHO) recommendations.

**Conclusions:** To the best of our knowledge, a comparable adult FL grade 2 case that transformed to B-ALL associated with such a complex karyotype and loss of *TP53* was not previously reported. Most of complex aberrations were found simultaneously in approximately 85% of studied malignant cells and the remained cells studied were non-clonal; mechanisms explaining this may be either multiple-step mechanisms or single step in sense of chromothripsis.

**Keywords:** Follicular lymphoma (FL), t(14;18)(q32;q21), Chromosomal aberration, Clonal evolution, FISH, Prognostic factors

* Correspondence: ascientific@aec.org.sy
[1]Human Genetics Division, Department of Molecular Biology and Biotechnology, Atomic Energy Commission of Syria, P.O. Box 6091, Damascus, Syria
Full list of author information is available at the end of the article

## Background

Follicular lymphoma (FL) is one of the most common B-cell non-Hodgkin's lymphoma (NHL) with a relatively indolent clinical course, accounting for 20–30% of all NHL cases. The overall survival rate in FL patients is 72–77% for 5 years, with a mean survival of 10 years [1]. A subset of FL cases may transform into more aggressive malignancies; most frequently observed is diffuse large B-cell lymphoma (DLBCL) [2]. Furthermore, lymphoblastic lymphoma and acute lymphoblastic leukemia (ALL) can result rarely from an FL [2–4]. During such processes a more virulent subclonal population of cells emerge, typically associated with the loss of the follicular growth pattern, a rapidly progressive clinical course refractory to treatment, and short survival (commonly of less than 2 years) [5, 6]. Also, this transformation is often associated with the occurrence of secondary chromosomal aberrations [7, 8].

The process of malignant transformation provides an important model for the study of oncogenesis and a number of recurring secondary events are recognized which may be of mechanistic significance [9]. These include acquisition of recurrent chromosomal aberrations like loss of 17p and gain of copy numbers at 12q, inactivation of *CDKN2A* and *CDKN2B*, dysregulation of *c-MYC* and translocations, gains and mutations involving *BCL-6* [9].

The most common cytogenetic abnormalities associated with FL are translocation t(14;18)(q32;q21) with *BCL2* rearrangements, being present in 80–90% of all FL. Other common cytogenetic aberrations are +7, +18, and abnormalities and gene rearrangements in 3q27–28 (*BCL6*), 6q23–26, and 17p [1]. However, the translocation t(14;18)(q32;q21) alone is insufficient to cause FL and those additional genomic events specifically leading to disease are still to be elucidated. Known common cytogenetic aberrations during transformation of FL to DLBCL are translocations and rearrangements of the *BCL2* and *MYC* genes [1].

Here we report a patient with an initial diagnosis of FL grade 2 that transformed to B-ALL. Cytogenetic and molecular cytogenetic analysis revealed a high complex karyotype including three yet unreported chromosomal aberrations, a stable dicentric derivative chromosome and monoallelic loss of the tumor suppressor genes (TSG) *TP53*. The patient was treated with hyper-CVAD but she relapsed many times.

## Case presentation

A 38-year-old female patient without any known personal or familial medical background presented with a 1 month history of fatigue, weakness, loss of weight and fever. Physical examination and CT scan showed mild splenomegaly (data not shown). Initial laboratory evaluation of peripheral blood revealed a white blood cell (WBC) of $3.1 \times 10^9$/l (15% were of blasts), red blood cells (RBC) $4.27 \times 10^6/mm^3$, hemoglobin level of 11.7 g/dl and a platelet count of $156 \times 10^9$/l. Biochemistry analyses revealed serum lactate dehydrogenase (LDH) value was 893.2 U/l (normal value up to 480 U/l); serum aspartate aminotrasferase (AST) level was 42 U/l (normal up to 45 U/l); and alanine aminotransferase (ALT) level was 122 U/l (normal up to 45 U/l). Total serum protein was within normal range at 7.1 gm/dl (normal value 6.4–8.3 gm/dl) but serum albumin was 4.2 gm/dl (normal value 3.2–5 gm/dl). Ferritin value was 1349 (13–150 ng/ml). Bone marrow aspiration revealed 95% of blasts. At this point the first cytogenetic and immunophenotypic data were determined; simultaneously she had been diagnosed as having B-ALL based on clinical and pathological data. Treatment with hyper-CVAD for overall 10 months was initiated. The patient did not respond to that treatment and suffered from hematuria, right eye vision deterioration, gastrointestinal bleeding, and fever; she received blood transfusion many times, and her peripheral blood (PB) showed pancytopenia. One month after initiation of hyper-CVAD treatment her PB reached a short amelioration of different cell counts (WBC, plt, RBC) together with severe diarrhea, fatigue and weakness. One week later the patient showed pancytopenia again with diarrhea, severe stomach heart burn and fever. After one month the BM smear showed less than 40% blats cells with hypocellularity and BM suppression. She received cortisone, and two months later BM revealed again / still pancytopenia, suppression and myelofibrosis. After another two months BM regenerated and WBC count was $66 \times 10^9$/l (90% were blasts). Nonetheless, the patient succumbed due to unknown causes whilst under treatment. Her cousin agreed with scientific evaluation of her case and the study was approved by the ethical committee of the Atomic Energy Commission, Damascus, Syria.

## Results

Banding cytogenetics defined a complex karyotype of 46,X,t(X;20)(?;?),t(2;9)(?;?),del(3)(q?),t(6;14)(?;?),t(X;9)(?;?), t(6;14)(?;?),del(14)(q?),+der(14)t(3;14)(?;?),+dic(17;18),-17, -18,t(3;20)(?;?)[13]/47,X,t(X;20)(?;?),t(2;9)(?;?),del(3)(q?), t(6;14)(?;?),t(X;9)(?;?),t(6;14)(?;?),del(14)(q?),+der(14)t(3;14) (?;?),t(3;20)(?;?)[4]/46,XX[3] (Fig. 1). Further studies were performed based on molecular cytogenetics (Fig. 1). Dual-color-FISH (D-FISH) using specific WCP probes for chromosomes 2, 3, 6, 9, 14, 17, 18, 20 and X (data not shown), m-FISH confirmed a highly complex karyotype (Fig. 1), CEP 17 and 18 probes showed a dicentric chromosome leading to deletions of parts of the short arms of the involved chromosomes (data not shown). The locus-specific probe 17p13 (*TP53*) confirmed the absence of the 17p on the dic(17;18) (Fig. 2). Finally, aMCB using probes for the corresponding chromosomes were performed; Fig. 3). Thus, the following final karyotype was determined:

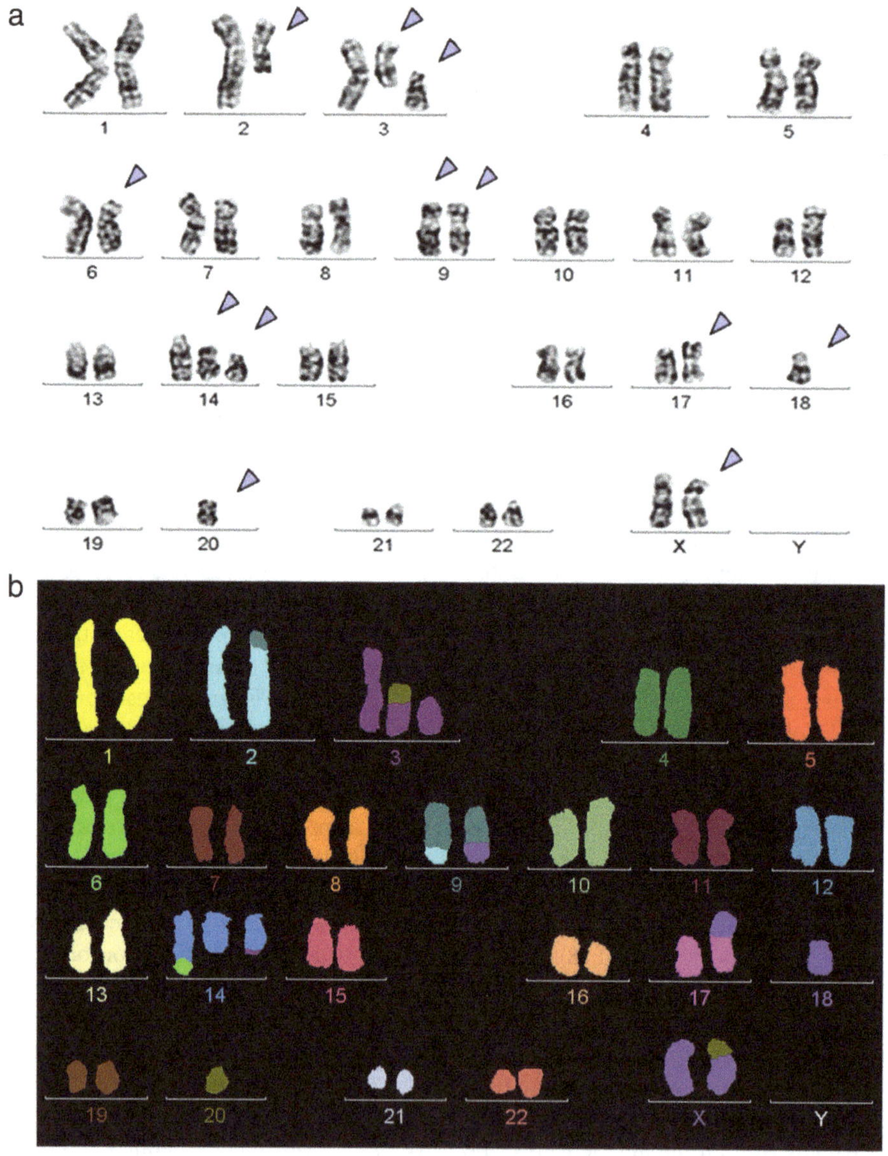


**Fig. 1** Karyotype and chromosomal aberrations were confirmed using molecular cytogenetic approaches. **a** GTG-banding revealed the following karyotype in 13/20 metaphases: 46,X,der(X)t(X;20)(?;?),t(2;9)(?;?),del(3)(q12),t(6;14)(?;?),der(9)t(X;9)(?;?),der(14)t(6;14)(?;?),del(14)(q?),+der(14)t(3;14)(?;?),+dic(17;18),-17,-18,t(3;20)(?;?). All derivative chromosomes are marked and highlighted by arrow heads. **b** M-FISH confirmed that complexity of the karyotype

46,X,t(X;20)(p21.3;q11.2),t(2;9)(p21;q22.3),del(3)(q26.2),t(6;14)(p22.3;q32),t(X;9)(p21.3;q22.3),t(6;14)(p22.3;q32),del(14)(q23),+der(14)(14pter->14q23::3q26.1 ~ 2:),+dic(17;18)(18qter->18p11.21::17p11.2->17qter),-17,-18,t(3;20)(q26.2;q12)[13]/47,X,t(X;20)(p21.3;q11.2),t(2;9)(p21;q22.3),del(3)(q26.2),t(6;14)(p22.3;q32),t(X;9)(p21.3;q22.3),t(6;14)(3p22.3;q32),del(14)(q23),+der(14)(14pter->14q23:: q26.1 ~ 2:),t(3;20)(q26.2;q12)[4]/46,XX[3].

Flow cytometric analysis of peripheral blood specimen characterized this case as B-lineage lymphoproliferative disorder most likely follicular center cell lymphoma according to WHO recommendations. The abnormal cell population (15%) was positive for CD45$^{dim}$, HLA-DR, CD19, CD20, CD10, CD79b, CD123, CD32, CD235a, Lambda and expressed CD7, CD117, CD22, CD23, and CD38 heterogeneously. This cell population was negative for CD34, CD103, CD5, CD11c, sIgD and sIgM.

## Conclusions

We report a cytogenetically highly complex adult FL grade 2 case that transformed to B-ALL with a karyotype involving eleven chromosomes, a dicentric derivative derived from parts of chromosomes 17 and 18 leading to partial monosomy 17p including TSG *TP53* and three yet

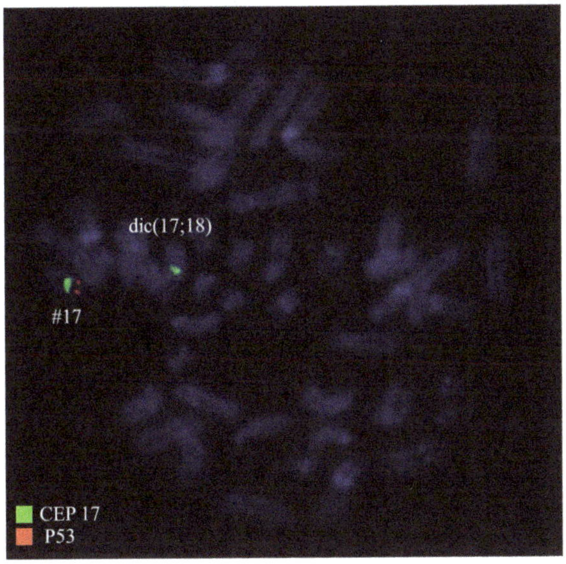


**Fig. 2** FISH using probes for CEP 17 (*green*) and *TP53* (*red*) showed one green and one red signals on normal chromosome 17; one green signal on der(17) that confirmed the absence of the *TP53* on dic(17;18). Abbreviations: # = chromosome; der = derivative chromosome

unreported chromosomal aberrations: t(X;20)(p21.3;q11.2), t(3;20)(q26.2;q12) and dic(17;18)(p11.2;p11.2).

Dicentric chromosomes are normally considered to be instable during mitosis; an idea that was not supported by this and previous own studies [10]. The role of dicentric chromosomes in cancer [11, 12] is still a field to be studied in more detail in future.

FL is regarded as a distinct entity by virtue of its characteristic cellular composition of follicle center cells (centroblasts and centrocytes), uniform immunophenotype ($CD10^{+}$), and common cytogenetic background displaying the translocation t(14;18)(q32;q21) in most of the cases [13]. Since this primary immortalizing event does not render the cells malignant, it is thought that additional secondary aberrations are necessary for tumorigenesis. In FL, the most frequently reported secondary changes are gains of chromosomes 7p or 7q, Xp, 12q and 18q, as well as losses on 6q and possibly mutations of *BCL2* and/or *BCL6* genes. The presence of additional genomic aberrations, in particular 17p and 6q deletions, is more frequent in grade 2 and 3 FL patients and correlated with shorter survival and a higher rate of transformation into DLBCL [14, 15].

The p53 protein, encoded by *TP53* tumor suppressor gene (17p13), lies at the point of convergence of a number of cellular stress pathways [16]. Activation induces cell cycle arrest, DNA repair and, in irreparably damaged cells, apoptosis [9]. Mutations of *TP53* are the most commonly

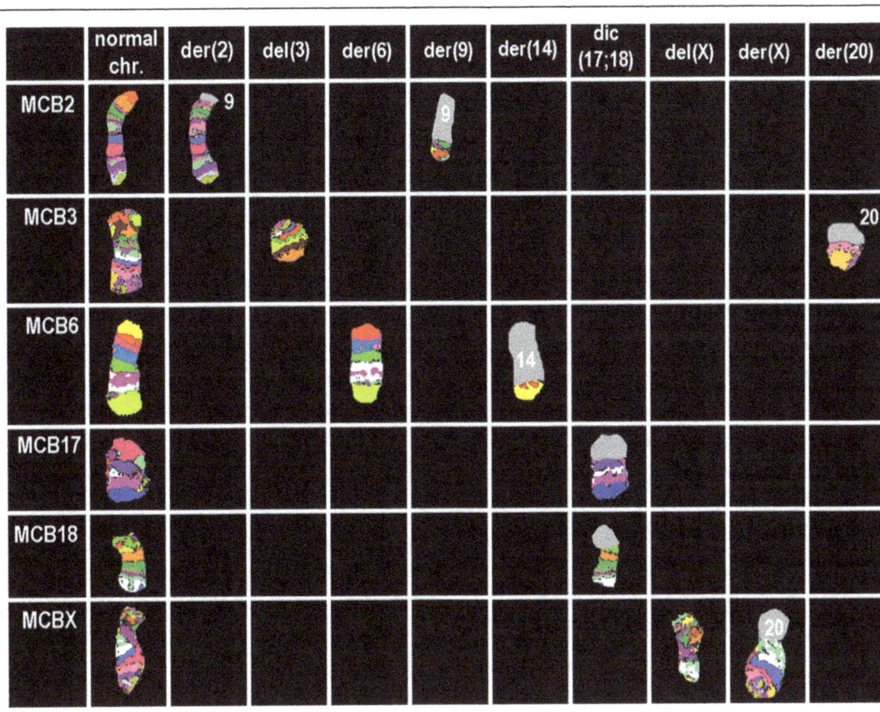


**Fig. 3** Array-proven multicolor banding (aMCB) results are shown. aMCB results are shown. The normal chromosomes (#) are depicted in the first column on the left side and the derivative of the other chromosomes on the right side of normal chromosomes. The unstained regions when suing chromosome-specific aMCB-probesets on the derivative chromosomes are shown in gray. Abbreviations: # = chromosome; der = derivative chromosome

observed in cancer [17]. In FL, mutations are infrequent, while in de novo DLBCL they are more common and may correlate with an adverse prognosis [18]. A recent study suggests that the detection of *TP53* mutations in primary diagnostic specimens of FL without signs of transformation also characterizes a patient subgroup with worse prognosis [19].

Approximately 10–60% of FL cases transform into DLBCL as well as Burkitt's lymphoma, precursor B lymphoblastic lymphoma and classical type of Hodgkin's lymphoma [2–4]. However, FL transforming into ALL has been documented in a limited number of cases [3, 4, 20–23]. Some chromosomal aberrations such as gains in chromosomes 2, 3q and 5 have been linked to higher grade transformations and inferior survival [24].

According to the literature, translocation t(2;9) involving short and/or long arms of these chromosomes has been reported in four FL cases to date [25]. Also, translocation t(X;9), deletion del(3)(q26), translocation t(6;14), deletion del(14)(q23), translocation t(3;14) and translocation t(17;18) were previously reported in 3, 3, 3, 1, 54 and 3 FL cases, respectively [25]. Interestingly, translocation t(X;20)(p21.3;q11.2), translocation t(3;20)(q26.2;q12) and dicentric chromosome dic(17;18) has never been described in FL cases. In addition, chromosomal bands such as 2p21, 3q26.2, 6p22.3, 9p22.3, 14q32, 17p11, 18p11, 20q12 and Xp21.3 are involved in chromosomal rearrangements in 14, 16, 5, 19, 1170, 36, 16, 1 and 8 cases, respectively [25]. To the best of our knowledge, a combination of all these rearrangements in one FL case was not previous reported [25]; the present case report is the first one to observe an adult FL transformed to B-ALL with high complexly karyotype.

Al-Tourah et al. [26] established a clinical diagnosis of transformation based on the presence of at least one of the following: sudden rise in LDH, rapid discordant localized nodal growth, new involvement of unusual extranodal sites, new B symptoms can be observed in 30–56% of FL patients and de novo hypercalcemia. However, clinical criteria may not correctly identify all the patients, since some of these symptoms may be associated with FL progression without histological evidence of transformation, while in other cases transformation may not be associated with any of these symptoms [27]. Moreover, FL transformation can also be diagnosed in the absence of all these clinical features at the time of a clinically asymptomatic FL relapse manifested by reappearance of enlarged lymph nodes [27].

The median time from diagnosis to transformation in the reported series ranges from 40 to 66 months, with the earliest transformation reported at 2 months and the latest at 25 years [26, 28, 29]. Transformation may occur at the time of the first or any of the subsequent progressions or recurrences in patients undergoing either expectant follow-up or during and after therapy [27]. Most studies have reported a poor prognosis after transformation with a median duration of survival ranging from 2.5 months to 2 years [27].

Chromothripsis represents one subtype of genomic chaos with highly rearranged chromosomes affecting one or a small number of chromosomes and it was detected in 1% of blood cancers [30]. Genome chaos likely plays a role in the evolution of most cancers [30]. Liu et al. [31] proposed that genome chaos is a common dynamic contributor to cancer progression. However, chromothripsis is not necessarily detectable in all tumors at all stages, it likely occurs during transitional phases (immortalization, transformation, tumor formation, metastasis, and drug resistance) of cancer evolution and is often eliminated or reduced during or after these transitions [32].

In conclusion, we described here a de novo adult FL grade 2 that transformed to B-ALL at diagnosis with a unique complex karyotype involving monosomy TSG *TP53* and three novel uncommon chromosomal aberrations t(X;20)(p21.3;q11.2), t(3;20)(q26.2;q12) and dic(17;18)(p11.2;p11.2). The patient was treated with hyper-CVAD but she relapsed many times. All findings including monosomy of 17p are considered to be an adverse prognostic factor in FL.

## Methods

### Chromosome analysis

Chromosome analysis using GTG-banding according to standard procedures [33] was performed before the treatment started. 20 metaphase cells derived from unstimulated bone marrow culture were analyzed. Karyotype was described according to the International System for Human Cytogenetic Nomenclature (ISCN 2013) [34].

### Molecular cytogenetics

Fluorescence *in situ* hybridization (FISH) using whole chromosome painting (WCP) probes for chromosomes 2, 3, 6, 9, 14, 17, 18, 20 and X (MetaSystems, Altlussheim, Germany), centromere-specific probes (CEP) for chromosomes 17 and 18 (Abbott Molecular/Vysis, USA), and a specific probe for 17p13 (*TP53*) (Q-Biogene, USA) were applied according to manufacturer's instructions [33]. Multicolor FISH (m-FISH) and FISH using the corresponding chromosome 2, 3, 6, 17, 18 and X specific array-proven multicolor banding (aMCB) probe sets was performed as previously reported [35]. A minimum of 10 metaphase spreads was analyzed, using a fluorescence microscope (AxioImager.Z1 mot, Carl Zeiss Ltd., Hertfordshir, UK) equipped with appropriate filter sets to discriminate between a maximum of five fluorochromes plus the counterstain DAPI (4′,6-diamino-2-phenylindole). Image capture and processing were performed using an ISIS imaging system (MetaSystems).

### Flow cytometric immunophenotype

Immunophenotyping was done using a general panel of fluorescent antibodies against the following antigens typical for different cell lineages and cell types: CD1a, CD2, CD3, CD4, CD5, CD8, CD10, CD11b, CD11c, CD13, CD14, CD15, CD16, CD19, CD20, CD22, CD23, CD32, CD33, CD34, CD38, CD41a, CD45, CD56, CD57, CD64, CD103, CD117, CD123, CD138, CD209, CD235a and CD243; in addition antibodies to Kappa and Lambda light Chains, IgD, sIgM, and HLADr were tested. All antibodies were purchased from BD Biosciences. Samples were analyzed on a BD FACSCalibur™ flow cytometer. Autofluorescence, viability, and isotype controls were included. Flow cytometric data acquisition and analysis were conducted by BD Cellquest™ Pro software.

#### Abbreviations

ALL: Acute lymphoblastic leukemia; ALT: Alanine aminotransferase; aMCB: Array-proven multicolor banding; AST: Aspartate aminotransferase; B-ALL: B-acute lymphoblastic leukemia; CEP: Centromeric probe; D-FISH: Dual-color-FISH; DLBCL: Diffuse large B-cell lymphoma; FISH: Fluorescence *in situ* hybridization; FL: Follicular lymphoma; ISCN: International System for Human Cytogenetic Nomenclature; LDH: Lactate dehydrogenase; NHL: Non-Hodgkin's lymphoma; PB: Peripheral blood; RBC: Red blood cells; TSG: Tumor suppressor genes; WBC: White blood cell; WCP: Probes whole chromosome painting probes; WHO: World Health Organization

#### Acknowledgements

We thank Prof. I. Othman, the Director General of Atomic Energy Commission of SYRIA (AECS) and Dr. N. Mirali, Head of Molecular Biology and Biotechnology Department for their support. This work was supported by the AECS.

#### Funding

This work was supported by the Atomic Energy Commission of SYRIA (AECS).

#### Authors' contributions

AW, FM and WA provided the case and/or did primary cytogenetic and main part of the FISH-tests; AA did the flow cytometry analysis; AW, SB and TL did detailed FISH studies. WA supervised the cytogenetic analysis as Head of HGD. AW and TL drafted the paper and all authors read and approved the final manuscript.

#### Competing interests

The authors declare that they have no competing interests. Funding there was no funding for this stud.

#### Author details

[1]Human Genetics Division, Department of Molecular Biology and Biotechnology, Atomic Energy Commission of Syria, P.O. Box 6091, Damascus, Syria. [2]Jena University Hospital, Institute of Human Genetics, Kollegiengasse 10, D-07743 Jena, Germany. [3]Molecular Biology and Biotechnology Department, Mammalians Biology Division, Flow-cytometry Laboratory, Atomic Energy Commission of Syria, P.O. Box 6091 Damascus, Syria.

#### References

1. Swerdlow SH, Campo E, Harris NL, Jaffe ES, Pileri SA, Stein H, et al., editors. WHO classification of tumours of haematopietic and lymphoid tissues. 4th ed. Lyon: WHO Press; 2008. p. 224–5.
2. de-Jong D, de-Boer JP. Predicting transformation in follicular lymphoma. Leuk Lymphoma. 2009;50:1406–11.
3. De-Jong D, Voetdijk BM, Beverstock GC, Van-Ommen GJ, Willemze R, Kluin PM. Activation of the c-myc oncogene in a precursor-B-cell blast crisis of follicular lymphoma, presenting as composite lymphoma. N Engl J Med. 1988;318:1373–8.
4. Gauwerky CE, Haluska FG, Tsujimoto Y, Nowell PC, Croce CM. Evolution of B-cell malignancy: pre-B-cell leukemia resulting from MYC activation in a B-cell neoplasm with a rearranged BCL2 gene. Proc Natl Acad Sci U S A. 1988;85:8548–52.
5. Hubbard SM, Chabner BA, DeVita VT, Simon R, Berard CW, Jones RB, et al. Histologic progression in non-Hodgkin's lymphoma. Blood. 1982;59:258–64.
6. Oviatt DL, Vousar JB, Collins RD, Flexner JM, Stein RS. Malignant lymphomas of follicular center cell origin in humans. V. Incidence, clinical features, and prognostic implications of transformation of small cleaved cell nodular lymphoma. Cancer. 1984;53:1109–14.
7. Johansson B, Mertens F, Mitelman F. Cytogenetic evolution patterns in non-Hodgkin's lymphoma. Blood. 1995;86:3905–14.
8. Horsman DE, Connors JM, Pantzar T, Gascoyne RD. Analysis of secondary chromosomal alterations in 165 cases of follicular lymphoma with t(14;18). Genes Chromosomes Cancer. 2001;30:375–82.
9. Davies AJ, Lee AM, Taylor C, Clear AJ, Goff LK, Iqbal S, et al. A limited role for TP53 mutation in the transformation of follicular lymphoma to diffuse large B-cell lymphoma. Leukemia. 2005;19:1459–65.
10. Ewers E, Yoda K, Hamid AB, Weise A, Manvelyan M, Liehr T. Centromere activity in dicentric small supernumerary marker chromosomes. Chromosome Res. 2010;18:555–62.
11. Camps J, Mrasek K, Prat E, Weise A, Starke H, Egozcue J, et al. Molecular cytogenetic characterisation of the colorectal cancer cell line SW480. Oncol Rep. 2004;11:1215–8.
12. Heller A, Trifonov V, Rubtsov N, Sauerbrey A, Starke H, Loncarevic IF, et al. Complex chromosomal rearrangements in a secondary acute myeloblastic leukemia after chemotherapy in TRAPS. Oncol Rep. 2003;10:1789–92.
13. Harris NL, Jaffe ES, Stein H, Banks PM, Chan JK, Cleary ML, et al. A revised European-American classification of lymphoid neoplasms: a proposal from the International Lymphoma Study Group. Blood. 1994;84:1361–92.
14. Tilly H, Rossi A, Stamatoullas A. Prognostic value of chromosomal abnormalities in follicular lymphoma. Blood. 1994;84:1043–9.
15. Viardot A, Barth TF, Moller P, Dohner H, Bentz M. Cytogenetic evolution of follicular lymphoma. Semin Cancer Biol. 2003;13:183–90.
16. Junttila MR, Evan GI. p53–a Jack of all trades but master of none. Nat Rev Cancer. 2009;9:821–9.
17. Olivier M, Eeles R, Hollstein M, Khan MA, Harris CC, Hainaut P. The IARC TP53 database: new online mutation analysis and recommendations to users. Hum Mutat. 2002;19:607–14.
18. Ichikawa A, Kinoshita T, Watanabe T, Kato H, Nagai H, Tsushita K, et al. Mutations of the p53 gene as a prognostic factor in aggressive B-cell lymphoma. N Engl J Med. 1997;337:529–34.
19. O'Shea D, O'Riain C, Taylor C, Waters R, Carlotti E, Macdougall F, et al. The presence of TP53 mutation at diagnosis of follicular lymphoma identifies a high-risk group of patients with shortened time to disease progression and a poorer overall survival. Blood. 2008;112:3126–9.
20. Kroft SH, Domiati-Saad R, Finn WG, Dawson DB, Schnitzer B, Singleton TP, et al. Precursor B-lymphoblastic transformation of grade I follicle center lymphoma. Am J Clin Pathol. 2000;113:411–8.
21. Kobrin C, Cha S-C, Qin H, Raffield M, Fend F, Quintanilla-Martinez L, et al. Molecular analysis of light-chain switch and acute lymphoblastic leukemia transformation in two follicular lymphomas: Implications for lymphomagenesis. Leuk Lymphoma. 2006;47:1523–34.
22. Ning Y, Foss A, Kimball AS, Neill N, Matz T, Schultz R. Characterization of a case of follicular lymphoma transformed into B-lymphoblastic leukemia. Mol Cytogenet. 2013;6:34.
23. Sun X, Gordon LI, Peterson LC. Transformation of follicular lymphoma to acute lymphoblastic leukemia. Arch Pathol Lab Med. 2002;126:997–8.

24. Eide MB, Liestøl K, Lingjaerde OC, Hystad ME, Kresse SH, Meza-Zepeda L, et al. Genomic alterations reveal potential for higher grade transformation in follicular lymphoma and confirm parallel evolution of tumor cell clones. Blood. 2010;116:1489–97.
25. Mitelman F, Johansson B, Mertens F, editors. Mitelman database of chromosome aberrations and gene fusions in cancer. 2015. http://cgap.nci.nih.gov/Chromosomes/Mitelman [accessed 11.12.2015].
26. Al-Tourah AJ, Gill KK, Chhanabhai M, Hoskins PJ, Klasa RJ, Savage KJ, Sehn LH, et al. Population-based analysis of incidence and outcome of transformed non-Hodgkin's lymphoma. J Clin Oncol. 2008;26:5165–9.
27. Lossos IS, Gascoyne RD. Transformation of follicular lymphoma. Best Pract Res Clin Haematol. 2011;24:147–63.
28. Bastion Y, Sebban C, Berger F, Felman P, Salles G, Dumontet C, Bryon PA, et al. Incidence, predictive factors, and outcome of lymphoma transformation in follicular lymphoma patients. J Clin Oncol. 1997;15:1587–94.
29. Montoto S, Davies AJ, Matthews J, Calaminici M, Norton AJ, Amess J, et al. Risk and clinical implications of transformation of follicular lymphoma to diffuse large B-cell lymphoma. J Clin Oncol. 2007;25:2426–33.
30. Stephens PJ, Greenman CD, Fu B, Yang F, Bignell GR, Mudie LJ, et al. Massive genomic rearrangement acquired in a single catastrophic event during cancer development. Cell. 2011;144:27–40.
31. Liu G, Stevens J, Horne S, Abdallah B, Ye K, Bremer S, et al. Genome chaos: Survival strategy during crisis. Cell Cycle. 2014;13:528–37.
32. Heng HH, Stevens JB, Liu G, Bremer SW, Ye KJ, Reddy PV, et al. Stochastic cancer progression driven by nonclonal chromosome aberrations. J Cell Physiol. 2006;208:461–72.
33. AL-achkar W, Wafa A, Nweder MS. A complex translocation t(5;9;22) in Philadelphia cells involving the short arm of chromosome 5 in a case of chronic myelogenous leukemia. J Exp Clin Cancer Res. 2007;26:411–5.
34. Shaffer LG, McGowan-Joran J, Schmid MS. ISCN 2013: an international system of human cytogenetic nomenclature. Unionville: S. Karger Publications, Inc; 2013.
35. Liehr T, Heller A, Starke H, Rubtsov N, Trifonov V, Mrasek K, et al. Microdissection based high resolution multicolor banding for all 24 human chromosomes. Int J Mol Med. 2002;9:335–9.

# 16

# *MYB* deregulation from a *EWSR1-MYB* fusion at leukemic evolution of a *JAK2*$^{V617F}$ positive primary myelofibrosis

Tiziana Pierini†, Danika Di Giacomo†, Valentina Pierini, Paolo Gorello, Gianluca Barba, Anair Graciela Lema Fernandez, Fabrizia Pellanera, Tamara Iannotti, Franca Falzetti, Roberta La Starza and Cristina Mecucci*

**Abstract**

**Background:** Although Philadelphia-negative myeloproliferative neoplasms (Ph-MPN) are usually not aggressive, the type and the number of molecular lesions impact greatly on leukemic transformation. Indeed, the molecular background underlying progression is still largely unexplored even though *ASXL1, IDH1/2, SRSF2*, and *TP53* mutations, together with adverse karyotypic changes, place the patient at high risk of leukemic transformation.

**Case presentation:** Our patient, a 64-year old man with a diagnosis of *JAK2*$^{V617F}$ primary myelofibrosis (PMF) had an unusually rapid leukemic transformation. Genomic profiling showed that *TET2* and *SRSF2* mutations were also present. At leukemic transformation, the patient developed a complex chromosome rearrangement producing a *EWSR1-MYB* fusion. Remarkably, the expression of *MYB* and of its target *BCL2* was, respectively, ≥4.7 and ≥2.8 fold higher at leukemic transformation than after chemotherapy, when the patient obtained the hematological remission. At this time point, the *EWSR1-MYB* fusion disappeared while *JAK2*$^{V617F}$, *TET2*, and *SRSF2* mutations, as well as PMF morphological features persisted.

**Conclusions:** Rapid leukemic transformation of *JAK2*$^{V617F}$ PMF was closely linked to a previously undescribed putative EWSR1-MYB transcription factor which was detected only at disease evolution. We hypothesize that the EWSR1-MYB contributed to leukemia transformation through at least two mechanisms: 1) it sustained *MYB* expression, and consequently deregulated its target *BCL2*, a putative onco-suppressor gene; and 2) ectopic *EWSR1-MYB* expression probably fulfilled its own oncogenic potential as demonstrated for other *MYB*-fusions. As our study confirmed that *MYB* is recurrently involved in chronic as well as leukemic transformation of PMF, it appears to be a valid molecular marker for tailored treatments.

**Keywords:** PMF, Leukemic transformation, *MYB*

**Abbreviations:** AML, Acute myeloid leukemia; BM, Bone marrow; DBD, DNA binding domain; DHPLC, Denaturing high performance liquid chromatography; ET, Essential thrombocytopenia; FISH, Fluorescence in situ hybridization; Hb, Haemoglobin; I-FISH, Interphase-FISH; MCV, Mean corpuscular volume; Ph-MPN, Philadelphia negative myeloproliferative neoplasia; PMF, Primary myelofibrosis; PV, Polycythemia vera; qRT-PCR, Quantitative reverse transcription-polymerase chain reaction; RT-PCR, Reverse transcription-polymerase chain reaction; SNPa, Single nucleotide polymorphism array; TAD, Transcriptional-activating domain; WBC, White blood cell

* Correspondence: cristina.mecucci@unipg.it
†Equal contributors
Hematology and Bone Marrow Transplantation Unit, University of Perugia, C.R.E.O., Piazzale Menghini n.9, 06132 Perugia, Italy

## Background

Ph-MPN are usually not aggressive malignancies. Evolution into Acute Myeloid Leukemia (AML) occurs in ~2 % of Polycythemia Vera (PV), 1 % of Essential Thrombocytopenia (ET), and 10–20 % of PMF, considering the first decade of disease. Although, transformation rates increase with genotoxic therapy, leukemic transformation is part of the natural history of these disorders as AML also occurs in treatment-naive patients [1, 2].

Genomic profiling of Ph-MPN is useful for understanding the pathobiology of leukemic transformation and improving prognostic stratification of patients and treatment. During leukemic transformation very few new mutations are acquired and the majority of somatic mutations are already present in the chronic phase. Two or more mutations affecting *ASXL1, IDH1/2, SRSF2*, and *TP53*, are considered high-risk events. Besides mutations, unfavourable (chromosome 3, 5 or 7 rearrangements), and very unfavourable (chromosome 17 abnormalities) karyotypic changes impact upon prognosis [3, 4]. In any case, the molecular mechanisms underlying the progression from Ph-MPN to AML are not yet completely understood [5–9].

Longitudinal genomic investigation into a unique case of $JAK2^{V617F}$ positive PMF with rapid leukemic evolution, detected a leukemia-specific complex rearrangement involving chromosomes 6, 9 and 22 which produced an aberrant EWSR1-MYB transcription factor. *EWSR1-MYB* ectopic expression, as well as high expression of *MYB* and its target *BCL2*, likely contributed to the leukemia phenotype. It is worth mentioning that, high level of *MYB* expression blocks differentiation and confers self-renewal properties to leukemic cells, whereas the expression of the anti-apoptotic BCL2 protein inhibits leukemic cell death [10–12].

## Case presentation

In January 2011, a 64-year-old man was referred to our Department with leukocytosis (WBC 20.100/uL with 71.8 % neutrophils), macrocytic anemia (Hb 11,5 g/dL; MCV 104 fl), splenomegaly, and hepatomegaly. Bone marrow (BM) biopsy revealed PMF with grade 1 fibrosis; karyotype was normal. The $JAK2^{V617F}$ mutation was found at 60 % allelic burden. After 4 months the patient developed an acute myeloid leukemia (AML; M2 morphology) and acquired an ins(6;22)(q23.3;q11) in the 20 metaphases analyzed (Fig. 1a). He was treated according to the FLAI protocol [13] and obtained hematologic and cytogenetic remission. Myeloproliferative features, including $JAK2^{V617F}$, persisted. Demethylating treatment with 5-azacytidine (5-AZA) was administered for 8 cycles, reducing anemia and splenomegaly, but treatment was discontinued because the patient developed a gastric adenocarcinoma. He died 30 months after PMF was diagnosed.

## Methods

### Molecular-cytogenetic and mutational analyses

All molecular and cytogenetic studies were carried out on BM samples. Multi-FISH (24XCyte Multi-colour probe kit, MetaSystems), whole chromosome paints for chromosomes 6, 9 and 22 (Cytocell, Milan, Italy), and metaphase FISH with DNA clones for *MYB* (G248P8686G9 and G248P89100B2), *EWSR1* (G248P89991F7 and G248P80286D12), 9q33.1-q33.3, and 22q11-q12 regions, were done at leukemic transformation (Additional file 1 and Additional file 2: Tables S1, S2, S3). A *EWSR1-MYB* FISH assay (RP1-32B1 for *MYB* and RP11-367E7 for *EWSR1*) was performed at leukemic transformation, diagnosis and post-chemotherapy. The *EWSR1-MYB* assay was also applied to a cohort of 7 PMF and 3 leukemia groups (Additional file 1). Single Nucleotide Polymorphism array (SNPa) experiments were performed at initial PMF and at leukemic transformation; targeted mutational analysis of *DNMT3A, SETBP1, EZH2, IDH1, IDH2, SRSF2, ASXL1, NRAS, TET2* and *TERT* promoter was done at diagnosis, leukemic transformation, and after chemotherapy by DHPLC and Sanger's Sequencing. For details of experiments see Additional file 1 and Additional file 2: Table S4.

### Reverse transcription-polymerase chain reaction (RT-PCR) and cloning of *EWSR1-MYB*

cDNA from each patient sample was amplified using primers *EWSR1*_400F (5′-GCCCACTCAAGGATATGCAC-3′) and *MYB*_561R (5′-TGCTTGGCAATAACAGACCA-3′), for the first amplification round; nested PCR was set up with primers *EWSR1*_515F (5′-CAGACCGCCTATGCAACTTC-3′) and *MYB*_433R (5′-GCACTGCACATCTGTTCGAT-3′). PCR products were cloned and sequenced (Additional file 1).

### Quantitative reverse transcription PCR (qRT-PCR) for *MYB* and *BCL2*

*MYB* expression was investigated in our patient, at all time points, and in 7 PMF cases (four at leukemic transformation and three in paired chronic phase/leukemic transformation) (TaqMan assay probe Hs00920556_m1; Applied Biosystems, Foster City, CA). Negative controls were four healthy BM samples. Positive controls were 12 acute leukemias with high *MYB* expression (4 *RUNX1-RUNX1T1* AML, 4 AML with *MLL* translocations, and 4 *BCR-ABL1*-positive B-cell ALL) [14]. Expression of *BCL2*, a known MYB target, was also investigated in our case (TaqMan assay probe Hs00608023_m1, Applied Biosystems). Amplifications were normalized to the endogenous reference control *ABL1* (Hs00245445_m1, Applied Biosystems) (Additional file 1).

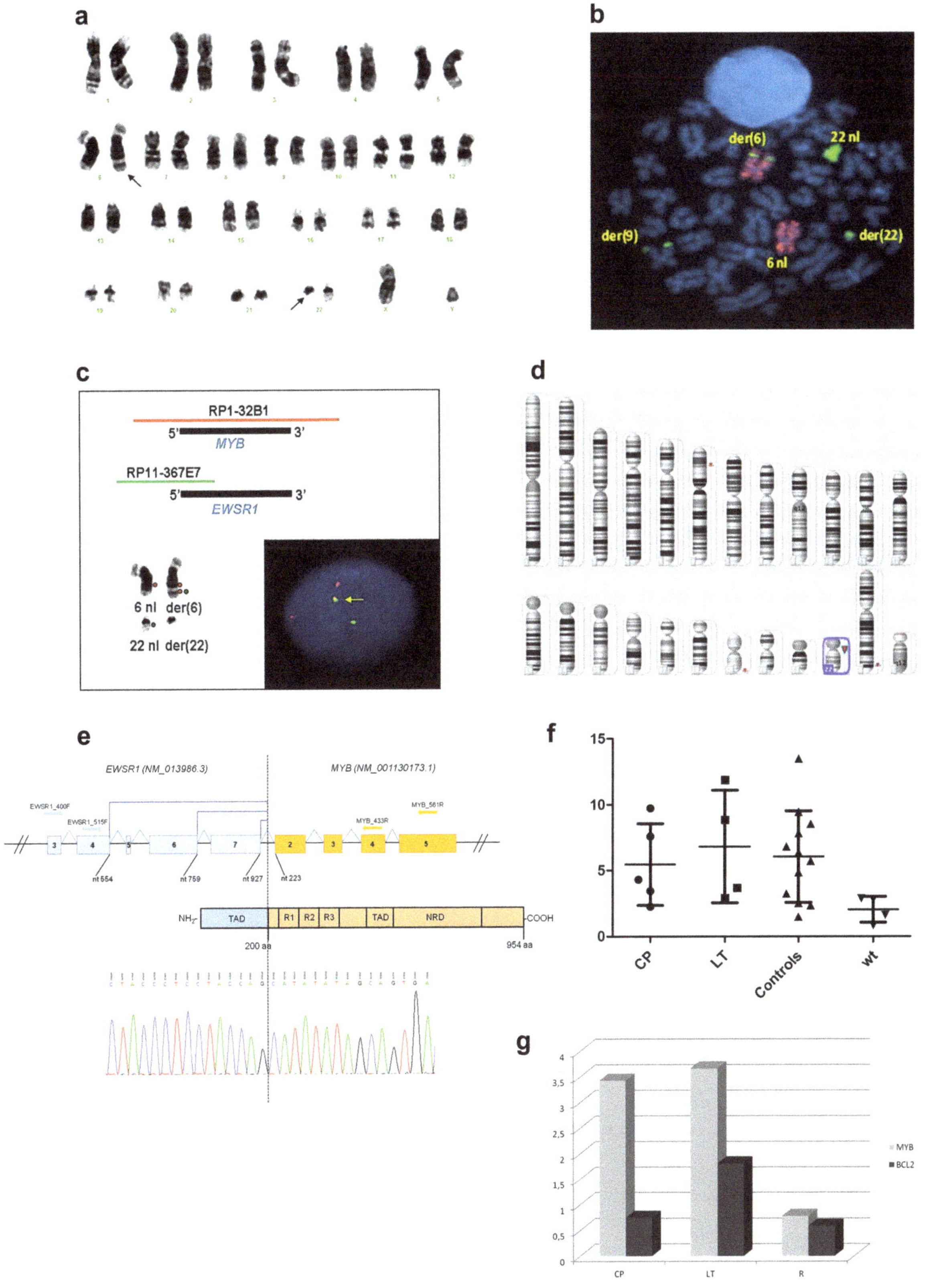


**Fig. 1** (See legend on next page.)

(See figure on previous page.)
**Fig. 1 a**) G-banded karyotype bone marrow cells at leukemic transformation showed ins(6;22)(q23.3;q11) and der(22q) (*black arrows*). **b**) Metaphase FISH experiment with Whole Chromosome Paint (WCP) 6 (*Texas Red*) and WCP 22 (FITC). Genomic material of chromosome 22 was present on der(6) and der(9) long arms. **c**) Schema of clones RP1-32B1 (*MYB*) (*Spectrum Orange*) and RP11-367E7 (*EWSR1*) (*Spectrum Green*) and their mapping. Normal and derivative chromosomes 6 and 22 hybridization patterns; a green/orange fusion signal was present on der(6). A fusion signal was found in interphase nuclei (*yellow arrow*). **d**) SNPa analysis detected loss at 22q (*red triangle*) in BM sample at leukemic transformation. **e**) Schema of the *EWSR1-MYB* fusion gene and putative protein. **f**) *MYB* expression analysis in four combined cases at chronic phase and leukemic transformation and in a positive control group (4 *RUNX1-RUNX1T1* AML, 4 *MLL*-positive AML, and 4 *BCR-ABL1*-positive B-cell ALL). **g**) Longitudinal expression of *MYB* and *BCL2* in the index case. Data are reported for one representative of three independent experiments. Abbreviations: der, derivative chromosome; nl, normal; TAD, transcriptional-activating domain; R1, R2, R3, imperfect aminoacidic repeats; NRD, negative regulatory domain; CP, chronic phase; LT, leukemic transformation; wt, wild-type; R, relapse

## Results

### Molecular cytogenetic and mutational analyses

Multi-FISH and whole chromosome paints showed chromosome 22q11-q12 material inserted into chromosome 6q23 and revealed an additional rearrangement between der(22) and an apparently normal chromosome 9 (Fig. 1b) (Additional file 3: Figure S1). The breakpoint occurred at 6q23 within the *MYB* oncogene (Additional file 3: Figure S2). Fosmids for *EWSR1* and the *EWSR1-MYB* assay showed that the 5'*EWSR1* was inserted into the *MYB* locus (Fig.1c) (Additional file 3: Figure S2). The *EWSR1-MYB* rearrangement was not detected at chronic phase or in 3 consecutive samples analyzed after chemotherapy and during treatment with 5-AZA (Table 1).

SNPa detected a 96 Mb copy neutral loss of heterozygosity (cnLOH) at 12q11-12q24.33 at chronic phase and leukemic transformation. Lack of germinal material precluded definition as a congenital or acquired event. Applying a 50 Kb filter revealed a 99 kb loss at 22q11.1 (cytostart 17585764 - cytoend 17684472) only at leukemic transformation (Fig. 1d) (Additional file 3: Figure S3). *SRSF2* (c.284C > A; p.P95H) and *TET2* (c.3781C > T; p.R1261C) (c.2732_2733insC; p.A912Cfs*12) mutations were found, and confirmed, at all disease stages (Table 1).

### RT-PCR and qRT-PCR

At leukemic transformation an in-frame fusion transcript *EWSR1-MYB* with breakpoint in *EWSR1* exon 7 (nt 927) (NM_013986.3) and *MYB* exon 2 (nt 223) (NM_001130173.1) was detected. The 954 aminoacids predicted fusion protein retained the EWSR1 transcriptional-activating domain (TAD) at the N-terminal and all MYB functional domains at the C-terminal (Fig. 1e). After chemotherapy, at hematological and cytogenetic remission, the *EWSR1-MYB* fusion disappeared. At leukemic phase, *MYB* and *BCL2* expression was respectively ≥4.7 and ≥2.8 fold higher than at remission. High *MYB* expression was detected in 7 PMF and in the 3 groups of acute leukemia used as positive controls (Fig. 1f).

## Discussion

This case of *JAK2*-positive PMF with very rapid evolution to AML had a specific mutational profile at diagnosis bearing mutations of *JAK2, SRSF2* and *TET2.* A complex rearrangement involving chromosomes 6, 9, and 22, which produced a previously undescribed *EWSR1-MYB* fusion, underlies the leukemic transformation.

EWSR1 is a member of the TET (TLS, EWSR1, TAFII68) protein family which acts as multifunctional protein and

**Table 1** Longitudinal cytogenetic and molecular studies in our patient with rapidly evolving PMF

| | PMF diagnosis | Leukemic transformation | Post-consolidation therapy | *Monitoring +3 months | *Monitoring +14 months |
|---|---|---|---|---|---|
| Karyotype | 46,XY [20] | 46,XY,ins(6;22)(q23q11q12),del(22)(q11) [20] | 46,XY [20] | 46,XY [20] | 46,XY [20] |
| *JAK2* $^{V617F}$ allele burden | 60 % | 63 % | 70 % | n.d. | 36 % |
| *TET2* c.2732_2733insC, p.A912Cfs*12; .c.3781C>T, p.R1261C | yes | yes | yes | n.d. | n.d. |
| *SRSF2* c.284C>A p.P95H | yes | yes | yes | n.d. | n.d. |
| SNPa | cnLOH 12q11-12q24.33 | cnLOH: 12q11-12q24.33<br>LOSS: 22q11.1 | n.d. | n.d. | n.d. |
| I-FISH: *EWSR1-MYB* | negative | positive | negative | negative | negative |
| RT-PCR: *EWSR1-MYB* | negative | positive | negative | n.d. | n.d. |

n.d. not done
*from leukemia transformation

regulates transcription and mRNA splicing to maintain cellular homeostasis. Although well known in soft tissue sarcoma, *EWSR1* fusions have only occasionally been detected in leukemia [15–19]. Interestingly, all EWSR1 fusions retained the TAD portion at the N-terminal and the partner DNA Binding Domain (DBD) at the C-terminal. Since EWSR1-FLI1, the most frequent sarcoma-associated fusion, acted as an aberrant transcription factor, deregulating several targets [20], one might speculate that the EWSR1-MYB fusion in our patient also acted as an aberrant transcription factor, altering the *MYB* transcriptional program.

MYB is a leucin zipper transcription factor which plays a key role in cell proliferation and differentiation [21–23]. High level of *MYB* is common in AML associated with *BCR-ABL1, RUNX1-RUNX1T1, MYST3-CREBBP*, or *MLL*-rearrangements [11, 12, 24]. Chromosomal aberrations placing *MYB* under the promoter of a partner gene, such as *TCRB-MYB* in T-cell ALL [14, 25] or in close proximity of super-enhancer regions, such as *MYB-NFIB* in adenoid cystic carcinoma [26], caused *MYB* over-expression. It is worth noting, however, that besides promoting tumour growth through *MYB* over-expression, the *MYB* fusions might have their own oncogenic potential as demonstrated for the *MYB-QKI* in pediatric angiocentric glioma, which drives tumor development in vitro and in vivo models [27].

High *MYB* level confers self-renewal properties on leukemic cells and blocks differentiation, thus it has been regarded as a putative therapeutic target [11, 12]. Indeed, in vitro and in vivo studies showed that a slight *MYB* drop is enough to block leukemic cell proliferation without affecting normal haematopoiesis [28]. The present study confirmed two previous reports of high *MYB* expression in PMF [29, 30] as it was detected in all cases at chronic phase with a rising trend at leukemic transformation (Fig. 1f).

In determining whether and how the aberrant EWSR1-MYB transcription factor played a role in rapid disease progression, paired longitudinal studies showed that the *EWSR1-MYB* fusion was closely linked to leukemic transformation, as it was not detected at diagnosis and disappeared after treatment. As a functional consequence of *MYB* deregulation we investigated *BCL2* expression as it is a well-known MYB target which acts as an anti-apoptotic onco-suppressor. Recent findings in leukemia xenograft models showed that sustained *MYB* expression maintained high *BCL2* expression and consequently, inhibited leukemic cell death [10]. In line with these data, we found that *MYB* as well as *BCL2* expression was higher at leukemic transformation than after treatment (Fig. 1g).

Our patient responded to treatment by regressing from AML to PMF maintaining *JAK2, TET2* and *SRSF2* mutations. Therefore, the *JAK2*-positive clone, showed a constant allele burden in all disease phases, marking the PMF stem line which persisted throughout disease, while the *EWSR1-MYB* fusion was the hallmark of the leukemic clone. Whether *EWSR1-MYB* affected a *JAK2*$^{V617F}$ cell or developed as an independent clone, could not be established. Interestingly Engle E.K. et al. [31], identified *MYB* mutations in a complex PMF subclonal branching.

## Conclusion

We report a unique case of *JAK2*$^{V617F}$ PMF. Rapid leukemia transformation, due to complex cytogenetic rearrangement, produced a previously undescribed EWSR1-MYB fusion that appeared to act as an aberrant transcription factor deregulating *BCL2*. Our study provided new insights to point to MYB as a good molecular target in patients presenting with high-risk PMF [11, 32].


#### Acknowledgements

The authors would like to thank Dr G A Boyd for assistance in preparing the manuscript.

#### Funding

This work was funded by Associazione Italiana per la Ricerca sul Cancro (AIRC, IG-15525), Fondo per gli Investimenti della Ricerca di Base (FIRB 2011 RBAP11TF7Z_005), Programmi di Ricerca scientifica di rilevante Interesse Nazionale (PRIN), Associazione Sergio Luciani, Fabriano, Italy and Fondazione Cassa di Risparmio di Perugia (2014.0265.021).


#### Authors' contributions

RLS and CM conceived and designed the study, analyzed the data, and wrote the manuscript; TP and DDG wrote the paper; TP and VP performed and analyzed FISH experiments; GB performed and analyzed SNP array; DDG and PG performed and analyzed RT-PCR and qRT-PCR; AGLF, FP, TI performed targeted mutational analysis and analyzed results; FF determined *JAK2*$^{V617F}$ allelic burden. All Authors approved the manuscript.

#### Competing interests

Authors declare that they have no competing interests.

#### References


1. Kennedy JA, Atenafu EG, Messner HA, et al. Treatment outcomes following leukemic transformation in Philadelphia-negative myeloproliferative neoplasms. Blood. 2013;121(14):2725–33.
2. Finazzi G, Caruso V, Marchioli R, et al. Acute leukemia in polycythemia vera: an analysis of 1638 patients enrolled in a prospective observational study. Blood. 2005;105(7):2664–70.
3. Tam CS, Abruzzo LV, Lin KI, et al. The role of cytogenetic abnormalities as a prognostic marker in primary myelofibrosis: applicability at the time of diagnosis and later during disease course. Blood. 2009;113(18):4171–8.
4. Tefferi A, Pardanani A, Gangat N, et al. Leukemia risk models in primary myelofibrosis: an International Working Group study. Leukemia. 2012;26(6):1439–41.
5. Abdel-Wahab O, Manshouri T, Patel J, et al. Genetic analysis of transforming events that convert chronic myeloproliferative neoplasms to leukemias. Cancer Res. 2010;70(2):447–52.
6. Harutyunyan A, Klampfl T, Cazzola M, Kralovics R. p53 lesions in leukemic transformation. N Engl J Med. 2011;364(5):488–90.

7. Klampfl T, Harutyunyan A, Berg T, et al. Genome integrity of myeloproliferative neoplasms in chronic phase and during disease progression. Blood. 2011; 118(1):167–76.
8. Lundberg P, Karow A, Nienhold R, et al. Clonal evolution and clinical correlates of somatic mutations in myeloproliferative neoplasms. Blood. 2014;123(14):2220–8.
9. Quintás-Cardama A, Kantarjian H, Pierce S, Cortes J, Verstovsek S. Prognostic model to identify patients with myelofibrosis at the highest risk of transformation to acute myeloid leukemia. Clin Lymphoma Myeloma Leuk. 2013;13(3):315–18.
10. Jing D, Bhadri VA, Beck D, et al. Opposing regulation of BIM and BCL2 controls glucocorticoid-induced apoptosis of pediatric acute lymphoblastic leukemia cells. Blood. 2015;125(2):273–83.
11. Uttarkar S, Dassé E, Coulibaly A, et al. Targeting acute myeloid leukemia with a small molecule inhibitor of the Myb/p300 interaction. Blood. 2016; 127(9):1173–82.
12. Lieu YK, Reddy EP. Conditional c-myb knockout in adult hematopoietic stem cells leads to loss of self-renewal due to impaired proliferation and accelerated differentiation. Proc Natl Acad Sci U S A. 2009;106(51):21689–94.
13. Russo D, Pricolo G, Michieli M, et al. Fludarabine, arabinosyl cytosine and idarubicin (FLAI) for remission induction in poor-risk acute myeloid leukemia. Leuk Lymphoma. 2001;40(3-4):335–43.
14. Lahortiga I, De Keersmaecker K, Van Vlierberghe P, et al. Duplication of the MYB oncogene in T cell acute lymphoblastic leukemia. Nat Genet. 2007; 39(5):593–5.
15. Schlaak M, Renner R, Treudler R, et al. CD30+ anaplastic lymphoma kinase-positive anaplastic large cell lymphoma with an unusual translocation t(11; 22). Br J Dermatol. 2008;159(1):240–2.
16. Martini A, La Starza R, Janssen H, et al. Recurrent rearrangement of the Ewing's sarcoma gene, EWSR1, or its homologue, TAF15, with the transcription factor CIZ/NMP4 in acute leukemia. Cancer Res. 2002;62(19): 5408–12.
17. Jakovljević G, Nakić M, Rogosić S, et al. Pre-B-cell acute lymphoblastic leukemia with bulk extramedullary disease and chromosome 22 (EWSR1) rearrangement masquerading as Ewing sarcoma. Pediatr Blood Cancer. 2010;54(4):606–9.
18. Hawkins JM, Craig JM, Secker-Walker LM, Prentice HG, Mehta AB. Ewing's sarcoma t(11;22) in a case of acute nonlymphocytic leukemia. Cancer Genet Cytogenet. 1991;55(2):157–62.
19. Cantile M, Marra L, Franco R, et al. Molecular detection and targeting of EWSR1 fusion transcripts in soft tissue tumors. Med Oncol. 2013;30(1):412.
20. Uren A, Toretsky JA. Ewing's sarcoma oncoprotein EWS-FLI1: the perfect target without a therapeutic agent. Future Oncol. 2005;1(4):521–8.
21. Sandberg ML, Sutton SE, Pletcher MT, et al. Myb and p300 regulate hematopoietic stem cell proliferation and differentiation. Dev Cell. 2005; 8(2):153–66.
22. Mucenski ML, McLain K, Kier AB, et al. A functional c-myb gene is required for normal murine fetal hepatic hematopoiesis. Cell. 1991;65(4):677–89.
23. Malaterre J, Carpinelli M, Ernst M, et al. Myb is required for progenitor cell homeostasis in colonic crypts. Proc Natl Acad Sci U S A. 2007;104(10):3829–34.
24. Pattabiraman DR, McGirr C, Shakhbazov K, et al. Interaction of c-Myb with p300 is required for the induction of acute myeloid leukemia (AML) by human AML oncogenes. Blood. 2014;123(17):2682–90.
25. Clappier E, Cuccuini W, Kalota A, et al. The C-MYB locus is involved in chromosomal translocation and genomic duplications in human T-cell acute leukemia (T-ALL), the translocation defining a new T-ALL subtype in very young children. Blood. 2007;110(4):1251–61.
26. Drier Y, Cotton MJ, Williamson KE, et al. An oncogenic MYB feedback loop drives alternate cell fates in adenoid cystic carcinoma. Nat Genet. 2016;48(3): 265–72.
27. Bandopadhayay P, Ramkissoon LA, Jain P, et al. MYB-QKI rearrangements in angiocentric glioma drive tumorigenicity through a tripartite mechanism. Nat Genet. 2016;48(3):273–82.
28. Zuber J, Rappaport AR, Luo W, et al. An integrated approach to dissecting oncogene addition implicates a Myb-coordinated self-renewal program as essential for leukemia maintenance. Genes Dev. 2011;25(15):1628–40.
29. Steensma DP, Pardanani A, Stevenson WS, et al. More on Myb in myelofibrosis: molecular analyses of MYB and EP300 in 55 patients with myeloproliferative disorders. Blood. 2006;107(4):1733–5.
30. Guglielmelli P, Tozzi L, Pancrazzi A, et al. MicroRNA expression profile in granulocytes from primary myelofibrosis patients. Exp Hematol. 2007;35(11): 1708–18.
31. Engle EK, Fisher DA, Miller CA, et al. Clonal evolution revealed by whole genome sequencing in a case of primary myelofibrosis transformed to secondary acute myeloid leukemia. Leukemia. 2015;29(4):869–76.
32. Amaru Calzada A, Todoerti K, Donadoni L, et al. The HDAC inhibitor Givinostat modulates the hematopoietic transcription factors NFE2 and C-MYB in JAK2(V617F) myeloproliferative neoplasm cells. Exp Hematol. 2012;40(8):634–45.

# Molecular characterization and evaluation of complex rearrangements in a case of ring chromosome 15

Stuti Tewari[1], Naznin Lubna[1], Raju Shah[2], Ahmed B. H. Al-Rikabi[3], Krati Shah[1], Jayesh Sheth[1] and Frenny Sheth[1*]

**Abstract**

**Background:** Ring chromosome 15 is a rare genetic entity. Only a few cases have been reported with characterization using molecular techniques. The clinical presentation is quite variable, as a result of differences in the breakpoints, haploinsufficiency of genes involved in deleted segment/s, level of mosaicism and ring instability resulting in a variability of rearrangement of genetic material.

**Case presentation:** The proband, a 2 months old boy, presented with small head size and facial dysmorphism. On examination microcephaly, triangular face, small anterior frontanelle, micrognathia, hypotonia, unilateral simian crease, hypertelorism, umbilical hernia, micropenis with mild phimosis were noted. Karyotype revealed 46,XY,r(15)(p11.2q26). Array-comparative genomic hybridization (aCGH) and targeted gene sequencing for microcephaly was carried out for genotype phenotype correlation. Array-CGH detected a 2.8 Mb terminal deletion at 15q26.3 along with a 496 kb interstitial micro-duplication, encompassing the *IGF1R* gene, in the affected genomic region, which was otherwise missed on conventional karyotype.

**Conclusion:** The present study highlights the importance of aCGH in not only delineating specific phenotypes through accurate genotypic correlation but also in detection and evaluation of ring chromosome with unexpected complex rearrangements.

**Keywords:** Ring chromosome 15, Array-comparative genomic hybridization (aCGH), Duplication/deletion, IGF-1R gene, Microcephaly

## Background

Ring chromosome 15 is associated with a rare disorder that was first described by Jacobsen in 1966 [1]. Around 50 cases with r(15) have been reported till date, with only a few cases being comprehensively characterized using molecular cytogenetic techniques [2, 3]. Major clinical features include severe pre- and postnatal growth delay, microcephaly, triangular face, hypertelorism, intellectual disability, clinodactyly and brachydactyly of the fifth finger, small hands and feet, and cafe-au-lait spots [2, 4, 5]. Moreover, more severe phenotypes may include congenital heart defects, renal anomalies, hypotonia, hydrocephaly, retinal abnormalities, ear anomalies, behavioral disorders and speech delay [2]. The varying degree of phenotypic severity can be attributed to differences in the breakpoints, haploinsufficiency of genes involved in the deleted segments, level of mosaicism and ring instability resulting in a variability of other genetic material rearrangements [6, 7].

In the present case report, we attempted to do a precise genotype and phenotype correlation in a male proband with ring chromosome 15 using array comparative genomic hybridization (aCGH) and targeted gene sequencing. The report also aims to highlight the utility of aCGH in the detection and evaluation of complex rearrangements in atypical ring chromosomes. Furthermore, the case was studied by banding and molecular cytogenetics.

* Correspondence: fshethad1@googlemail.com
[1]FRIGE's Institute of Human Genetics, FRIGE House, Jodhpur Gam Road, Satellite, Ahmedabad 380009, India
Full list of author information is available at the end of the article

## Case presentation

The proband, a 2 months old boy, was born full term to 33-year-old non-consanguineous parents, by Caesarian section. The child had an APGAR score of ten with a birth weight of 2.8 kg. At the time of presentation, the proband was 2 months old; his length and weight were at the 3rd centile while the head circumference being significantly less than the 3rd centile, according to WHO (i.e.: 54 cm, 4.15 kg and 34 cm respectively). The proband had microcephaly, triangular face, small anterior frontanelle, micrognathia, hypertelorism unilateral simian crease, umbilical hernia and micropenis with mild phimosis. On neurological examination, the child presented hypotonia with oromotor delay. Ophthalmologic, auricular and cardiac examinations were normal. MRI brain revealed oligogyria with normal myelination in accordance with age suggesting the possibility of microcephaly with simplified gyral-pattern (MSG Group-1).

The proband was the second child of his parents (mother G2P2). His elder brother was apparently normal. The family history was unremarkable; the parents had a normal phenotype. The baby was referred to our centre for karyotyping and genetic counseling. Sample collection and written informed consent was obtained according to the regulations of the institutional ethics committee working according to the Helsinki declaration.

Chromosome analysis performed on proband's 72-h lymphocyte cultures revealed an apparently stable non-mosaic ring chromosome 15, instead of one normal chromosome 15 [46,XY,r(15)(p11.2q26)] (Fig. 1). None of the 100 metaphases showed secondary aberrations. The karyotypes of the parents were normal. Array-CGH was carried out to characterize possible additional submicroscopic rearrangements associated with ring chromosome 15. DNA was extracted from the patient's peripheral white blood cells using salting out method [8]. aCGH was performed by Affymetrix CytoScan™ 750 K array and obtained data was analyzed using Chromosome Analysis Suite (ChAS) based on the Human reference genome (GRCh37/hg19). It revealed according to ISCN 2016 [9] as arr[GRCh37] 15q26.3(99550797_102429040)×1,15q26.3(99049746_99546177)×3, indicating for a 496 kb gain encompassing *IGF1R* gene, and for a loss of 2.8 Mb, both in 15q26.3, and the latter encompassing genes like *MEF2A, CHSY1, ADAMTS17, ADLH1A3* (Fig. 2). The genomic imbalance was later confirmed by fluorescence in situ hybridization (FISH) as well. For FISH various probes were applied, like a microdissection derived probe for all acrocentric p-arms (midi54 [10]), the locus-specific probe RP11-654A16 in 15q26.3 (GRCh37: 99338019_99529036), and two commercially available probes (Abbott/Vysis, Wiesbaden, Germany) for subtelomeric region in 15qter and a centromere-specific probe for 15p11.1-q11.1 (Fig. 3). No other relevant genomic imbalance was found, however; by aCGH not addressable short arm of ring chromosome 15 was also lost, as visualized by probe midi54.

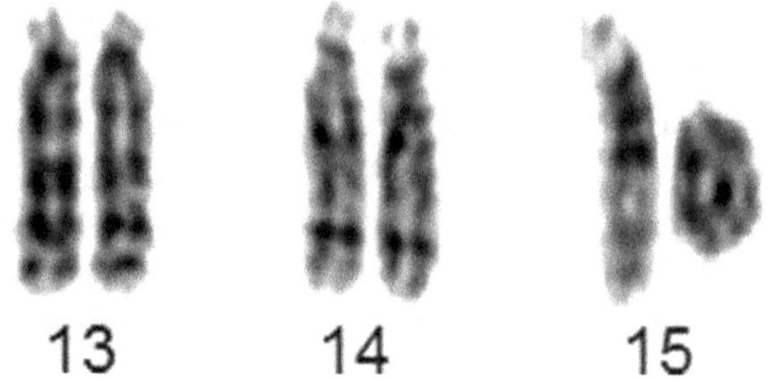


**Fig. 1** Partial karyotype showing ring chromosome 15, i.e. r(15)(p11.2q26)

Both parents were also investigated using aCGH and by quantitative polymerase chain reaction (qPCR) to rule out the inheritance of either duplication or deletion in the proband using following primers:

-to address *LRR28* gene, exon 5 [for deleted region]
5′ TTG AAG CCA TTG GGT CTC TT 3′
5′ CCT GGA GGT AGG AAT TGC AG 3′
-to address *IGF1R* gene, exon 13 [for duplicated region]
5′ ATC AGC GAG AAT GTG TGT CC-3′
5′ TTG GCC TGG ACA TAG AAG AA 3′.

qPCR established a de novo origin of deletion and duplication in the proband.

Selective capture and sequencing of the protein coding regions of the genes of the microcephaly panel (Additional file 1) was also performed, wherein no pathogenic and likely pathogenic variants causative of the reported phenotype was detected.

## Discussion and conclusion

Ring chromosome 15 is a rare finding, generally occurring as a de novo event [11]. Here, we report one of the few cases of a ring chromosome 15 that have been characterized using molecular cytogenetic technique – FISH and aCGH, which not only helped determine the exact breakpoints, enabling precise genotype-phenotype correlation, but also offered an insight into the plausible mechanisms of ring formation. Simultaneously, targeted gene sequencing of the microcephaly panel ruled out the presence of other causative mutations that could have possibly given rise to microcephaly with simplified gyral-pattern (MSG Group-1).

The results of aCGH showed a 2.8 Mb terminal deletion at 15q26.3 along with a 496 kb interstitial microduplication in the adjacent region. The findings were

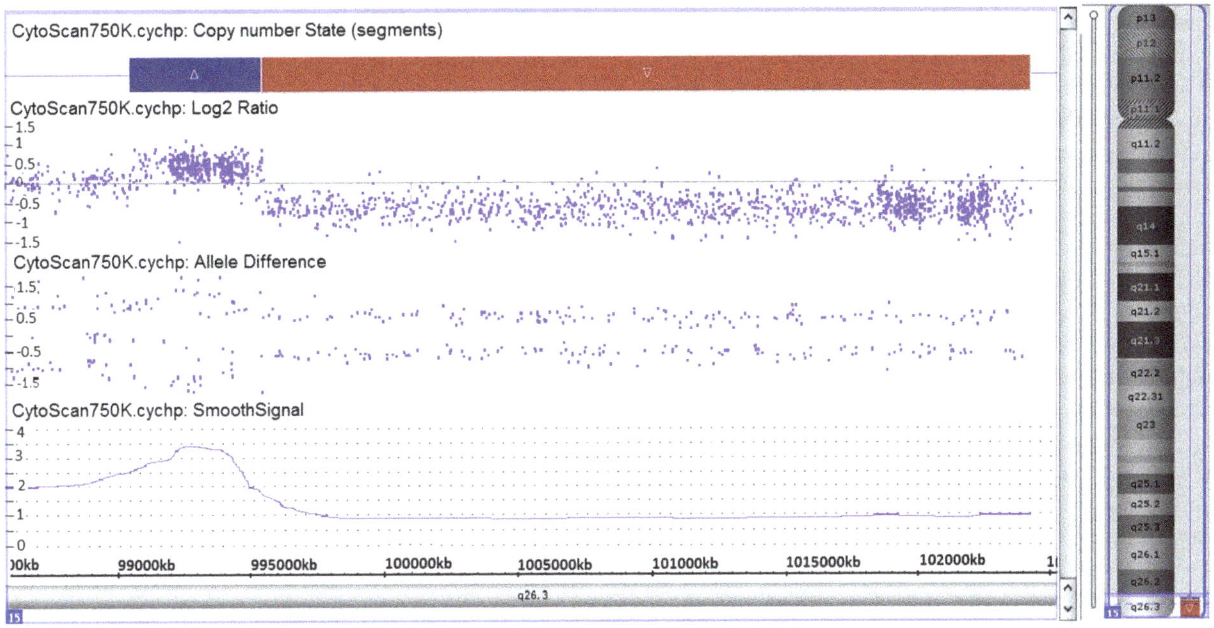


**Fig. 2** Array-CGH profile of the patient showing a 2.8 Mb loss at 15q26.3 and 496 kb gain at 15q26.3 i.e. arr[GRCh37] 15q26.3(99550797_102429040)×1,15q26.3(99049746_99546177)×3

further confirmed and refined for breakpoint in short arm by FISH analysis. Recent studies have discovered that a small proportion of ring chromosomes with terminally deleted segments are found to have a contiguous duplicated genomic segment [12, 13]. Knijnenburg et al. [12] and Rossi et al. [13] in their respective studies highlighted the presence and the underlying mechanisms of duplicated segments in ring chromosomes with terminal deletions and hypothesized that inverted duplication deletion rearrangements may have been stabilized by circularization that result into ring formation. Guilherme et al. [6] further concluded that phenotypic correlation in patients with ring chromosome cannot be done by assuming a simple deletion without excluding the detection of additional duplicated segments, thereby resulting in not just partial monosomy but also a partial trisomy [6]. They emphasized the importance of molecular genetic testing in detecting complex rearrangements like these, which are otherwise easily missed on conventional karyotyping. The present case, to the best of our knowledge, is only the second case of ring chromosome 15 with terminal deletion and a contiguous duplication at 15q26.3. The first one was reported by Rossi et al. in 2008 [13]. However, we could not determine the inverted/tandem nature of duplication due to its small size.

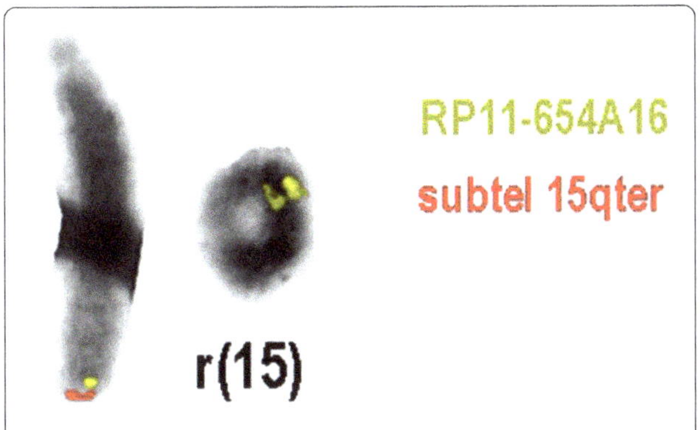


**Fig. 3** Partial karyotype showing comprehensive characterization of the chromosome ring15 in the proband's karyotype and was identified as 46,XY,r(15)(p11.2q26),ish r(15)(p11.2q26)(RP11-654A16++)(subtel15qter-)

In general, clinical phenotypes of patients with ring chromosomes may be related with different factors, including gene haploinsufficiency, gene duplications, ring instability and level of mosaicism [6, 7]; also, loss of ring chromosomes may lead for some chromosomes to mosaic karyotypes with 45 chromosomes [14]. The proband under report presented with primary observation of small head size and facial dysmorphism. On examination microcephaly, triangular face, micrognathia, small anterior frontanelle, slanted skull, hypotonia, unilateral simian crease, hypertelorism, umbilical hernia, micropenis with mild phimosis were noteworthy. Many patients with ring chromosome 15 syndrome frequently present with pre- and postnatal growth retardation, developmental delay, microcephaly, craniofacial dysmorphism, hypertelorism, café-au-lait spots and brachydactyly [4, 5]. The specific pattern of microcephaly with simplified gyral-pattern observed in the present case is being reported for the first time.

Only a couple of genes have been mapped to date in the distal part of chromosome 15, 15q26.3, one of which is Insulin like Growth Factor 1 Receptor gene (*IGF-1R*). Other morbid genes include *MEF2A* (*600660), *ADAMTS17* (*607511), *CERS3* (*615276), *CHSY1* (*608183), *ALDH1A3* (*600463) (DECIPHER database, https://decipher.sanger.ac.uk/). Apart from ring instability, marked growth deficiency in cases of ring chromosome 15 has been attributed to loss of *IGF-1R* [2, 3, 15–17]. Interestingly, a microduplication at 15q26.3 was detected in the current case, resulting in three copies of *IGF-1R*, which in turn has been linked to overgrowth and mental retardation [18]. However, the case under report had mild growth deficiency. Considering that the ring chromosome 15 was apparently stably transmitted during cell division, the plausible explanation for growth retardation could be the reduced level of expression of the *IGF1R* gene. The mechanisms responsible for the reduction of *IGF1R* expression are not clear but could have resulted from haploinsufficiency of a gene or genes within the deleted region that modifies *IGF1R* expression or the mechanism of gene silencing taking place due to a telomere position effect in which the 15p telomere silences nearby gene(s) on the q-arm or a spread of the heterochromatin-inactivated state of the centromere and short-arm (15p) DNA to the adjacent long arm (15q), also known as position effect variegation (PEV) [6, 19, 20]. In a recent paper Leffler et al. [19] proposed the possibility of *LRRK1* as being another growth regulating gene located at the distal region of 15q [19]. Few other authors too have questioned the role of *IGF-1R* gene as the sole growth determining factor [4, 15].

There is still a paucity of literature on ring chromosome 15 and further studies on genotype phenotype correlation are indicated. The case reported here, together with clinical and molecular findings highlights the importance of aCGH in detection and systematic evaluation of atypical ring chromosomes, especially in distinguishing rings with a duplication/deletion from those with a deletion only and thereby helping to delineate precise genotype-phenotype correlation. We would like to add that further expression studies of candidate genes located at 15q26.3 are essential to prove their biological significance in human growth and development.

**Abbreviations**

aCGH: Array based comparative genomic hybridization;
DNA: Deoxyribonucleic acid; FISH: Fluorescence In Situ Hybridization;
MRI: Magnetic Resonance Imaging;

**Acknowledgments**

We thank the patient and the parents for their cooperation. Special thanks to Dr. Sunil Trivedi for valuable suggestions and to Mr. Akhil Gupta and Ms. Priya Pandey for helping preparation of one of the figures.

**Funding**

This work is partly supported by Gujarat State Biotechnology Mission (GSBTM) [grant no.: GSBTM/MD/PROJECTS/SSA/505/4865/2016–17]. The funding agency was not involved in the study design, specimen collection, analysis, interpretation and preparation of the manuscript.

**Authors' contributions**

Conceived and designed the experiments: FS, JS. Clinical analysis: RS and FS. Cytogenetic and Molecular analysis: ABHA-R, FS. Wrote the first draft of the manuscript: ST, NL, FS. Made critical revisions and approved final version: FS, ST, KS and JS. All authors reviewed and approved of the final manuscript.

**Competing interests**

The authors declare that they have no competing interests (financial or non-financial).

**Author details**

[1]FRIGE's Institute of Human Genetics, FRIGE House, Jodhpur Gam Road, Satellite, Ahmedabad 380009, India. [2]Ankur Institute of Child Health, Ashram Road, Ahmedabad 380009, India. [3]Institute of Human Genetics, Am Klinikum 1, 07747 Jena, Germany.

**References**

1. Jacobsen P. A ring chromosome in the 13-15 group associated with microcephalic dwarfism, mental retardation and emotional immaturity. Hereditas. 1966;55:188–91.
2. Guilherme RS, Meloni Vde F, Takeno SS, Pellegrino R, Brunoni D, Kulikowski LD, et al. Twenty-year cytogenetic and molecular follow-up of a patient with ring chromosome 15: a case report. J Med Case Rep. 2012;6:283. doi:10.1186/1752-1947-6-283.
3. Gediya SG, Poswal L, Sanadhya A, Goyal S. Ring chromosome 15 presenting as short stature, intellectual disability and café-au-lait spots. Int J Res Med Sci. 2016;4(11):5087–9. DOI: http://dx.doi.org/10.18203/2320-6012.ijrms20163825
4. Nuutinen M, Kouvalainen K, Knip M. Good growth response to growth hormone treatment in the ring chromosome 15 syndrome. J Med Genet. 1995;32:486–8.
5. Butler MG, Fogo AB, Fuchs DA, Collins FS, Dev VG, Phillips JA. Brief clinical report and review. Two patients with ring chromosome 15 syndrome. Am J Med Genet. 1988;29:149–54.
6. Guilherme RS, Meloni VF, Kim CA, Pellegrino R, Takeno SS, Spinner NB, et al. Mechanisms of ring chromosome formation, ring instability and clinical consequences. BMC Med Genet. 2011;12:171. doi:10.1186/1471-2350-12-171.
7. Yip MY. Autosomal ring chromosomes in human genetic disorders. Transl Pediatr. 2015;4(2):164–74.
8. Miller SA, Dykes DD, Polesky HF. A simple salting out procedure for extracting DNA from human nucleated cells. Nucleic Acids Res. 1998;16(3):1215.
9. McGowan-Jordan J, Simons A, Schmid M. An international system for human cytogenetic nomenclature. Basal: S. Kager; 2016.
10. Starke H, Seidel J, Henn W, Reichardt S, Volleth M, Stumm M, Behrend C, Sandig KR, Kelbova C, Senger G, Albrecht B, Hansmann I, Heller A, Claussen U, Liehr T. Homologous sequences at human chromosome 9 bands p12

and q13-21.1 are involved in different patterns of pericentric rearrangements. Eur J Hum Genet. 2002;10(12):790–800.

11. Kosztolanyi G. Does "ring syndrome" exist? An analysis of 207 case reports on patients with a ring autosome. Hum Genet. 1987;75:174–9.
12. Knijnenburg J, van Haeringen A, Hansson KB, Lankester A, Smit MJ, Belfroid RD, et al. Ring chromosome formation as a novel escape mechanism in patients with inverted duplication and terminal deletion. Eur J Hum Genet 2007;15:548-555.
13. Rossi E, Riegel M, Messa J, Gimelli S, Maraschio P, Ciccone R, et al. Duplications in addition to terminal deletions are present in a proportion of ring chromosomes: clues to the mechanisms of formation. J Med Genet. 2008;45:147–54.
14. Koç A, Kan D, Karaer K, Ergün MA, Karaoğuz MY, Gücüyener K, Hinreiner S, Liehr T, Perçin EF. An unexpected finding in a child with neurological problems: mosaic ring chromosome 18. Eur J Pediatr. 2008;167(6):655–9.
15. Xu F, Zou CC, Liang L, Huang XM, Shao YN. Ring chromosome 15 syndrome: case report and literature review. HK J Paediatr (new series). 2011;16:175–9.
16. Tümer Z, Harboe TL, Blennow E, Kalscheuer VM, Tommerup N, Brøndum-Nielsen K. Molecular cytogenetic characterization of ring chromosome 15 in three unrelated patients. Am J Med Genet A. 2004;130A(4):340–4.
17. Kitatani M, Takahashi H, Ozaki M, Okino E, Maruoka T. A case of ring chromosome 15 accompanied by almost normal intelligence. Hum Genet. 1990;85:138–9.
18. Faivre L, Gosset P, Cormier-Daire V, Odent S, Amiel J, Giurgea I, et al. Overgrowth and trisomy 15q26.1-qter including the IGF1 receptor gene: report of two families and review of the literature. Eur J Hum Genet. 2002; 10:699–706.
19. Leffler M, Puusepp S, Žilina O, Zhu Y, Kuuse K, Bain N, et al. Two familial microduplications of 15q26.3 causing overgrowth and variable intellectual disability with normal copy number of IGF1R. Eur J Med Genet. 2016;59(4):257–62.
20. Kleinjan D, van Heyningen V. Position effect in human genetic disease. Hum Mol Genet 1998; 7(10):1611-1618.DOI: https://doi.org/10.1093/hmg/7.10.1611.

18

# Analysis of the accuracy of Z-scores of non-invasive prenatal testing for fetal Trisomies 13, 18, and 21 that employs the ion proton semiconductor sequencing platform

Yuan Tian[1], Linlin Zhang[1], Weifang Tian[1], Jinshuang Gao[1], Liting Jia[1*] and Shihong Cui[2]


## Abstract

**Background:** Non-invasive prenatal testing (NIPT) is frequently being used to screen for trisomies 13, 18 and 21 for prenatal diagnosis. However, NIPT performs poorly when compared with invasive testing and thus should not be used to diagnose trisomies. The result of NIPT for an individual woman in most genome-wide methods is calculated as a Z-score. The aim of this study was to assess the correlation between Z-scores of NIPT results and the accuracy of non-invasive prenatal testing.

**Results:** We evaluated 108 pregnant women with positive NIPT results, which were validated through karyotype analysis of amniotic fluid puncture by means of sequencing, bioinformatics analysis, and follow-up. Utilizing the ion proton semiconductor sequencing platform, we report a performance evaluation of NIPT-positive results at Third Affiliated Hospital of Zhengzhou University of Henan Province, China, by classifying Z-scores as $3 \leq Z<5$, $5 \leq Z < 9$ and $Z \geq 9$. The findings indicate that positive NIPT results at $Z \geq 9$ have a higher accuracy compared with positive NIPT results at $5 \leq Z < 9$ and $3 \leq Z<5$.

**Conclusions:** The findings show that Z-scores of NIPT results are closely related to the accuracy of non-invasive prenatal testing. However, false-positive NIPT results at $3 \leq Z<5$ may occur due to confined placental mosaicism (CPM).


**Keywords:** Non-invasive prenatal testing (NIPT), False positive, Confined placental mosaicism (CPM), Trisomies

## Background

Non-invasive prenatal testing (NIPT) is frequently being applied to screen for trisomies 13, 18 and 21 for prenatal diagnosis. Due to its simple operation and avoidance of amniocentesis, NIPT, as opposed to invasive procedures (chorionic villus sampling (CVS) or amniotic fluid), is regarded as the first choice when screening is required for fetal assessment in pregnant women. Indeed, NIPT is an attractive option because it is procedurally safe for both mother and fetus, can be conducted as early as 10 weeks of gestation, and is highly accurate [1]. Nonetheless, NIPT performs poorly when compared with invasive testing and thus should not be used to diagnose trisomies [2]. Confined placental mosaicism (CPM), which can occur through a mitotic nondisjunction event or through aneuploidy rescue, has one of the greatest obstacles on NIPT result confirmation [3]. CPM is a phenomenon whereby a cytogenetic abnormality, most often trisomy, is confined to the placenta [4]. False-positive NIPT results can occur due to CPM.

Recent NIPT technologies are predominantly based on next-generation sequencing (NGS) [5]. NGS enables rapid and effective clinical testing such as the IONA® test, which uses the Ion proton semiconductor sequencing platform, has a turnaround time, from the start of sample processing to the result, of 3 days [6]. For most genome-wide methods, the result of NIPT for an individual woman is calculated as a Z-score, where the

* Correspondence: jialiting@sina.com
[1]Department of Clinical Laboratory, The Third Affiliated Hospital of Zhengzhou University, No. 7 Front Kangfu Street, Er'qi District, Zhengzhou 450052, China
Full list of author information is available at the end of the article

individual sample is compared with a control group of normal (diploid) samples. In some research, an a posteriori risk (PPR) calculator is used to more accurately express the true likelihood of carrying a fetus with a trisomy. For an individual woman, a positive NIPT result with a sensitivity and specificity of more than 99% does not necessarily indicate that she actually has more than a 99% chance of carrying a fetus with a trisomy. The true likelihood depends not only on the NIPT result but also on the prevalence of the anomaly in the population to which she belongs [7], which is expressed as an a priori risk. Thus, to properly counsel women about a positive result by cell-free fetal DNA screening, it can be useful to express the result as a personalized PPR, which takes the woman's a priori risk into account. Research shows that PPR is effectively independent under all conditions for Z-scores above 6, and high PPR for low a priori risk can only be reached at Z-scores> 5 [8].

In the present study, we report a performance evaluation of NIPT-positive results in our hospital by classifying Z-scores as $3 \leq Z<5$, $5 \leq Z < 9$ and $Z \geq 9$. The results of our study indicate that positive NIPT results with Z-scores of $Z \geq 9$ have higher accuracy compared with positive NIPT results with Z-scores of $3 \leq Z<5$ and $5 \leq Z < 9$.

## Methods

### Patients

Written informed consent was obtained from each patient. The study was a retrospective analysis of NIPT-positive results in singleton pregnancies from January 2015 to December 2017 at Third Affiliated Hospital of Zhengzhou University of Henan Province, China. Positive NIPT results would be validated through postpartum follow-up of patients, involving the results of karyotype analysis via amniotic fluid puncture, including trisomies 13, 18, and 21 (T21, T18 and T13); 108 cases were validated in this manner.

### Sequencing process

Maternal peripheral blood (5 ml) was collected into an ethylenediaminetetraacetic acid (EDTA) tube at 12 + 0 to 25 + 6 weeks of gestation. The blood samples were stored at 4 °C immediately after collection. Plasma was isolated within 8 h through a two-step centrifugation protocol, after which the samples were stored at − 80 °C. Cell-free DNA extraction, library construction, sequencing, and bioinformatics analysis were performed according to a previous study [6].

### Bioinformatics analysis

Sequencing data were analyzed by using the ion proton semiconductor sequencing platform and software from Capitalbio Corporation. The binary hypothesis Z-score of particular chromosomes in each sample was determined, as reported previously [7]. To assess fetal risk of T21, T18 and T13, sample with a Z-score $\geq 3$ for these chromosomes was classified as positive. We classified the positive samples into three groups according to Z-score = 5 and Z = 9 among them. Group 1 contained samples with NIPT results of $3 \leq Z<5$. Group 2 contained samples with NIPT results of $5 \leq Z<9$. Group 3 contained samples with NIPT results of $Z \geq 9$.

### Karyotype analysis and amniotic fluid puncture

For those with positive NIPT results, karyotype analysis and amniotic fluid puncture were recommended for validation. Amniotic fluid puncture was performed as routinely described; karyotype analysis was performed according to the International System for Human Cytogenetic Nomenclature guidelines [9].

### Follow-up

Follow-up for NIPT-positive cases was performed via telephone. The follow-up duration was 56 days after delivery.

## Results

### Patient characteristics

A total of 21,114 pregnant women were tested by NIPT from 2015 to 2017, with 202 having positive results. According to follow-up, cases of induced labor that was not validated through other invasive methods were removed. Overall, 108 NIPT-positive women who were validated via karyotype analysis and amniotic fluid puncture, with a mean maternal age of 33.5 (19–48 years), were included in this study. Gestational age was from 12 weeks to 25 + 6 weeks at blood sample collection. Because the fetal DNA fraction in NIPT needs to be higher than 4% for a singleton and 8% for twins, pregnant women tend to accept NIPT at more than 16 weeks to obtain a higher fetal fraction. As cases of NIPT-positive results should be validated through karyotype analysis and amniotic fluid puncture, we would suggest that the patients accept NIPT within 20 weeks. The patient characteristics are listed in Table 1.

## Relationship of NIPT-positive results group 1 with karyotype analysis and amniotic fluid puncture

In total, 18 NIPT-positive cases were included in Group 1 ($3 \leq Z<5$); 15 cases with false-positive results were validated through karyotype analysis and amniotic fluid puncture. Conversely, 3 true-positive cases were validated through karyotype analysis and amniotic fluid puncture, with a positive predictive value (PPV) of only 16.67%. The NIPT-positive cases in Group 1 are listed in Table 2. By analyzing the data of the 3 true-positive NIPT cases, we found that the fetal DNA fraction

**Table 1** Basic Characteristics of 108 NIPT-Positive Patients

| Characteristics | Numbers |
|---|---|
| Maternal age(years) | |
| ≤ 20 | 1 |
| 20–24 | 5 |
| 25–29 | 31 |
| 30–34 | 21 |
| 35–39 | 35 |
| 40–45 | 13 |
| ≥ 45 | 2 |
| Mean | 33.5 |
| Range | 19–48 |
| Gestation at NIPT tests(weeks) | |
| 12–12 + 6 | 4 |
| 13–13 + 6 | 9 |
| 14–14 + 6 | 5 |
| 15–15 + 6 | 8 |
| 16–16 + 6 | 17 |
| 17–17 + 6 | 14 |
| 18–18 + 6 | 14 |
| 19–19 + 6 | 17 |
| 20–20 + 6 | 5 |
| 21–21 + 6 | 6 |
| 22–22 + 6 | 2 |
| 23–23 + 6 | 5 |
| 24–24 + 6 | 0 |
| 25–25 + 6 | 2 |

estimation for samples YC151439 and YC173711 was less than 4%; the fetal DNA fraction estimation for sample YC174141 was 6.4%, which was less than 8%.

## Relationship of NIPT-positive results for group 2 with karyotype analysis and amniotic fluid puncture

A total of 34 NIPT-positive cases were in Group 2 (5 ≤ Z<9). Four cases of false positivity were validated through karyotype analysis and amniotic fluid puncture. In contrast, 30 true-positive results were validated via karyotype analysis and amniotic fluid puncture, with a PPV of 88.24%. Table 3 lists the positive NIPT cases in Group 2.

Based on analysis of the data for the 4 false-positive cases, sample YC167160 was validated as CPM through karyotype analysis and amniotic fluid puncture (Table 3). Sample YC160356 was possibly affected by chromosome duplication from the maternal fragment (Fig. 1). The false-positive NIPT result for samples YC166422 and YC177345 might have resulted from a small region of chromosome duplication (Fig. 2 and Fig. 3).

**Table 2** The 18 NIPT-Positive Cases in Group 1 (3 ≤ Z<5)

| No. | Sample ID | Z-scores | NIPT results | Fetal karyotype |
|---|---|---|---|---|
| 1 | YC150550 | 3.330 | T21 | 46,XN |
| 2 | YC150816 | 4.342 | T13 | 46,XN |
| 3 | YC151439 | 3.643 | T21 | 47,XN + 21 |
| 4 | YC161217 | 4.056 | T13 | 46,XN |
| 5 | YC163341 | 4.778 | T13 | 46,XN |
| 6 | YC164267 | 3.968 | T13 | 46,XN |
| 7 | YC165157 | 3.392 | T21 | 46,XN |
| 8 | YC165602 | 3.362 | T18 | 46,XN |
| 9 | YC167031 | 3.075 | T21 | 46,XN |
| 10 | YC171503 | 3.207 | T21 | 46,XN |
| 11 | YC173711 | 4.951 | T21 | 47,XN + 21 |
| 12 | YC174141 | 3.242 | T21 | 47,XN + 21 |
| 13 | YC175988 | 3.713 | T21 | 46,XN |
| 14 | YC175996 | 4.111 | T18 | 46,XN |
| 15 | YC176477 | 3.351 | T18 | 46,XN |
| 16 | YC176775 | 3.620 | T21 | 46,XN |
| 17 | YC177355 | 3.263 | T21 | 46,XN |
| 18 | YC177383 | 3.697 | T13 | 46,XN |

## Relationship of NIPT-positive results for group 3 with karyotype analysis and amniotic fluid puncture

Group 3 (Z ≥ 9) comprised 56 cases of NIPT positivity. Only one false-positive case was validated by karyotype analysis and amniotic fluid puncture. For sample YC175377, a unique sample with a false-positive result, a unique sample with a false-positive result, the discordant NIPT result was caused by a vanished twin, as revealed by NIPT in the 4 weeks during follow-up. In total, 55 true-positive cases were validated through karyotype analysis and amniotic fluid puncture; the PPV was 98.12%. The positive NIPT cases in Group 3 are listed in Table 4.

Among all of the 21,114 patients accepting NIPT, two cases of false-negative NIPT results were found. However, those with false-negative NIPT results refused to accept further validation of aborted tissue.

## Discussion

NIPT has been widely used in the last few years for prenatal screening of T21, T18 and T13. Although PPR calculation suggests that high PPR for low a priori risk can only be reached at Z-scores> 5 [7], large-scale clinical studies to validate the hypothesis are lacking. The present study including 108 NIPT-positive cases was

**Table 3** The 34 NIPT-Positive Cases in Group 2 (5 ≤ Z<9)

| No. | Sample ID | Z-scores | NIPT results | Fetal karyotype |
|---|---|---|---|---|
| 1 | YC150539 | 5.570 | T21 | 47,XN + 21 |
| 2 | YC150431 | 5.960 | T18 | 47,XN + 18 |
| 3 | YC150725 | 7.463 | T21 | 47,XN + 21 |
| 4 | YC152284 | 8.249 | T21 | 47,XN + 21 |
| 5 | YC153184 | 8.532 | T21 | 47,XN + 21 |
| 6 | YC160356 | 8.830 | T21 | 46,XN |
| 7 | YC161880 | 8.188 | T21 | 47,XN + 21 |
| 8 | YC163276 | 5.467 | T18 | 47,XN + 18 |
| 9 | YC163808 | 6.104 | T21 | 47,XN + 21 |
| 10 | YC164065 | 5.219 | T18 | 47,XN + 18 |
| 11 | YC164811 | 8.489 | T21 | 47,XN + 21 |
| 12 | YC165074 | 6.677 | T21 | 47,XN + 21 |
| 13 | YC165729 | 5.944 | T21 | 47,XN + 21 |
| 14 | YC166180 | 6.150 | T21 | 47,XN + 21 |
| 15 | YC166202 | 6.220 | T18 | 47,XN + 18 |
| 16 | YC166253 | 5.931 | T21 | 46XX + 21, der(14;15)(q10,q10) |
| 17 | YC166422 | 8.945 | T13 | 46,XN |
| 18 | YC167160 | 5.710 | T18 | 46,XX/47,XX + 18(28:2) |
| 19 | YC167331 | 7.790 | T21 | 47,XN + 21 |
| 20 | YC168025 | 6.840 | T21 | 47,XN + 21 |
| 21 | YC170096 | 8.280 | T21 | 47,XN + 21 |
| 22 | YC171234 | 6.119 | T21 | 47,XN + 21 |
| 23 | YC171535 | 7.273 | T21 | 47,XN + 21 |
| 24 | YC171540 | 6.019 | T21 | 47,XN + 21 |
| 25 | YC173331 | 5.330 | T21 | 47,XN + 21 |
| 26 | YC173539 | 7.514 | T21 | 47,XN + 21 |
| 27 | YC173759 | 6.834 | T21 | 47,XN + 21 |
| 28 | YC175051 | 6.908 | T21 | 47,XN + 21 |
| 29 | YC175492 | 8.646 | T18 | 47,XN + 18 |
| 30 | YC175694 | 6.704 | T13 | 47,XN + 13 |
| 31 | YC176740 | 7.803 | T21 | 47,XN + 21 |
| 32 | YC177345 | 5.178 | T21 | 46,XN |
| 33 | YC176881 | 5.566 | T21 | 47,XN + 21 |
| 34 | YC177644 | 8.523 | T21 | 47,XN + 21 |

performed to investigate the relationship between NIPT Z-scores and accuracy of trisomy 13, 18, and 21 diagnosis.

The PPV is much more meaningful to clinicians and patients than the commonly reported measures of sensitivity and specificity [10]. The PPV referred to here is a population-based figure that reports the chance prior to testing that an abnormal test result is actually reflective of the karyotype of the fetus. Except for the PPV, neither sensitivity nor specificity reflects the prevalence of a disorder in the population [10]. Based on the results of the present study, a sample with Z ≥ 9 has higher accuracy than does a sample with 3 ≤ Z<5 or 5 ≤ Z<9. Although the PPV rate in Group 2 (88.24%) was apparently higher that of Group 1 (16.67%), this approach cannot be used for diagnosis because of the relatively high false-positive rate (11.76%). Nonetheless, positive results at Z ≥ 9 are significant for diagnosing trisomies 13, 18 and 21; However, karyotype analysis is necessary for validating trisomies due to the exist of sample YC175377, whose discordant NIPT result may be caused by a vanished twin. There are many biological reasons for discordant results that can be of either fetal or maternal origin. Contributing fetal factors include an insufficient or absent fetal fraction, confined placental mosaicism and the presence of a vanishing twin [11]. For example, Hall AL et al. reported a case that confirmed positive cell-free fetal DNA (cffDNA) testing for trisomy 13, revealing confined placental mosaicism [12]. In addition, Chen C et al. reported a pregnancy with discordant fetal and placental chromosome 18 aneuploidies, as revealed by invasive and noninvasive prenatal diagnoses [13].

CPM is one of the major factors causing false positivity. cffDNA originates from chorionic villi in the placenta, where the constant turnover of cytotrophoblasts induces apoptosis and cffDNA release into the maternal blood. The cytotrophoblast layer of chorionic villi is not always representative of the fetus, as it is derived from the trophoblast of the blastocyst; in contrast, the fetus is derived from the inner cell mass (epiblast) [14]. Postzygotic mitotic division errors in chromosomally normal

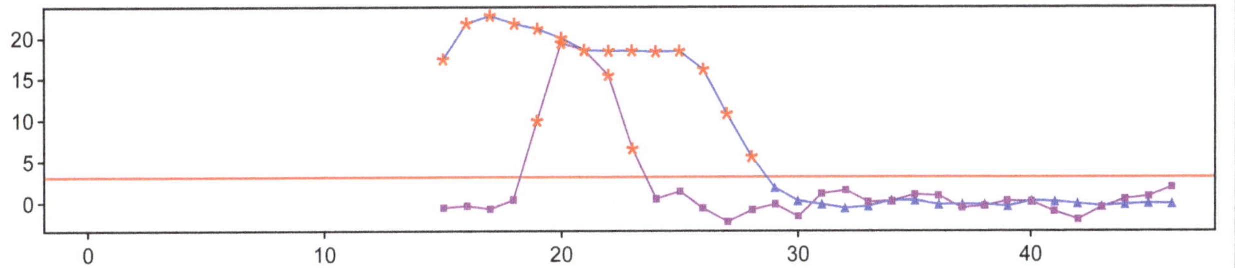


**Fig. 1** The Distribution Curve of Z-scores for Chromosome 21 of Sample YC160356

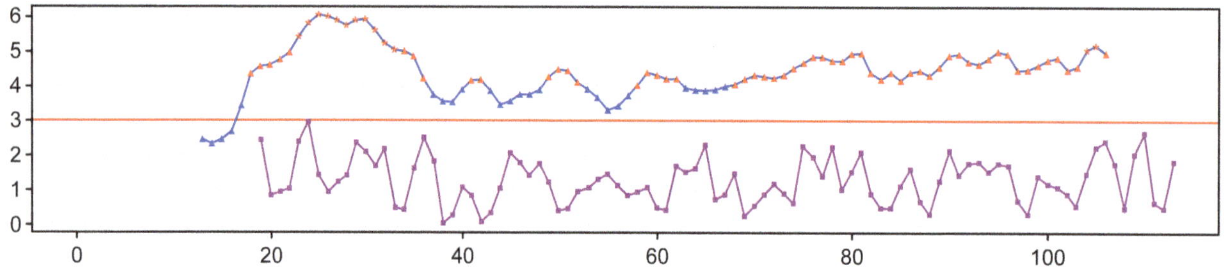


**Fig. 2** The Distribution Curve of Z-scores for Chromosome 13 of Sample YC166422

and abnormal conceptuses will lead to chromosomal mosaicism [15]. Most often, mosaicism is characterized as CPM, in which the abnormal cell line is confined to the cytotrophoblast and/or the mesenchymal core of the chorion villi, whereas the fetus has a normal karyotype [15]. If abnormal cells are restricted to the cytotrophoblast layer and are not present in the mesenchymal core or fetus, such a case is categorized CPM and depending on the extent of mosaicism, will possibly cause a false-positive NIPT result. According to the above, we suggest that the occurrence of CPM may slightly elevate a Z-score for NIPT, higher than 3 but lower than 5.

In addition, estimation of the fetal DNA fraction is important for the accuracy of NIPT results. The definition of the fetal fraction of circulating cell-free DNA in maternal blood is the amount of cffDNA divided by the amount of total cell-free DNA. The circulating cell-free DNA (cfDNA) in a pregnant woman is a mixture of predominant maternal DNA derived from her hematopoietic system and fetal DNA released through apoptosis of cytotrophoblast cells during fetal development [16]. A fetal DNA concentration of less than 4% in a maternal plasma sample would suggest a potential issue present in the quality control (QC) step [17]. Methods for calculating the fetal fraction differ between laboratories. We are aware of six different methods based on methylation [18], single-nucleotide polymorphisms [19], quantitative polymerase chain reaction of the Y-chromosome (only for male fetuses) [20], autosomal regional read counts calculated by SeqFF [21], differences in length between cffDNA and maternal cffDNA [21] and single reads nucleosome-based fetal fraction [22]. The fetal fraction is also related to maternal weight and body mass index. For example, the increased turnover of adipocytes in obese women increases the amount of maternal cell-free DNA and decreases the cffDNA fraction [23]. Furthermore, gestational age influences the fetal fraction. Some research has found that levels of cffDNA increase at 0.1% per week between 10 and 21 weeks of gestation and at 1% per week beyond 21 weeks of gestation [24]. Because the limited amount of fetal DNA molecules to be detected and analyzed may give rise to a false-negative result, we deduce that the Z-scores of samples YC151439, YC173711 and YC174141 were less than 5 because of the estimation of a low fetal DNA fraction.

Regardless, maternally derived chromosomal abnormalities (likely also submicroscopic abnormalities) constitute a rare case of maternal occult malignancy and usually cause false-positive results [25]. Our study validated the hypothesis regarding the false-positive NIPT result for sample YC160356 (Fig. 1).

## Conclusions

NIPT is feasible for prenatal screening of T13, T18 and T21, with higher sensitivity and specificity compared with conventional methods. However, Z-scores of NIPT results are closely related to the accuracy of non-invasive prenatal

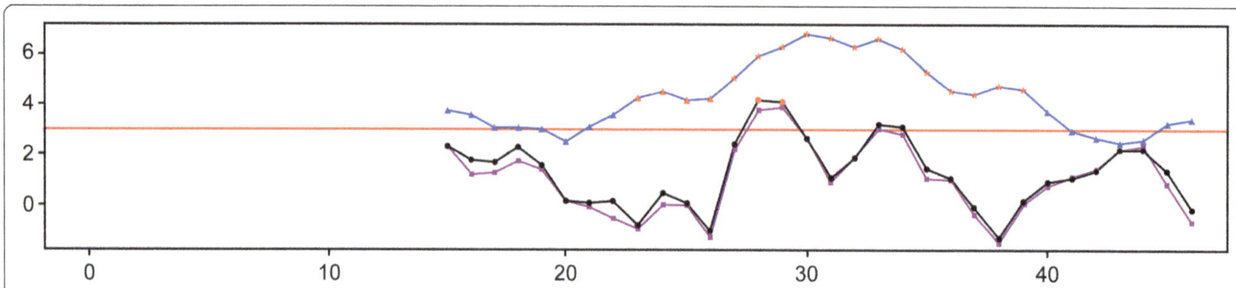


**Fig. 3** The Distribution Curve of Z-scores for Chromosome 21 of Sample YC177345

**Table 4** The 56 NIPT-Positive Cases in Group 2 (Z ≥ 9)

| No. | Sample ID | Z-scores | NIPT results | Fetal karyotype |
|---|---|---|---|---|
| 1 | YC151198 | 11.203 | T21 | 47,XN + 21 |
| 2 | YC151297 | 11.605 | T21 | 47,XN + 21 |
| 3 | YC151374 | 9.306 | T21 | 47,XN + 21 |
| 4 | YC151424 | 19.541 | T21 | 47,XN + 21 |
| 5 | YC151577 | 14.882 | T21 | 47,XN + 21 |
| 6 | YC151725 | 12.367 | T21 | 47,XN + 21 |
| 7 | YC152585 | 18.082 | T21 | 47,XN + 21 |
| 8 | YC153464 | 10.126 | T21 | 47,XN + 21 |
| 9 | YC153533 | 11.864 | T21 | 47,XN + 21 |
| 10 | YC160344 | 14.298 | T21 | 47,XN + 21 |
| 11 | YC161058 | 10.8 | T21 | 47,XN + 21 |
| 12 | YC161066 | 21.457 | T21 | 47,XN + 21 |
| 13 | YC161368 | 13.275 | T21 | 47,XN + 21 |
| 14 | YC162688 | 9.707 | T21 | 47,XN + 21 |
| 15 | YC162822 | 16.21 | T18 | 47,XN + 18 |
| 16 | YC162943 | 11.347 | T21 | 47,XN + 21 |
| 17 | YC163223 | 13.694 | T21 | 47,XN + 21 |
| 18 | YC163261 | 13.627 | T21 | 47,XN + 21 |
| 19 | YC163310 | 13.977 | T18 | 47,XN + 18 |
| 20 | YC163400 | 11.603 | T13 | 47,XN + 13 |
| 21 | YC164204 | 10.546 | T21 | 47,XN + 21 |
| 22 | YC164355 | 11.135 | T21 | 47,XN + 21 |
| 23 | YC164722 | 13.955 | T21 | 47,XN + 21 |
| 24 | YC164999 | 13.661 | T21 | 47,XN + 21 |
| 25 | YC165003 | 11.899 | T18 | 47,XN + 18 |
| 26 | YC165723 | 10.192 | T21 | 47,XN + 21 |
| 27 | YC165823 | 10.346 | T18 | 47,XN + 18 |
| 28 | YC165859 | 11.962 | T18 | 47,XN + 18 |
| 29 | YC166626 | 9.374 | T13 | 47,XN + 13 |
| 30 | YC167544 | 11.253 | T18 | 47,XN + 18 |
| 31 | YC168149 | 11.004 | T21 | 47,XN + 21 |
| 32 | YC170133 | 12.085 | T21 | 47,XN + 21 |
| 33 | YC170411 | 12.536 | T21 | 47,XN + 21 |
| 34 | YC170724 | 10.017 | T21 | 47,XN + 21 |
| 35 | YC170829 | 12.456 | T21 | 47,XN + 21 |
| 36 | YC170974 | 11.555 | T21 | 47,XN + 21 |
| 37 | YC171134 | 9.885 | T21 | 47,XN + 21 |
| 38 | YC171423 | 11.41 | T21 | 47,XN + 21 |
| 39 | YC172015 | 18.693 | T21 | 47,XN + 21 |
| 40 | YC172946 | 20.224 | T21 | 47,XN + 21 |
| 41 | YC173326 | 9.674 | T21 | 47,XN + 21 |
| 42 | YC173370 | 17.431 | T21 | 47,XN + 21 |
| 43 | YC173573 | 26.587 | T21 | 47,XN + 21 |
| 44 | YC173742 | 9.054 | T21 | 47,XN + 21 |
| 45 | YC174011 | 13.767 | T21 | 47,XN + 21 |
| 46 | YC174110 | 11.488 | T21 | 47,XN + 21 |
| 47 | YC174589 | 16.765 | T21 | 47,XN + 21 |
| 48 | YC175377 | 12.367 | T18 | 46,XN |
| 49 | YC175406 | 11.424 | T21 | 47,XN + 21 |
| 50 | YC175583 | 9.772 | T21 | 47,XN + 21 |
| 51 | YC175824 | 13.609 | T21 | 47,XN + 21 |
| 52 | YC175903 | 12.095 | T21 | 47,XN + 21 |
| 53 | YC176469 | 11.443 | T18 | 47,XN + 18 |
| 54 | YC177386 | 25.448 | T18 | 47,XN + 18 |
| 55 | YC176915 | 12.225 | T21 | 47,XN + 21 |
| 56 | YC178093 | 18.509 | T18 | 47,XN + 18 |

testing that employs the ion proton semiconductor sequencing platform. NIPT results with low Z-scores should not be used for diagnosis, which should be performed using invasive testing. However, the relationship between Z-scores of NIPT and CPM lacks validation by clinical trials due to the influence of chorionic villi in the placenta.

#### Abbreviations

cfDNA: Circulating cell-free DNA; CPM: Confined placental mosaicism; EDTA: Ethylenediaminetetraacetic acid; NIPT: Non-invasive prenatal testing; QC: Quality control

#### Author contributions

YT performed the bioinformatics analysis and drafted the manuscript. LZ performed karyotype analysis, amniotic fluid puncture and follow-up. WT recruited the patients, provided blood samples and clinical data for each participant and helped to draft the manuscript. JG performed the NIPT. LJ performed the statistical analysis and helped to draft the manuscript. SC took a plan for the research. All authors read and approved the final manuscript.

#### Funding

National Key Research and Development Program of China,2016YFC1000700,2016YFC1000703.

#### Competing interests

The authors declare that they have no competing interests.

#### Author details

[1]Department of Clinical Laboratory, The Third Affiliated Hospital of Zhengzhou University, No. 7 Front Kangfu Street, Er'qi District, Zhengzhou 450052, China. [2]Department of gynaecology and obstetrics, The Third Affiliated Hospital of Zhengzhou University, No. 7 Front Kangfu Street, Er'qi District, Zhengzhou 450052, China.

**References**

1. Minear MA, Lewis C, Pradhan S, et al. Global perspectives on clinical adoption of NIPT. Prenat Diagn. 2015;35(10):959–67.
2. Lau TK, Cheung SW, Lo PS, et al. Non-invasive prenatal testing for fetal chromosomal abnormalities by low-coverage whole-genome sequencing of maternal plasma DNA: review of 1982 consecutive cases in a single center. Ultrasound Obstet Gynecol. 2014;43(3):254–64.
3. Mardy A, Wapner RJ. Confined placental mosaicism and its impact on confirmation of NIPT results. Am J Med Genet C Semin Med Genet. 2016; 172(2):118–22.
4. Kalousek DK, Vekemans M. Confined placental mosaicism. J Med Genet. 1996;33(7):529–33.
5. Vrachnis N, Vlachadis N, Creatsas G. DNA sequencing versus standard prenatal aneuploidy screening. N Engl J Med. 2014;371(6):578.
6. Papageorghiou AT, Khalil A, Forman M, et al. Clinical evaluation of the IONA test: a non-invasive prenatal screening test for trisomies 21, 18 and 13. Ultrasound Obstet Gynecol. 2016;47(2):188–93.
7. Morain S, Greene MF, Mello MM. A new era in noninvasive prenatal testing. N Engl J Med. 2013;369(6):499–501.
8. Sikkema-Raddatz B, Johansson LF, de Boer EN, et al. NIPTRIC: an online tool for clinical interpretation of non-invasive prenatal testing (NIPT) results. Sci Rep. 2016;6:38359.
9. Gonzalez GJ, Meza-Espinoza JP. Use of the international system for human cytogenetic nomenclature (ISCN). BLOOD. 2006;108(12):3952–3.
10. Meck JM, Kramer DE, Matyakhina L, et al. Noninvasive prenatal screening for aneuploidy: positive predictive values based on cytogenetic findings. Am J Obstet Gynecol. 2015;213(2):211–4.
11. Grati FR. Implications of fetoplacental mosaicism on cell-free DNA testing: a review of a common biological phenomenon. Ultrasound Obstet Gynecol. 2016;48(4):415–23.
12. Hall AL, Drendel HM, Verbrugge JL, et al. Positive cell-free fetal DNA testing for trisomy 13 reveals confined placental mosaicism. GENET MED. 2013; 15(9):729–32.
13. Chen C, Cram DS, Xie F, et al. A pregnancy with discordant fetal and placental chromosome 18 aneuploidies revealed by invasive and noninvasive prenatal diagnosis. Reprod BioMed Online. 2014;29(1):136–9.
14. Bianchi DW, Wilkins-Haug LE, Enders AC, et al. Origin of extraembryonic mesoderm in experimental animals: relevance to chorionic mosaicism in humans. Am J Med Genet. 1993;46(5):542–50.
15. Malvestiti F, Agrati C, Grimi B, et al. Interpreting mosaicism in chorionic villi: results of a monocentric series of 1001 mosaics in chorionic villi with follow-up amniocentesis. Prenat Diagn. 2015;35(11):1117–27.
16. Peng XL, Jiang P. Bioinformatics Approaches for Fetal DNA Fraction Estimation in Noninvasive Prenatal Testing. Int J Mol Sci. 2017:18(2).
17. Canick JA, Palomaki GE, Kloza EM, et al. The impact of maternal plasma DNA fetal fraction on next generation sequencing tests for common fetal aneuploidies. Prenat Diagn. 2013;33(7):667–74.
18. Poon LL, Leung TN, Lau TK, et al. Differential DNA methylation between fetus and mother as a strategy for detecting fetal DNA in maternal plasma. Clin Chem. 2002;48(1):35–41.
19. Dar P, Curnow KJ, Gross SJ, et al. Clinical experience and follow-up with large scale single-nucleotide polymorphism-based noninvasive prenatal aneuploidy testing. Am J Obstet Gynecol. 2014;211(5):521–7.
20. Hudecova I, Sahota D, Heung MM, et al. Maternal plasma fetal DNA fractions in pregnancies with low and high risks for fetal chromosomal aneuploidies. PLoS One. 2014;9(2):e88484.
21. Kim SK, Hannum G, Geis J, et al. Determination of fetal DNA fraction from the plasma of pregnant women using sequence read counts. Prenat Diagn. 2015;35(8):810–5.
22. Straver R, Oudejans CB, Sistermans EA, et al. Calculating the fetal fraction for noninvasive prenatal testing based on genome-wide nucleosome profiles. Prenat Diagn. 2016;36(7):614–21.
23. Haghiac M, Vora NL, Basu S, et al. Increased death of adipose cells, a path to release cell-free DNA into systemic circulation of obese women. Obesity (Silver Spring). 2012;20(11):2213–9.
24. Wang E, Batey A, Struble C, et al. Gestational age and maternal weight effects on fetal cell-free DNA in maternal plasma. Prenat Diagn. 2013; 33(7):662–6.
25. Bianchi DW, Chudova D, Sehnert AJ, et al. Noninvasive prenatal testing and incidental detection of occult maternal malignancies. JAMA. 2015; 314(2):162–9.

19

# Cytogenetic/mutation profile of chronic lymphocytic leukemia/malignant melanoma collision tumors of the skin

Roberta La Starza[1†], Tiziana Pierini[1†], Lorenza Pastorino[2], Elisa Albi[1], Caterina Matteucci[1], Barbara Crescenzi[1], Paolo Sportoletti[1], Piero Covarelli[3], Franca Falzetti[1], Giovanni Roti[4], Stefano Ascani[5] and Cristina Mecucci[1*]

## Abstract

**Background:** Collision tumors are rare entities that consist of two histologically distinct tumor types arising in the same anatomic site. An association between chronic lymphocytic leukemia (CLL) and malignant melanoma (MM) has been already described. Up to now, they have been documented only at positive regional lymph nodes while we focused on collision tumor in a skin lesion.

**Case presentation:** We characterized the genomic profile of a skin CLL/MM collision tumor in a patient with a 9-years story of CLL. Typical high-grade genomic biomarkers featured the CLL: the immunoglobulin heavy variable genes were unmutated; a clonal del(11q), involving *ATM* and *BIRC3*, was present in the peripheral blood (PB) and skin lesion, while a subclonal large del(13q)/D13S319-*RB1* was detected only in the PB. Interestingly, the del(13q) clone, increased from 10% to 46% from diagnosis to relapse. *NOTCH1*, *SF3B1*, and *TP53* were wild type. The MM lesion carried a $BRAF^{V600E}$ and a *TERT* promoter mutation.
As the family story was consistent with a genetic predisposition to cancer, we performed mutational analysis of genes involved in familial melanoma and CLL, and of *BRCA1* and *BRCA2*. No germinal mutation known to predispose to CLL, MM, or breast cancer was found. Interestingly, conventional cytogenetic detected a constitutional t(12;17)(p13;p13).

**Conclusions:** Our data are consistent with distinct genetic landscape of the two tumors which were characterized by specific disease-related abnormalities. CLL cells carried poor prognostic imbalances, i.e. large deletions of the long arm of chromosomes 11 and 13, while in MM cells two functionally linked mutations, i.e. $BRAF^{V600E}$ and a *TERT* promoter occurred. Although, known germline variations predisposing to MM and/or CLL were ruled out, genetic counseling suggested the proband family was at high risk for MM.

**Keywords:** Collision tumor, CLL, Melanoma, Molecular cytogenetics, Mutational analysis

## Background

CLL, the most frequent hematological disease in adults, is characterized by a marked variable outcome, from an indolent clinical course to more aggressive forms with acquisition of chemo-resistance, after a benign onset. CLL evolution is largely dependent upon molecular and cytogenetic features which are well recognized prognostic markers [1, 2]. Of note, 30–35% of long-term CLL survivors are at high risk of developing secondary neoplasms mostly epithelial. This susceptibility do not appear to depend on anti-neoplastic treatment as the same incidence of leukemia was observed in treated and untreated patients [3]. Namely, CLL patients have a four-fold increase in the risk of developing MM compared with the general population.

MM and CLL collision tumors were reported, as occasional findings, in metastatic lymph nodes of patients with cutaneous MM [4, 5]. A collision tumor is defined as the occurrence of two neoplastic cell populations in

* Correspondence: cristina.mecucci@unipg.it
†Equal contributors
[1]Molecular Medicine Laboratory, Hematology and Bone Marrow Transplantation Unit, University of Perugia, Hospital S. Maria della Misericordia, Piazzale Menghini n.9, 06132 Perugia, Italy
Full list of author information is available at the end of the article

close proximity to each other, though maintaining separate boundaries. Combination of solid and hematological neoplasms, such as colon or breast carcinoma or MM, in conjunction with non-Hodgkin lymphoma or CLL, are the most frequent association [6, 7].

We report the molecular-cytogenetic characterization of a unique case of CLL and MM collision tumors. Our molecular findings are consistent with an independent origin of the two tumors and suggest that both a familial predisposition and the CLL-associated immune dysregulation might have played a role in their onset.

## Case presentation

At diagnosis of CLL (Rai stage I; Binet stage B), the patient, a 58 year-old male, had 20.150/mmc white blood cells with 75% lymphocytes. The bone marrow (BM) biopsy showed a diffuse pattern of infiltration by small CD20, CD5, CD23, CD38, and ZAP70 positive lymphoid elements with unmutated immunoglobulin heavy chain. The patient was treated with 6 cycles of fludarabine, cyclophosphamide, and rituximab, achieving hematological remission. He relapsed after 79 months from diagnosis with marked lymphocytosis (211.100/mmc) and widespread lymphadenopathy; PET scan assessed lymph nodes hyperactivity (SUV max 6.1). At this time, the patient presented a 17 × 13 mm skin lesion plus twenty-three ~5 mm lesions on the right side of the trunk. Histology and immunohistochemical features of the main lesion and in-transit metastasis were consistent with a diagnosis of collision CLL and MM tumors. The MM lesion infiltrated the epidermal layer and the reticulis dermis (Breslow thickness of 3,4 mm; mitosis 3/mm2) and showed pigmentation, regression, and ulceration. The MM was classified as stage T3N2M0. The underlying dermis, and partially the hypodermis, were infiltrated by small CD20, CD5, CD23 positive, CD3 and cyclin D1 negative lymphoid cells (Fig. 1).

MM treatment consisted of wide local excision of the primary lesion, surgical dissection of 71 axillary lymph nodes (all positive for CLL involvement), and electrochemotherapy with intravenous injection of bleomycin for three times, which elicit a short lasting complete remission (9 months) of skin lesions. CLL treatment consisted of 6 cycles of bendamustine and rituximab which induced the hematological remission of CLL.

At MM relapse, a combined treatment with BRAF (dabrafenib) and MEK (trametinib) inhibitors was started. He is still under treatment and in remission of MM skin lesions.

## Methods

### Genetic counseling

The family story satisfied the criteria of familial melanoma as two first-degree relatives, the proband and his brother developed MM [8]. In particular, the brother was affected by 4 cutaneous MM. Additionally, the proband's mother and sister had both suffered of breast cancer, at the age of 49 and 51, respectively (Fig. 2a). Genetic testing was performed by Ion Personal Genome Machine® (PGM™) Sequencer (Thermo Fisher Scientific Inc., Monza, Italy) using a custom familial melanoma panel including *BAP1*, *CDKN2A*, *CDK4*, *TERT* promoter (p*TERT*), *MITF* exon 10, *ATM*, *PALB2*, and *POT1*; *TERF2IP* and *ACD*, also known to be involved in familial CLL [9]. Sanger's sequencing investigated *BRCA1* and *BRCA2* and validated next generation sequencing findings (3500 Genetic Analyzer-Life Technologies, Monza, Italy). Constitutional karyotype of the proband and his brother and sister, was done on phytohaemagglutinin (PHA) stimulated peripheral blood (PB) T-lymphocytes.

### Molecular-cytogenetic studies

All studies were carried out in accordance with the Declaration of Helsinki. Written informed consent was obtained from the patient for publication of clinical history and any additional related information. The study was approved by the Bioethics Committee of the University of Perugia (prot. Number 2014–019).

A specific CLL panel probes (LSI ATM SO/CEP11 SG, LSI TP53 SO/CEP17 SG, LSI D13S319/LSI 13q34/CEP12 Multi-color probe set, LSI 13 RB1 SO, LSI D13S319 SO and LSI IgH dual color break-apart; Vysis Abbott, Milan, Italy), was applied on PB samples taken at diagnosis and relapse, and on formalin-fixed paraffin embedded skin lesion after marking the MM and CLL areas according to haematoxylin/eosin staining. Home-made probes were also used to investigate the 11q region, by *BIRC3*/11q22.2 (RP11-605B8) and *DDX10*/11q22.3 (RP11-244G23), and the *RB1*/13q14.2 (RP11-305D15, RP11-174I10) (UCSC Genome Browser, Human/Feb.2009 GRCh37/hg19). Analysis was carried out on 200 nuclei/100 cells per experiment with fluorescence microscopy using an Olympus BX61 (Olympus, Milan, Italy) equipped with a JAI camera (Copenhagen, Denmark) and CytoVision 4.5.4 software (Genetix, New Milton, Hampshire, UK). CLL and MM areas were analyzed separately.

Hot-spot mutations of *BRAF*, p*TERT*, *SF3B1*, *NOTCH1*, and the whole coding region of *TP53* were studied by Denaturing High Performance Liquid Chromatography (DHPLC) and/or Sanger's sequencing of genomic DNA samples extracted from skin biopsy after macro-dissection to separate MM from CLL.

## Results

FISH (fluorescent in situ hybridization) analysis of the CLL skin lesion detected a monoallelic del(11)(q23) with loss of a large 11q region, involving *ATM* and *BIRC3* (Fig. 2c). Besides del(11)(q23), PB samples also carried a del(13q). Double-color FISH assay combining probes for common

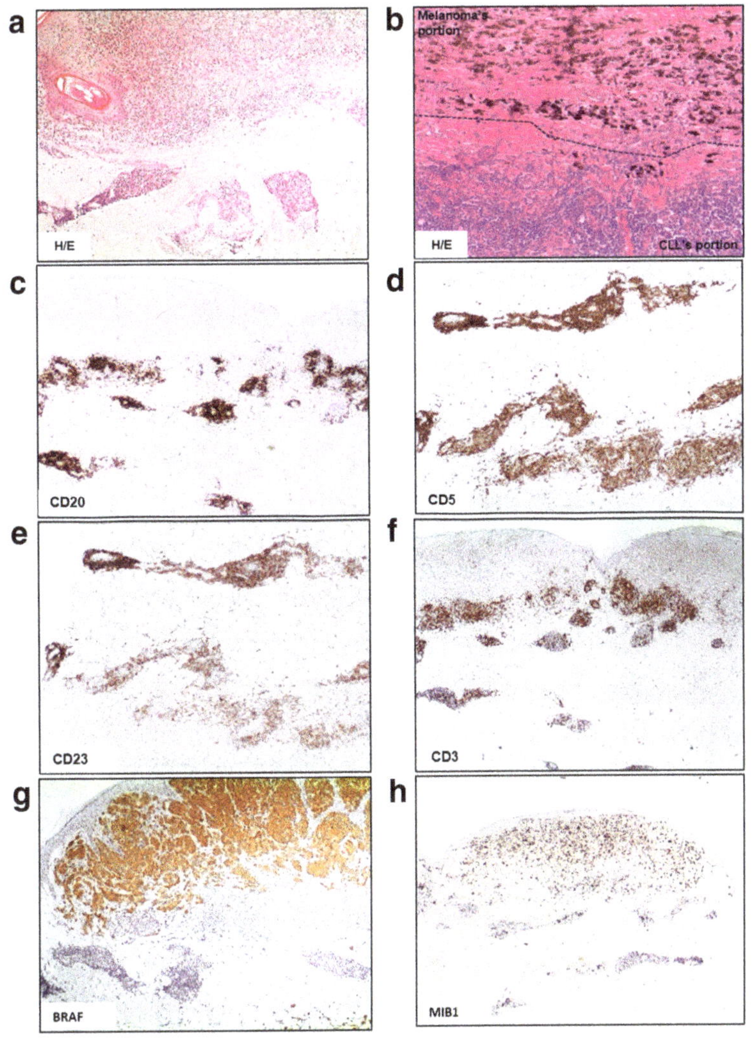


**Fig. 1** Immunohistochemical characterization of skin lesion. **a** Haematoxylin/eosin staining, ×4. **b** Haematoxylin/eosin staining, ×10, the dotted black line defines the border area between CLL and MM tumors. **c**, **d** and **e** Immunohistochemical positivity for CD20, CD5 and CD23 antigens. **f** Immunohistochemical negativity for CD3. **g** Presence of mutant BRAF only in MM lesion. **h** MIB1 expression to evaluate the neoplastic proliferation

deleted region D13S319 and *RB1* demonstrated that two distinct clones were present: 10% of cells had a small del(13q)/D13S319; 3% of cells had a large del(13q) involving both *RB1* and D13S319 (Fig. 2d, e). The two clones increased at relapse to 46% and 13%, respectively. The CLL-associated genomic rearrangements were not detected in the MM skin lesion. No mutations of *NOTCH1*, *SF3B1*, and *TP53* were found. The MM cells carried a $BRAF^{V600E}$ and a p*TERT* c.1–57 A > C mutation.

The familial melanoma panel did not detect known predisposing gene variations. *BRCA1* and *BRCA2* were wild type.

## Discussion

This study reports, for the first time, a collision CLL/MM tumor of the skin, and the molecular-cytogenetic background underlying the two tumors. Collision tumors occurr very rarely, and the association of CLL and MM have been sporadically found, at metastatic lymph nodes, of patients with MM [4, 5].

Our molecular and cytogenetic studies showed that the CLL and the MM had distinct genetic landscapes. The CLL skin lesion and PB samples were wild type for recurrent CLL associated mutations and shared high risk biomarkers. Namely, unmutated *IgH* variable regions and monoallelic del(11)(q23). *ATM* is known to be involved in DNA repair processes that are altered when deletion and/or *ATM* loss-of-function mutations occur; *BIRC3*, a negative regulator of alternative NFkB signaling pathway, is implicated in the modulation of different cellular processes, such as apoptosis, cell proliferation, invasion and metastasis, inflammatory and mitogenic kinase signaling. Several lines of evidence indicate that *ATM* biallelic deletions and/or loss-of-function mutations are poor prognostic markers

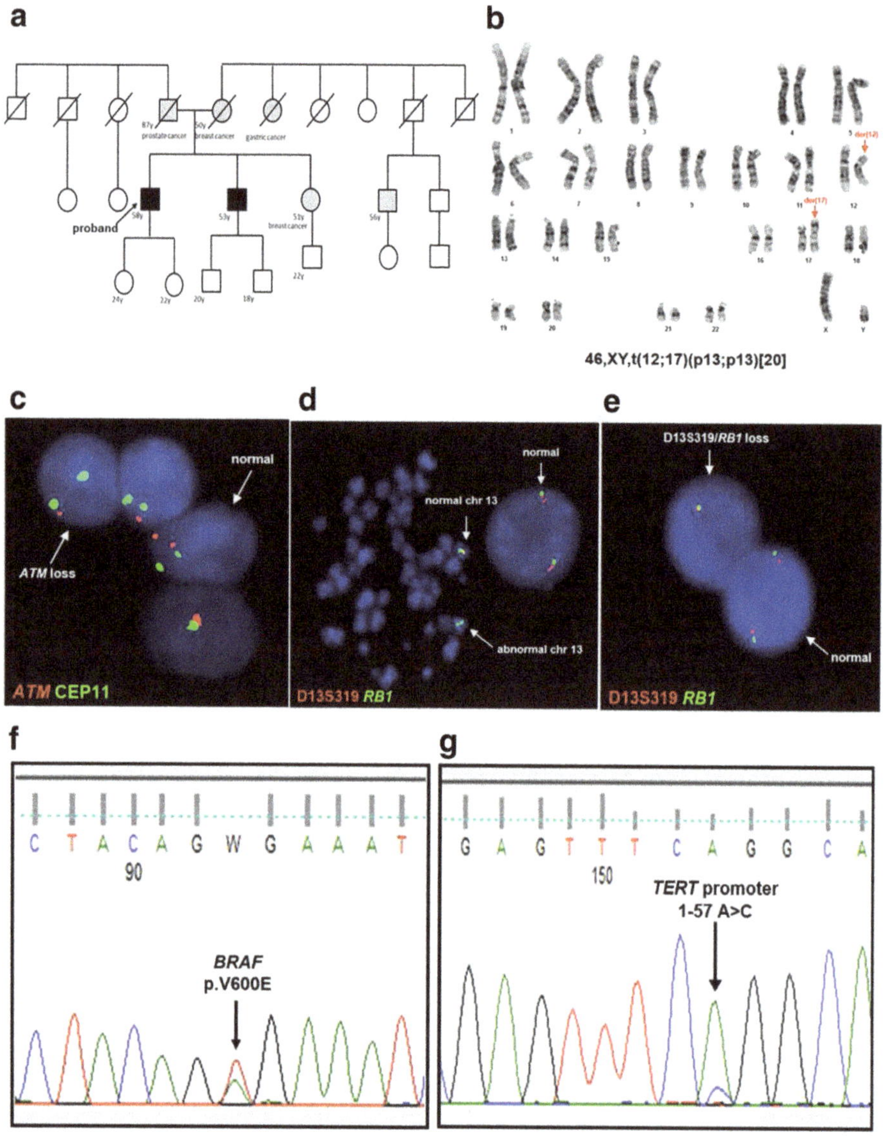


**Fig. 2** Clinical and molecular data of CLL/MM collision tumor. **a** Pedigree of patient's family. The proband is indicated by a black arrow. **b** Constitutional patient karyotype showed the t(12;17)(p13;p13) in all metaphases analyzed [20]. The 12 and 17 derivative chromosomes are indicated by red arrows. **c** Interphase FISH shows *ATM* monoallelic deletion (red signal referred to target gene and green signal referred to centromere 11). The abnormal and normal nucleus are indicated by white arrows. **d** Metaphase FISH of the 13q14 region (D13S319) (red signal) and the *RB1* gene (green signal). The arrows indicate the abnormal derivative chromosome 13 with loss of D13S319 region, and the normal chromosome 13. **e** Interphase FISH of the 13q14 region (D13S319) (red signal) and the *RB1* gene (green signal). The white arrows show a nucleus with loss of both D13S319 region and *RB1* gene, and a nucleus without deletion. **f** Nucleotidic sequence of *BRAF* (exon 15) with hot-spot mutation (p.V600E) on melanoma lesion (black arrow). **g** Nucleotidic sequence of *TERT* promoter mutation (1–57 A > C) on melanoma lesion (black arrow)

correlating with a significantly reduced overall survival, while *BIRC3* haplo-insufficiency does not appear to have a prognostic value [10].

Besides del(11)(q22-q23), PB samples also carried a del(13q), which is the most common cytogenetic aberration in CLL, occurring in ~40% of cases and, when isolated, and it's regarded as good prognostic marker. However, the amount of leukemic cells bearing the del(13q) as well as the extension of the deleted region, appeared to influence patient's outcome [11]. Moreover, large del(13q) which include the *RB1* oncosuppressor gene, called "type II" deletions, were associated with genome complexity [12]. In our case, FISH showed that both the D13S319 locus and *RB1* were lost as expected in cases with progressive disease and both clones increased at relapse (Fig. 2d, e).

Negative for CLL-associated genomic losses, the MM carried a *BRAF*$^{V600E}$ and a p*TERT* c.1–57 A > C mutation (Fig. 2f, g). It is worth mentioning that p*TERT* mutations occur as germline, in familial MM, or acquired in sporadic MM [13]. The majority of p*TERT* mutations occurr at c.1–124 C > T and c.1–146 C > T positions, and both generate binding motifs for the Ets/TCF transcription factors. The p*TERT* c.1–57 A > C mutation, of our case, was previously reported in familial MM and in bladder tumors [13].

The $BRAF^{V600E}$ is an early genomic lesion, occurring in melanocytic nevi, not sufficient to drive a full-blown malignant phenotype, while p*TERT* mutations emerge in intermediate lesions and melanoma in situ. A functional link between *BRAF* and p*TERT* mutations has been demonstrated since the RAS-ERK signaling, in $BRAF^{V600E}$ positive melanomas, is critical for regulating active chromatin state and recruitment of RNA polymerase II at mutant p*TERT*. Notably, the mutant p*TERT* is a key substrate downstream of the RAS-ERK pathway [14].

As expected, a combined treatment with dabrafenib and trametinib induced a complete regression of MM skin lesions, which is still maintained (after 12 months of treatment). Whether these inhibitors were also effective against CLL, could not be assessed in our patient, since he had already undergone chemotherapy. However, the use of BRAF/MEK inhibitors, in CLL, might be exploited as new therapeutic approach since *BRAF* exon 15 mutations have been found in ~3% of cases [15].

Seeking for inherited cancer predisposition, we uncovered that the proband's brother had suffered of multiple MM and both the mother and the sister of breast cancer. However, although genetic counseling suggested a family predisposition (Fig. 2a), we ruled out known germinal mutations of genes involved in these types of hereditary tumors. Interestingly, the patient had a constitutional t(12;17)(p13;p13), not detected in his brother and sister. Even though rare familial CLL were linked to chromosome translocations, the role of this new translocation in collision CLL/MM onset of our cases, could not be determined [16].

## Conclusions

In conclusion, we reported for the first time, a case of collision CLL/MM tumors in a skin lesion [17]. While our molecular-cytogenetic studies proved that specific and distinct genetic events selectively underlie the two lesions, i.e. 11q and 13q deletions for the CLL, and $BRAF^{V600E}$ and p*TERT* mutations for the MM, other reports have shown that the two tumors share the same lesion. Although, genetic counseling suggested a familial risk to MM, investigating known gene variations predisposing to MM was not informative. Thus, an inherited condition along with a long lasting story of immune dysregulation might have cooperated in the CLL/MM collision tumour onset of our case.

**Abbreviations**

BM: Bone marrow; CLL: Chronic lymphocytic leukemia; DHPCL: Denaturing high performance liquid chromatography; FISH: Fluorescent in situ hybridization; MM: Malignant melanoma; PB: Peripheral blood; PET: Positron emission tomography; PGM: Personal genome machine; PHA: Phyto hemagglutinin; p*TERT*: *TERT* promoter; SUV: Standardized uptake values; UCSC: University of California Santa Cruz

**Acknowledgements**

Not applicable.

**Funding**

This study was partially funded by Fondazione Cassa di Risparmio di Perugia (PL R.L.S. project code: 2015.0295.021). Paolo Sportoletti is a recipient of a My First AIRC Grant No. 17442, Associazione Italiana per la Ricerca sul Cancro (AIRC) Foundation and the Scientific Independence of young Researchers (SIR) 2014 Grant No. RBSI14GPBL, Ministero dell'Istruzione, dell'Università e della Ricerca. C.M. is supported by AIRC (IG15525). RF ricerca finalizzata I97E11000380001.

**Authors' contributions**

RLS, SA conceived and designed the study; TP, LP, CM, BC, GR did experimental work, acquired and interpreted data; EA, PS, FF, PC, managed the patient and did experimental work; RLS, TP, CM drafted the paper; all authors critically revised the paper. All authors read and approved the final manuscript.

**Competing interests**

The authors declare that they have no competing interests.

**Author details**

[1]Molecular Medicine Laboratory, Hematology and Bone Marrow Transplantation Unit, University of Perugia, Hospital S. Maria della Misericordia, Piazzale Menghini n.9, 06132 Perugia, Italy. [2]Department of Internal Medicine and Medical Specialties (DiMI), University of Genova and IRCCS AOU San Martino-IST, Viale Benedetto XV n.6, 16132 Genova, Italy. [3]Department of Surgery, University of Perugia, Piazzale Menghini n.1, 06132 Perugia, Italy. [4]C.S. Ematology and Center of bone marrow transplants, University and Hospital of Parma, Via Gramsci n.14, Parma 43126, Italy. [5]Institute of Pathology, University of Perugia and Hospital S. Maria di Terni, Viale Tristano di Joannuccio n.1, 05100 Perugia, Italy.

**References**

1. Malek SN. The biology and clinical significance of acquired genomic copy number aberrations and recurrent gene mutations in chronic lymphocytic leukemia. Oncogene. 2013;32:2805–17.
2. Sportoletti P, Baldoni S, Del Papa B, Aureli P, Dorillo E, Ruggeri L, et al. A revised NOTCH1 mutation frequency still impacts survival while the allele burden predicts early progression in chronic lymphocytic leukemia. Leukemia. 2014;28:436–9.
3. Falchi L, Vitale C, Keating MJ, Lerner S, Wang X, Elhor Gbito KY, et al. Incidence and prognostic impact of other cancers in a population of long-term survivors of chronic lymphocytic leukemia. Ann Oncol. 2016;27:1100–6.
4. Gero D, Queiros da Mota V, Boubaker A, Berthod G, de Leval L, Demartines N, et al. Accuracy of sentinel lymph node dissection for melanoma staging in the presence of a collision tumour with a lymphoproliferative disease. Melanoma Res. 2014;24:371–6.
5. Famenini S, Martires KJ, Zhou H, Xavier MF, Wu JJ. Melanoma In patients with chronic lymphocytic leukemia and non-Hodgkin lymphoma. J Am Acad Dermatol 2015;72:78–84.
6. Cheung KJ, Tam W, Chuang E, Osborne MP. Concurrent invasive ductal carcinoma and chronic lymphocytic leukemia manifesting as a collision tumor in breast. Breast J. 2007;13:413–7.
7. Bhattacharya A, Saha R, Biswas J, Biswas J, Ghosh B. Collision tumors in the gastrointestinal tract: a rare case series. Int Med Case Rep J. 2012;5:73–7.
8. Leachman SA, Carucci J, Kohlmann W, Banks KC, Asgari MM, Bergman W, et

al. Selection criteria for genetic assessment of patients with familial melanoma. J Am Acad Dermatol. 2009;61:e1–14.
9. Speedy HE, Kinnersley B, Chubb D, Broderick P, Law PJ, Litchfield K, et al. Germline mutations in shelterin complex genes are associated with familial chronic lymphocytic leukemia. Blood. 2016;128:2319–26.
10. Nabhan C, Raca G, Wang YL. Predicting prognosis in chronic lymphocytic leukemia in the contemporary era. JAMA Oncol. 2015;1:965–74.
11. Dal Bo M, Rossi FM, Rossi D, Deambrogi C, Bertoni F, Del Giudice I, et al. 13q14 deletion size and number of deleted cells both influence prognosis in chronic lymphocytic leukemia. Genes Chromosomes Cancer. 2011;50: 633–43.
12. Ouillette P, Fossum S, Parkin B, Ding L, Bockenstedt P, Al-Zoubi A, et al. Aggressive chronic lymphocytic leukemia with elevated genomic complexity is associated with multiple gene defects in the response to DNA double-strand breaks. Clin Cancer Res. 2010;16:835–47.
13. Rachakonda PS, Hosen I, de Verdier PJ, Fallah M, Heidenreich B, Ryk C, et al. TERT promoter mutations in bladder cancer affect patient survival and disease recurrence through modification by a common polymorphism. Proc Natl Acad Sci U S A. 2013;110:17426–31.
14. Li Y, Cheng HS, Chng WJ, Tergaonkar V. Activation of mutant TERT promoter by RAS-ERK signaling is a key step in malignant progression of BRAF-mutant human melanomas. Proc Natl Acad Sci U S A. 2016;113: 14402–7.
15. Jebaraj BMC, Kienle D, Bühler A, Winkler D, Döhner H, Stilgenbauer S, et al. BRAF mutations in chronic lymphocytic leukemia. Leuk & Lymph. 2013;54: 1177–82.
16. Eclache V, Benzacken B, Kettaneh A, Fain OA. Constitutional translocation t(1;4)(p21;p15) in a case of chronic lymphocytic leukemia. Ann Genet. 2002; 45:169–71.
17. Farma JM, Zager JS, Barnica-Elvir V, Puleo CA, Marzban SS, Rollison DE, et al. A collision of diseases: chronic lymphocytic leukemia discovered during lymph node biopsy for melanoma. Ann Surg Oncol. 2013;20:1360–4.

# 20

# Derivative chromosomes involving 5p large rearranged segments went unnoticed with the use of conventional cytogenetics

Emiy Yokoyama[1], Victoria Del Castillo[1], Silvia Sánchez[2], Sandra Ramos[2], Bertha Molina[2], Leda Torres[2], María José Navarro[1], Silvia Avila[3], José Luis Castrillo[3], Benilde García-De Teresa[2], Bárbara Asch[4] and Sara Frías[2,5*]

**Abstract**

**Background:** In countries where comparative genomic hybridization arrays (aCGH) and next generation sequencing are not widely available due to accessibility and economic constraints, conventional 400–500-band karyotyping is the first-line choice for the etiological diagnosis of patients with congenital malformations and intellectual disability. Conventional karyotype analysis can rule out chromosomal alterations greater than 10 Mb. However, some large structural abnormalities, such as derivative chromosomes, may go undetected when the analysis is performed at less than a 550-band resolution and the size and banding pattern of the interchanged segments are similar. Derivatives frequently originate from inter-chromosomal exchanges and sometimes are inherited from a parent who carries a reciprocal translocation.

**Case presentation:** We present two cases with derivative chromosomes involving a 9.1 Mb 5p deletion/14.8 Mb 10p duplication in the first patient and a 19.9 Mb 5p deletion/ 18.5 Mb 9p duplication in the second patient. These long chromosomal imbalances were ascertained by aCGH but not by conventional cytogenetics. Both patients presented with a deletion of the Cri du chat syndrome region and a duplication of another genomic region. Each patient had a unique clinical picture, and although they presented some features of Cri du chat syndrome, the phenotype did not conclusively point towards this diagnosis, although a chromosomopathy was suspected.

**Conclusions:** These cases highlight the fundamental role of the clinical suspicion in guiding the approach for the etiological diagnosis of patients. Molecular cytogenetics techniques, such as aCGH, should be considered when the clinician suspects the presence of a chromosomal imbalance in spite of a normal karyotype.

**Keywords:** Derivate chromosomes, Translocations, Intellectual disability, Congenital malformations, 5p deletion, 10p15 duplication, 9p22 duplication

## Background

In Mexico and other developing countries, the genetic approach for patients with intellectual disability (ID) and congenital malformations (CM) uses conventional G-banded karyotyping as the first-choice diagnostic test. It is usually performed at a 500-band level that allows the detection of 5–10 Mb abnormalities and results in an etiological diagnosis in approximately 3–10% of patients with a suspected chromosomopathy [1–3]. However, some structurally abnormal chromosomes with rearrangements larger than 5 Mb may go unnoticed by conventional cytogenetics. This may occur with derivative chromosomes, which are unbalanced intra- or inter-chromosomal rearrangements, in which the exchanged segments share a similar size and banding pattern, making them difficult to identify by conventional karyotyping [3, 4].

When a patient presents with a derivative chromosome, phenotypic evaluation and chromosome analysis of the parents are mandatory to rule out the presence of a balanced translocation in one of them [1]. In fact, 70% of derivatives are inherited and this information has a

* Correspondence: sarafrias@biomedicas.unam.mx
[2]Laboratorio de Citogenética, Departamento de Genética Humana, Instituto Nacional de Pediatría, Ciudad de México, México
[5]Departamento de Medicina Genómica y Toxicología Ambiental, Instituto de Investigaciones Biomédicas, Universidad Nacional Autónoma de México, Avenida IMAN no. 1, Torre de Investigación, Colonia Insurgentes Cuicuilco, Coyoacán, Ciudad de México, Mexico
Full list of author information is available at the end of the article

significant impact on genetic counseling [5, 6]. Comparative Genomic Hybridization arrays (aCGH) may uncover this type of abnormalities, because the finding of a combined deletion/duplication in the same patient points towards the presence of a derivative chromosome. Here, we describe the cytogenetic and clinical findings of two patients in whom a clinical phenotype consisting of ID and CM prompted the completion of aCGH despite having a normal 450-band karyotype. The two patients presented here, were ascertained through aCGH during the study of a cohort of 152 patients that presented with ID or CM and a normal conventional karyotype (manuscript in preparation).

Genomic DNA from the two patients and their parents was amplified and labeled using the CGH-labeling kit for oligo arrays (Enzo Life Sciences, New York, USA) and then analyzed with a 60 K oligonucleotide arrays according to the manufacturer's protocol (Agilent, Santa Clara, USA). The slides were scanned using a microarray scanner with Surescan High Resolution Technology (Agilent, Santa Clara, USA). Image quantification, array quality control and aberration detection were performed using the Agilent Feature Extraction and DNA Analytics software (Agilent, Santa Clara, USA) according to the manufacturer's instructions. Changes identified in the samples were visualized using the UCSC Genome Browser online tool (http://genome.ucsc.edu) and were compared to the Database of Genomic Variants (http://projects.tcag.ca/variation) to exclude copy number changes considered to be benign variants. The DECIPHER (Database of Chromosomal Imbalance and Phenotype in Humans using Ensembl Resources) (https://decipher.sanger.ac.uk/) and ECARUCA (European Cytogeneticists Association Register of Unbalanced Chromosome Aberrations) (http://umcecaruca01.extern.umcn.nl:8080/ecaruca/ecaruca.jsp) databases were used to assist with the genotype-phenotype correlation.

The rearrangements were validated using Fluorescence in situ hybridization (FISH) probes (Sure-FISH, Agilent, Santa Clara, USA). Molecular cytogenetic techniques, and GTG-banded karyotypes were performed on patients and their first-degree relatives to establish the origin (inherited or sporadic) of the chromosomal rearrangement and provide appropriate genetic counseling.

## Case presentation

Both patients were males, born to non-consanguineous parents. There was no family history of congenital diseases, intellectual disability, autism, seizures, neurological disorders, metabolic diseases, infertility or recurrent pregnancy loss. Physical examination revealed that both patients had weight, height and head circumference below the 5th percentile. An informed consent letter for each patient was obtained from the parents.

### Patient 1

Eight years old boy, born from the fourth pregnancy of a 33 years old mother and a 40 years old father; he has 3 healthy sisters. During pregnancy, decreased fetal movements were noted, and two ultrasound studies (USG) were reported as normal. He was delivered by cesarean section due to breech presentation at 37 weeks of gestation. He weighed 2800 g (between the 10th and 50th percentile), his height was 48 cm (50th percentile), and he received an Apgar score of 7/8. He required hospitalization for hypoglycemia and seizures. Delayed psychomotor development was noted at 9 months of age. Physical examination at the age of 3 years showed that the patient had posterior flattening of the skull, carp-shaped mouth (downturned corners of mouth), low-set ears, short neck, appendicular hypotonia, hands with prominent finger pads and multiple palmar creases, and a non-palpable right testicle. The computed tomography (CT) and magnetic resonance imaging (MRI) of the brain were normal. He also had brainstem auditory evoked potentials (BAEP), with bilateral severe hearing loss. USG of gonads reported both testes at the proximal third of the inguinal canal. Conventional karyotype at 450-band resolution was reported as normal, however, aCGH demonstrated the presence of a 9.1 Mb deletion of chromosome 5 and a 14.8 Mb duplication of chromosome 10 [Fig. 1a-e]. FISH analysis showed a normal pattern of the probes in the father's sample, while a balanced translocation was observed in the mother and in two of his sisters. Following the 2016 International System for Human Cytogenomic Nomenclature (ISCN 2016) [7], the patient's karyotype was 46,XY,der(5)t(5;10)(p15.2;p13)mat. ish der(5)t(5;10)(p15.2;p13)(wcp5+,wcp10+).arr [GRCh37/hg19]5p15.33p15.2(151737_9215425)× 1, 10p15.3p13(148,206_14,869,993)× 3 mat.

### Patient 2

Seven years old boy, he is the first child of 30 years old parents. Two USGs were performed during the second trimester of pregnancy and intrauterine growth retardation was detected. Delivered at term by vaginal childbirth with a weight of 2175 g (below the 3th percentile). Birth height and Apgar score are unknown. He did not spontaneously breathe and required supplemental oxygen and hospitalization for 20 days. At the age of 8 months he was diagnosed with developmental delay. Physical examination revealed disproportion at the craniofacial-body level, round face, telecanthus, epicanthus, ears with posterior rotation, prominent helix and antihelix, short and wide philtrum, downturned corners of the mouth, micrognathia, heart murmur, abdomen with gastrostomy catheter, axial hypertonia, upper limbs with hypoplastic nails and bilateral clinodactyly of the 5th fingers, bilateral transversal palmar crease, and male genitalia but neither testis was palpable. Renal ultrasound reported left renal

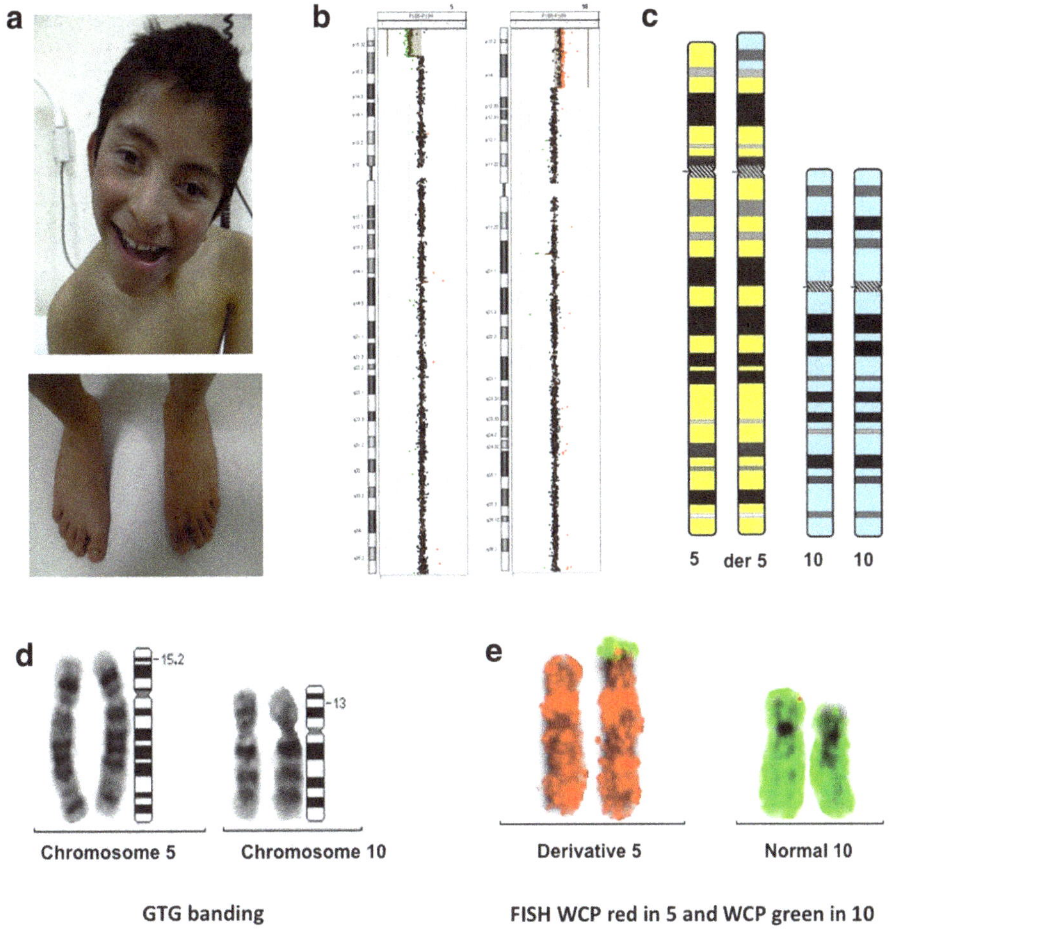


**Fig. 1 a.** Long face, left eye strabismus, bilateral hallux valgus and hammertoes. **b.** Array CGH and FISH: 46,XY,der(5)t(5;10)(p15.2;p13)mat. ish der(5)t(5;10)(p15.2;p13)(wcp5+,wcp10+).arr[GRCh37/hg19] 5p15.33p15.2(151737_9215425)× 1, 10p15.3p13(148,206_14,869,993)× 3 mat. **c.** Ideogram with the two chromosomes involved (normal and translocated). **d.** GTG-banding of derivative chromosomes 5 and normal chromosome 10. Note the similar pattern of banding between the derivative chromosome 5 and the corresponding normal chromosome. **e.** FISH with WCP5 in red and WCP10 in green

ectopia and crossed fused renal ectopia; BAEP indicated severe right hearing loss and moderate left hearing loss. Conventional GTG karyotype was reported to be normal but aCGH showed a 19.9 Mb deletion of chromosome 5 and an 18.5 Mb duplication of chromosome 9 [Fig. 2a-e]. The patient's karyotype was defined following ISCN 2016 [7] as: 46,XY,der(5)t(5;9)(p14.3;p22.1). ish der(5)t(5;9)(p14.3;p22.1)(PDCD6-,AHRR-,C5orf55-,EXOC3-,PP7080-, SLC9A3-,C9orf66+,DOCK8+,KANK1+).arr[GRCh37/hg19]5p15.33p14.3(151737_20049770)× 1, 9p22.3p22.1(271,257_18,681,089)× 3 dn.

In Fig. 2d, it is evident that the derivative chromosome 5 shows a very similar G-band pattern than the normal chromosome 5, which explains why it was not detected in the conventional karyotype despite the large segment involved in the rearrangement. FISH with the specific probes did not show a balanced chromosomal rearrangement in either parent.

## Discussion

The prevalence of derivative chromosomes is unknown, although the estimated frequency of balanced reciprocal translocations ranges from 1 in 500 to 1 in 1000 in live births [4, 6]. The carriers of a balanced rearrangement may have decreased fertility, miscarriages and children with ID and CM. All of these are consequences of pregnancies with genomic imbalances due to the fertilization with a gamete that received the derivative chromosome during meiotic segregation [8–10].

### Genotype-phenotype correlation

We describe two patients with derivative chromosomes that despite having large chromosomal imbalances were not identified by conventional karyotyping. Furthermore, even though these rearrangements resulted in a 5p deletion, the patients did not present a phenotype in which the Cri-du-chat syndrome was readily recognized. The

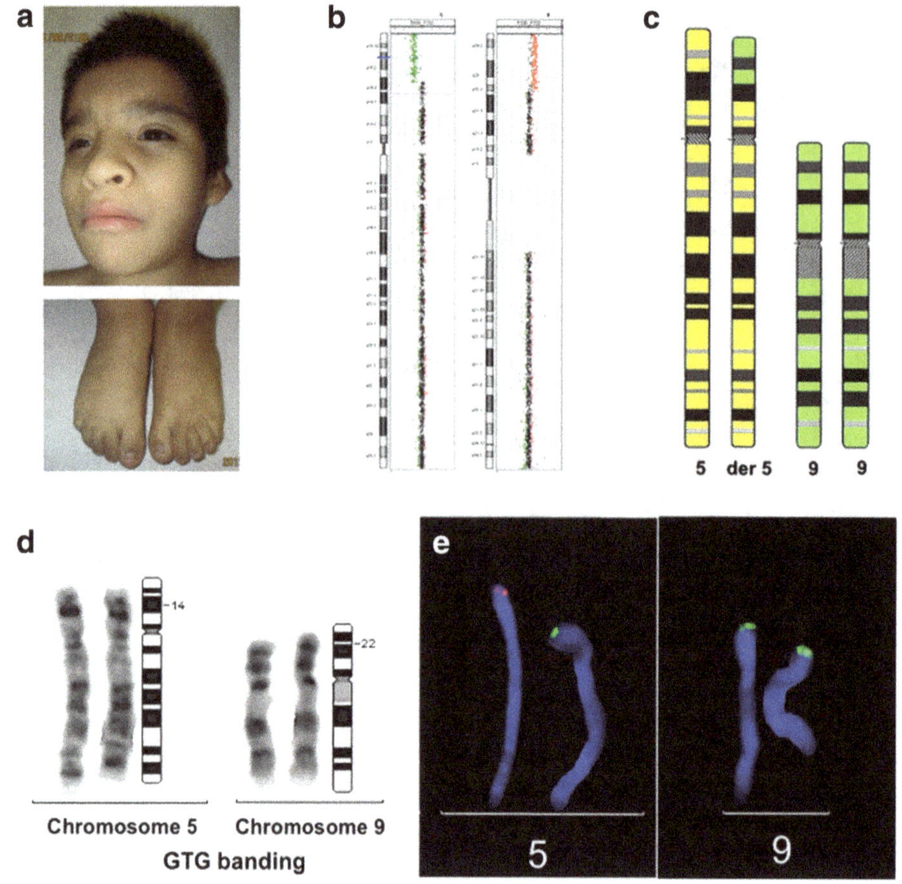


**Fig. 2** **a**. Long palpebral fissures, prominent antihelix, nail hypoplasia of toes and clinodactyly of the fifth finger. **b**. Array CGH with FISH: 46,XY,der(5)t(5;9)(p14.3;p22.1). ish der(5)t(5;9)(p14.3;p22.1)(PDCD6-,AHRR-,C5orf55-,EXOC3-,PP7080-,SLC9A3-,C9orf66+,DOCK8+,KANK1+).arr[GRCh37/hg19] 5p15.33p14.3(151737_20049770)× 1, 9p22.3p22.1(271,257_18,681,089)× 3 dn; **c**. Ideogram with the two chromosomes involved (normal and translocated); **d**. GTG-banding of chromosome 5 and 9 pairs; one of these chromosomes is the derivative 5 and the normal chromosome 9 from the patient, indicating the involved bands. **e**. FISH with probe located in 5p15.33 in red and probe located in 9p24.3 in green, showing the single dose of 5p and three doses of 9p

first patient's karyotype is 46,XY,der(5)t(5;10)(p15.2;p13) mat carrying a chromosome 5 derivative that arose from a t(5;10)(p15.2;p13). The derivative chromosome results in a partial monosomy of 5p15.2 → pter, producing haploinsufficiency of the *SDHA* (5p15.33) and *SEMA5A* (5p15.31) genes that have been related to psychomotor retardation, microcephaly, pachygyria and microgyria. All these symptoms were present in our patient [11]. The der(5)t(5;10)(p15.2;p13) also results in partial chromosome 10 trisomy 10p13 → pter. This region contains the *AKR1C3* gene (10p15.1) that is involved in male gonadal development [12] although its overexpression is yet to be related to an altered function. Thus, it is possible that the cryptorchidism found in this patient is a phenotype due to the 5p deletion [13]. In addition, the *GATA3* gene (10p14) is involved in ear development, and abnormalities at this level have been linked to ear defects [14]. Our patient shares ID, growth delay, microcephaly, low-set ears, downturned corners of mouth, cryptorchidism and abnormal palmar creases with previously reported 5p deletion patients [13]. Patients with the 10p duplication present with ID, microcephaly, low-set ears, hearing impairment, cryptorchidism and abnormal palmar creases [15, 16].

The second patient also has a chromosome 5 derivative with a karyotype 46,XY,der(5)t(5;9)(p14.3;p22.1)dn leading to a partial monosomy of 5p14.3 → pter. This karyotype explains why this patient shared clinical manifestations with Cri du chat syndrome such as microcephaly, round face, epicanthus, telecanthus, downturned corners of mouth and dysplastic pinnae [17]. This derivative also results in partial trisomy of 9p22.1 → pter and the patient presents with clinical manifestations that have been previously reported in patients with a 9p duplication. These include ID, growth delay, microcephaly, hypertelorism, epicanthic folds, low-set ears, transverse fold, short stature, hearing loss, and nail hypoplastic [18, 19].

Cri du chat syndrome due to a translocation is rare (10–15%) [13] and the typical phenotype of this syndrome also depends on the extent and composition of the trisomic region involved. Both our patients have some clinical manifestations of Cri du chat syndrome, which was not initially suspected, because the phenotype was modified by the combination of the trisomic segments and the deletion. Therefore, we reviewed the literature and compared our patients' phenotype with clinical manifestations of classical Cri du chat syndrome, and with those of dup(10)(p13p15.3) and dup(9)(p22.1p22.3) (Table 1). We found that, when the case is not detected neonatally, the classical phenotype is masked by the clinical manifestations of the trisomic regions, and the deletion of Cri du chat region is detected only when aCGH is done [20–23]. It is worth mentioning that we could not find other cases reported in the literature in which partial trisomies 10p13 → p15.3 or 9p22.1 → p22.3 coexisted with deletion 5p14.3 → pter or 5p15.2 → pter.

## Genetic counseling

We were able to offer precise genetic counseling to these two families regarding the origin of these derivative chromosomes. It has been reported that 62% of rearrangements are paternal in origin, and only 38% are maternal [24]. However, when we analyzed the parents and siblings of patient 1 with specific FISH probes, we found that his mother and two of his sisters were carriers of a balanced translocation. This poses them at an increased risk of having offspring with ID and CM, as well as recurrent abortions, due to the generation of a gamete with an unbalanced rearrangement. In this family with identified carriers, knowing the breakpoints of the chromosomes involved in the rearrangement allowed us to build a pachytene cross (Fig. 3) and determine the percentages of possible normal, balanced, and unbalanced gametes. In addition to complement the medical history, it was possible to anticipate the viability of the unbalanced products and the products of the 2:2 segregation [8]. In this family, the theoretical risk of having a healthy child is 2 out of 6 (33%), with the healthy child receiving either the normal chromosomes or the balanced translocation

**Table 1** Comparison of the phenotype of patients 1 and 2 vs Cri du chat syndrome and clinical manifestations in patients with trisomy 10p or 9p

| Clinical Manifestations | dup10p[15,16] | Patient 1 | Cri du chat[13] | Patient 2 | dup9p[18] |
|---|---|---|---|---|---|
| Intellectual Disability | + | + | + | + | + |
| Short stature/Growth delay | | + | + | + | + |
| Nasal speech | + | | | | |
| High pitched | | | + | | |
| Typical cry | | | + | | |
| Microcephaly | + | + | + | + | + |
| Craneosynostosis | | | | | + |
| Seizures | + | | | | |
| Disgenesis of corpus callosum | | | | | + |
| Short neck | | + | | | |
| Abnormality of the face | | | | | + |
| Round face | | | + | + | |
| Prominent forehead | + | | | | |
| Hypertelorism | + | | + | + | + |
| Epicanthic folds | | | + | + | + |
| Downward palpebral fissures | | | + | | |
| Abnormal eyes | + | | | | |
| Large nasal bridge | | | + | | |
| Low-set ears | + | + | + | + | + |
| Hearing impairment | + | + | | + | + |
| Preauricular tags | | | + | | |
| Downturned corners of mouth | | + | + | + | |
| Micrognatia | | | + | + | |
| Cleft palate | + | | | | |
| Cardiovascular defects | + | | + | | |
| Renal alterations | + | | + | + | |
| Cryptorchidism | + | + | + | + | |
| Hypospadias | + | | + | | |
| Abnormal palmar creases | + | + | + | + | + |
| Nail dystrophy/hypoplastic | | | | + | + |
| Syndactyly | + | | + | | |

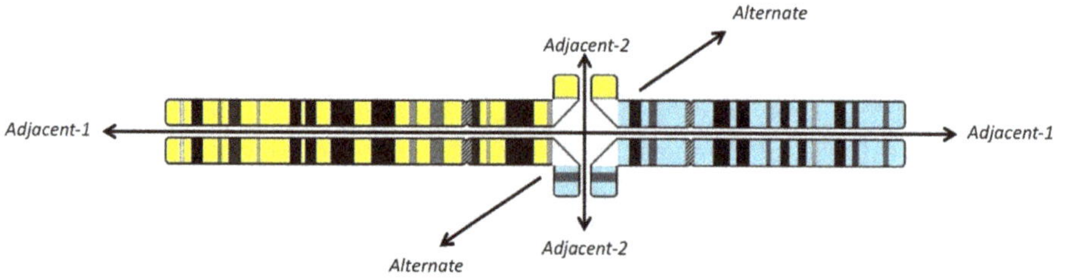


| Type of segregation | Unbalanced | Products |
|---|---|---|
| *Alternate* | Normal | Healthy |
| | Balanced carrier | Healthy |
| *Adjacent-1* | 5p15.2 to 5pter partial trisomy and 10p13 to 10pter partial monosomy | malformed |
| | 10p13 to 10pter partial trisomy and 5p15.2 to 5pter partial monosomy | malformed (Patient 1) |
| *Adjacent-2* | 5p15.2 to 5qter partial trisomy and 10p13 to 10qter partial monosomy | malformed, more frequently not viable |
| | 10p13 to 10qter partial trisomy and 10p13 to 10qter partial monosomy | malformed, more frequently not viable |

**Fig. 3** Pachytene cross between chromosomes 5 and 10. Possible gametes according to the type of segregation, as well as the expected manifestations and viability of the products

(Fig. 3), and the empiric risk is 2 out of 4 (50%), considering only the viable products.

Genetic counseling for the second family is different because neither parent are carriers. Thus, the theoretical risk of recurrence is zero. However, we cannot rule out the presence of germline mosaicism in one of the parents or a non-paternity situation.

### The use of molecular cytogenetics methodology should be mandatory in patients with intellectual disability and multiple congenital malformations

Currently, it is well accepted that conventional karyotyping is an excellent and non-expensive methodology for detecting aneuploidies, low-level mosaicism and large -more than 10 Mb- rearrangements; however, detection of chromosomal structural abnormalities largely depends on the skills and experience of the cytogeneticist and yet, some alterations may go unnoticed [25]. To improve the detection of chromosomal abnormalities, molecular methodologies such as FISH or Multiplex Ligation-dependent Probe Amplification (MLPA) and chromosomal microarrays have been used [1]. Several groups have highlighted the economical and medical convenience of using microarrays as a first-line diagnostic test for detecting constitutional genomic imbalances [26–33]. The high cost of microarrays keeps these methodologies from being the first-line diagnostic tests in some developing countries, forcing a careful selection of patients in whom such studies are performed. Often, the few available microarrays are used in patients in whom a submicroscopic alteration is suspected, overlooking other patients who could also benefit from these types of analyses. Our cases support the benefit of offering microarray analysis to patients with a more severe phenotype such as ID and developmental delay, dysmorphic features or multiple CM, and when the clinical picture does not point toward a specific target region of the genome. A high rate of detection of unbalanced rearrangements using microarray methodology has been observed in patients with these referral indications [32]. It should be noted that microarrays can only detect unbalanced genomic regions, while the chromosomal locations of the duplicated or deleted regions material cannot be defined. In order to do so, the analysis must be complemented with the use of FISH to localize the segments in the karyotype.

## Conclusions

The phenotype of the patients with a derivative chromosome are unique, since it combines the clinical features of both the partial deletion and the partial duplication.

Noticeably, only when the clinical geneticist makes a detailed phenotype-genotype correlation, it becomes evident that the patient has clinical manifestations of the specific syndrome, such as Cri du chat syndrome in this study. The typical gestalt is modified by non-classical manifestations resulting from the new genome created by the chromosomal rearrangement, and the clinical diagnosis is not apparent.

Patients presented here are clear examples in which large chromosomal rearrangements go unnoticed by experienced cytogeneticists when using conventional cytogenetics. These cases highlight the importance of performing complementary analyses in patients with developmental delay or ID associated with CM using molecular cytogenetics techniques. The clinician's suspicion of a chromosomal etiology for the patient's condition, despite a normal conventional karyotype, is fundamental to support the need and demand the funding to perform further molecular cytogenetic testing that could positively impact the patient's diagnosis, and to provide information regarding the biology of the disease.


#### Acknowledgements
The aCGH was carried out at Genetadi Laboratory (Bilbao, Spain). Many thanks to Dr. Ariadna Gonzalez del Angel and Dr. Esther Lieberman for the referral of patients.

#### Funding
This study was partially supported by CONACYT FOSSIS-S0008–2008-C01–87792 and Fondos Federales 2013, project 2009/06, Instituto Nacional de Pediatría (México). The funding body did not participate in the design of the study, collection, analysis, or interpretation of data, or in writing the manuscript. EY received a fellowship, CONACYT-176523 (Doctorado en Ciencias Médicas, Odontológicas y de la Salud, UNAM).


#### Authors' contributions
EY and SF contributed to the design and development of the protocol, analyzed the results, wrote the manuscript, and designed the figures. VC contributed to the design of the protocol, clinical description and analyzed results. BM, SS and SR performed the G-banded karyotype and FISH technique. LT contributed with the analysis of the aCGH results. MJN wrote the first draft of the manuscript and interpreted results. SA and JLC performed the aCGH. BGT and BA contributed in the clinical description and revised the manuscript for the English language. All authors read and approved the final version and are responsible for all aspects of the manuscript.

#### Competing interests
The authors declare that they have no competing interests.


#### Author details
[1]Departamento de Genética Humana, Instituto Nacional de Pediatría, Ciudad de México, México. [2]Laboratorio de Citogenética, Departamento de Genética Humana, Instituto Nacional de Pediatría, Ciudad de México, México. [3]Laboratorio GENETADI, Bilbao, Spain. [4]Laboratorio Diagen, Hospital ABC Santa Fe, Cuidad de México, México. [5]Departamento de Medicina Genómica y Toxicología Ambiental, Instituto de Investigaciones Biomédicas, Universidad Nacional Autónoma de México, Avenida IMAN no. 1, Torre de Investigación, Colonia Insurgentes Cuicuilco, Coyoacán, Ciudad de México, Mexico.


#### References

1. Jehee FS, Takamori JT, Medeiros PF, Pordeus AC, Latini FR, Bertola DR, et al. Using a combination of MLPA kits to detect chromosomal imbalances in patients with multiple congenital anomalies and mental retardation is a valuable choice for developing countries. Eur J Med Genet. 2011;54(4):e425–32.
2. Yokoyama-Rebollar E, Frias S, Del Castillo-Ruiz V. Cytogenetic and cytogenomic approach of patients with intellectual disability and congenital malformations. Acta Pediatra Mex. 2017;38(6):433–41.
3. Puri RD, Tuteja M, Verma IC. Genetic approach to diagnosis of intellectual disability. Indian J Pediatr. 2016;83(10):1141–9.
4. Kaiser-Rogers K, Rao K. Structural chromosome rearrangements. In: Gersen SL, Keagle MB, editors. The principles of clinical cytogenetics. New Jersey: Humana Press Inc; 2005. p. 165–206.
5. Sharkey FH, Maher E, FitzPatrick DR. Chromosome analysis: what and when to request. Arch Dis Child. 2005;90(12):1264–9.
6. Wellesley D, Dolk H, Boyd PA, Greenlees R, Haeusler M, Nelen V, et al. Rare chromosome abnormalities, prevalence and prenatal diagnosis rates from population-based congenital anomaly registers in Europe. Eur J Hum Genet. 2012;20(5):521–6.
7. McGowan-Jordan J, Simons A, Schimd M. ISCN: an international system for human Cytogenomic nomenclature. Basel: Karger; 2016.
8. Hu L, Cheng DH, Gong F, Lu CF, Tana YQ, Luo KL, et al. Reciprocal translocation carrier diagnosis in preimplantation human embryos. EBioMedicine. 2016;14:139–47.
9. Keify F, Zhiyan N, Mirzaei F, Tootian S, Ghazaey S, Abbaszadegan MR. Two novel familial balanced trans locations t(8;11)(p23;q21) and t(6;16)(q26;p12) implicated in recurrent spontaneous abortion. Arch Iran Med. 2012;15(4):249–52.
10. Gardner RJM, Sutherland GR, Shaffer LG. Autosomal reciprocal translocations. In: Chromosome abnormalities and genetic counseling. 4th ed. New York: Oxford University Press; 2004.
11. Chen CP, Huang MC, Chen YY, Chern SR, Wu PS, Su JW, et al. Cri-du-chat (5p-) syndrome presenting with cerebellar hypoplasia and hypospadias: prenatal diagnosis and aCGH characterization using uncultured amniocytes. Gene. 2013;524(2):407–11.
12. Ashley RA, Yu ZX, Fung KM, Frimberger D, Kropp BP, Penning TM, et al. Developmental evaluation of aldo-keto reductase 1C3 expression in the cryptorchid testis. Urology. 2010;76(1):67–72.
13. Nguyen JM, Qualmann KJ, Okashah R, Reilly A, Alexeyev MF, Campbell DJ. 5p deletions: current knowledge and future directions. Am J Med Genet C Semin Med Genet. 2015;169(3):224–38.
14. Melis D, Genesio R, Boemio P, Del Giudice E, Cappuccio G, Mormile A, et al. Clinical description of a patient carrying the smallest reported deletion involving 10p14 region. Am J Med Genet A. 2012;158A(4):832–5.
15. DECIPHER. Sanger Institute, England. https://decipher.sanger.ac.uk/browser#q/10:148206-14869993/location/10:23206-14994993. Accessed 28 Feb 2018.
16. Slinde S, Hansteen IL. Two chromosomal syndromes in the same family: monosomy and trisomy for part of the short arm of chromosome 10. Eur J Pediatr. 1982;139:153–7.
17. Fang JS, Lee KF, Huang CT, Syu CL, Yang KJ, Wang LH, et al. Cytogenetic and molecular characterization of a three-generation family with chromosome 5p terminal deletion. Clin Genet. 2008;73(6):585–90.
18. Di Bartolo DL, El Naggar M, Owen R, Sahoo T, Gilbert F, Pulijaal VR, et al. Characterization of a complex rearrangement involving duplication and deletion of 9p in an infant with craniofacial dysmorphism and cardiac anomalies. Mol Cytogenet. 2012;5(1):31.
19. DECIPHER. Sanger Institute, England. https://decipher.sanger.ac.uk/browser#q/9:271257-18681089/location/9:146257-18806089
20. Fukushi D, Kurosawa K, Suzuki Y, Suzuki K, Yamada K, Watanabe S, et al. Clinical and molecular genetic characterization of two siblings with trisomy 2p24.3-pter and monosomy 5p14.3-pter. Am J Med Genet A. 2017;173(8):2201–9.
21. Elmakky A, Carli D, Lugli L, Torelli P, Guidi B, Falcinelli C, et al. A three-generation family with terminal microdeletion involving 5p15.33-32 due to a whole-arm 5;15 chromosomal translocation with a steady phenotype of atypical cri du chat syndrome. Eur J Med Genet. 2014;57(4):145–50.
22. Masri A, Gimelli S, Hamamy H, Sloan-Béna F. Microarray delineation of familial chromosomal imbalance with deletion 5q35 and duplication 10q25 in a child showing multiple anomalies and dysmorphism. Am J Med Genet A. 2014;164A(5):1254–61.
23. Sharma P, Gupta N, Chowdhury MR, Sapra S, Shukla R, Lall M, et al. Inherited 5p deletion syndrome due to paternal balanced translocation: phenotypic heterogeneity due to duplication of 8q and 12p. J Pediatr Genet. 2013;2(3):163–9.
24. Thomas NS, Morris JK, Baptista J, Ng BL, Crolla JA, Jacobs PA. De novo apparently balanced translocations in man are predominantly paternal in origin and associated with a significant increase in paternal age. J Med Genet. 2010;47(2):112–5.
25. Shaffer LG, Rosenfeld JA. Microarray-based prenatal diagnosis for the identification of fetal chromosome abnormalities. Expert Rev Mol Diagn. 2013;13(6):601–11.
26. Regier DA, Friedman JM, Marra CA. Value for money? Array genomic hybridization for diagnostic testing for genetic causes of intellectual disability. Am J Hum Genet. 2010;86(5):765–72.
27. Ahn JW, Bint S, Bergbaum A, Mann K, Hall RP, Ogilvie CM. Array CGH as a first line diagnostic test in place of karyotyping for postnatal referrals - results from four years' clinical application for over 8,700 patients. Mol Cytogenet. 2013;6(1):16.

# 21

# Microduplication in the 2p16.1p15 chromosomal region linked to developmental delay and intellectual disability

Luca Lovrecic[1*], Chiara Gnan[2], Federica Baldan[3], Alessandra Franzoni[2], Sara Bertok[4], Giuseppe Damante[5], Bertrand Isidor[6] and Borut Peterlin[1]

## Abstract

**Background:** Several patients with the 2p16.1p15 microdeletion syndrome have been reported. However, microduplication in the 2p16.1p15 chromosomal region has only been reported in one case, and milder clinical features were present compared to those attributed to 2p16.1p15 microdeletion syndrome. Some additional cases were deposited in DECIPHER database.

**Case presentation:** In this report we describe four further cases of 2p16.1p15 microduplication in four unrelated probands. They presented with mild gross motor delay, delayed speech and language development, and mild dysmorphic features. In addition, two probands have macrocephaly and one a congenital heart anomaly. Newly described cases share several phenotype characteristics with those detailed in one previously reported microduplication case.

**Conclusion:** The common features among patients are developmental delay, speech delay, mild to moderate intellectual disability and unspecific dysmorphic features. Two patients have bilateral clinodactyly of the 5th finger and two have bilateral 2nd-3rd toes syndactyly. Interestingly, as opposed to the deletion phenotype with some cases of microcephaly, 2 patients are reported with macrocephaly. The reported cases suggest that microduplication in 2p16.1p15 chromosomal region might be causally linked to developmental delay, speech delay, and mild intellectual disability.

**Keywords:** 2p16.1p15, Molecular karyotyping, Array CGH, microduplication, Duplication, Developmental delay, Macrocephaly

## Background

The implementation of molecular karyotyping (array CGH; aCGH) into the routine genetic diagnostics of children with intellectual disability/developmental delay with or without various congenital anomalies and dysmorphic features has considerably increased the diagnostic utility of genetic testing, as well as the pace of identification of novel microdeletion and microduplication syndromes [1, 2]. In parallel, it enabled us to further delineate genes or groups of genes whose deletion or duplication is associated with a specific phenotype; the recurrent microdeletion and microduplication syndromes.

Herein reported region of 2p16.1p15 was identified as a new microdeletion syndrome (OMIM #612513) already in 2007, when two patients with 4.5 Mb and 5.7 Mb de novo deletions were reported [3]. Since then more than 10 additional patients with different deletion sizes and breakpoints were reported in the literature, with the clinical phenotype including different levels of intellectual disability and developmental delay, speech delay, microcephaly, structural brain anomalies, neuromotor deficits, visual

* Correspondence: lucalovrecic@gmail.com
[1]Clinical Institute of Medical Genetics, University Medical Center Ljubljana, Ljubljana, Slovenia
Full list of author information is available at the end of the article

impairment, strabismus, renal anomalies, camptodactyly, and dysmorphic features [4–10].

On the other hand, the microduplication of the same region 2p16.1p15 has only been recently described in one case [11]. The authors report a relatively milder clinical phenotype as compared to the above mentioned clinical features of the individuals with the deletion in this chromosomal region. As only one case has been extensively described, the phenotype associated to the 2p16.1p15 microduplication has not been delineated as a specific disorder.

**We present four further cases of microduplication 2p16.1p15 and** compare the clinical features of our patients with those previously described. In addition, some patients are described in DECIPHER and ClinGen databases and are included in the report as well (Fig. 2/Table 1). With growing number of patients further evidence is provided that 2p16.1p15 microduplication might be linked to developmental delay, speech delay, and mild intellectual disability.

## Cases presentation

### Patient 1

The first patient is a male child of healthy non consanguineous parents. He was born at term after an uneventful pregnancy with birth weight 3.244 g (25-50P), birth length 50.3 cm (25-50P) and head circumference 38.5 cm (97P). At birth he presented mild jaundice, reduced movements and some initial feeding difficulties. Thoracic and abdominal ultrasound were normal.

The developmental milestones in the boy were delayed - he was able to sit independently at 11 months of age and he started to walk at 21 months. The first sounds and signs of speech/language development were described after 14 months of age. At 4 years of age he was not able to generate complete sentences. A mild intellectual disability was present. His growth parameters were within the normal range. Mild dysmorphic features were described - receding forehead, broad and high nasal bridge, sparse eyebrows, epicanthal folds, straight eyelashes and pronounced philtrum (Fig. 1a). He has bilateral clinodactyly of the 5th finger and bilateral 2nd-3rd toes syndactyly. He was referred to genetic counseling for delayed global development. Informed consent for the study was obtained from the parents.

Microarray analysis (180 K CGH array, Agilent Technologies-Fig. 1b) revealed a de novo microduplication of 2,00 Mb in chromosome 2p16.1p15 region (arr[GRCh37] 2p16.1p15(60113626_62111114)× 3 dn). No other pathogenic genomic imbalance was detected in the proband's sample.

### Patient 2

The second patient is a 5-year old boy, born as a first child to healthy non-consanguineous parents. The mother reported two previous early spontaneous abortions. Otherwise, the family history is unremarkable. He was born after an uneventful pregnancy in the 37th week of gestation after a spontaneous start of the delivery. The boy's birth weight was 2430 g (10-25P), birth length 46 cm (10-25P), and head circumference 34.5 cm (75-90P). He had gastroesophageal reflux in the first few months, the abdominal ultrasound was normal. Due to apnoic attacks the boy was administered to hospital at the age of 5 months. The pH-metry confirmed gastroesophageal reflux, ECG and CMCRF were normal. The neurologist described a mild hypertonus and related mild motor delay. He sat independently at 9 months of age and he started walking at 20 months of age. The parents noted shortness of breath and tiredness after simple physical tasks, therefore, he was evaluated by a paediatric cardiologist. Two haemodynamically significant ASDs were noted and a slightly dilated right ventricle; corrective surgery is planned. The tests of acylcarnitine profiles and aminoacids in blood and organic acid in urine were normal. At the age of four his height and weight were in the normal range (height 99.2 cm (17P), weight 16.1 kg (46P)), however, the head circumference showed macrocephaly - 53.8 cm (>97P).

Microarray analysis (180 K CGH array, Agilent Technologies- Fig. 1b) revealed a de novo microduplication of 2.06 Mb in chromosome 2p16.1p15 region (arr[GRCh37] 2p16.1p15(60308869_62368583)× 3 dn). No other pathogenic genomic imbalance was detected in the proband's sample.

### Patient 3 - DECIPHER ID323264

This male patient was born after an uneventful pregnancy in the 36th week of gestation with birth weight 2820 g (50P), birth length 51 cm (90P), and head circumference 36.5 cm (97P). He walked at 18 months and showed speech delay. He has learning difficulties and attends a special education program. At 15 years his growth parameters were in the normal range (weight 60 kg (50-75P), height 165 cm (25-50P), head circumference 55 cm (25P). Microarray analysis revealed a microduplication of 1.61 Mb in chromosome 2p16.1p15 region, confirmed by FISH (arr[GRCh37] 2p16.1p15(60236241–61,848,845)× 3 mat). Also, his mother was a carrier of the duplication with learning difficulties, epilepsy and obesity. No further details about her phenotype were available.

### Patient 4 - DECIPHER ID258333

This male patient was born at term after an uneventful pregnancy. He displayed early hypotonia and neonatal feeding difficulties. He walked at 20 months and showed

**Table 1** Clinical characteristics of previously reported cases with overlapping duplications

| Case ID | Our case 1 | Our case 2 | DECIPHER 323264 | DECIPHER 258333 | Mimouchi-Bloch A, et al. (ref) | DECIPHER 1570 | DECIPHER 265052 |
|---|---|---|---|---|---|---|---|
| Coordinates of duplications (hg19) | Chr2:60113626_62111114 | Chr2:60308869_62368583 | Chr2:60236241–61,848,845 | Chr2:59938734–62,025,519 | Chr2:60150427_61816209 | Chr2:60648296–61,568,645 | Chr2:60541781–61,952,880 |
| Chromosome band | 2p16.1p15 | 2p16.1p15 | 2p16.1p15 | 2p16.1p15 | 2p16.1p15 | 2p16.1p15 | 2p16.1p15 |
| Gender* | M, 3y | M, 5y | F, 15y | M | M, 5y | F, 3y | F, 7y |
| Developmental delay | +** | + | + | + | + | + | + |
| Speech delay | + | + | + | + | + | + | + |
| Intellectual disability | + | + | + | + | mild | + | - |
| Autism | - | - | - | - | - (ADHD) | - | - |
| Craniofaci al signs | | Macrocephaly | | Macrocephaly | | | |
| Forehead | Receding forehead | | - | | | Frontal bossing | - |
| Eyes | Epicanthal folds<br>Straight eyelashes, sparse eyebrows | Upslanted palpebral fissures | - | | Puffy eyelids | Blepharophimosis<br>Upslanted palpebral fissures | -<br>- |
| Nose | Broad and high nasal bridge | Concave nasal bridge | - | | | Wide nasal bridge | - |
| Ears | | | - | | Right earlobe | | |
| Mouth | Pronounced philtrum<br>Pronounced Cupid's bow | Pronounced philtrum<br>Pronounced Cupid's bow | - | Small ears | sinus<br>Broad philturm | Low-set ears<br>Thin upper<br>and lower lip vermilion<br>Micrognathia | |
| Other Cardiovascular | – | Atrial septum defect | – | – | – | Atrial septum defect | – |
| Hypotonia | + | + | - | + | - | - | - |
| Other | Clinodactyly of the 5th finger, bilaterally<br>2nd-3rd toes syndactyly | Clinodactyly of the 5th finger | Epilepsy<br>Obesity | Recurrent infections<br>Abnormality of erythrocytes<br>Small hands | Visual impairment | Short stature<br>Short palm<br>Tapered fingers<br>2nd-3rd toe syndactyly | Obesity<br>Arthritis<br>Precocious puberty |

* *M* male, *F* female, ** + present, – not reported

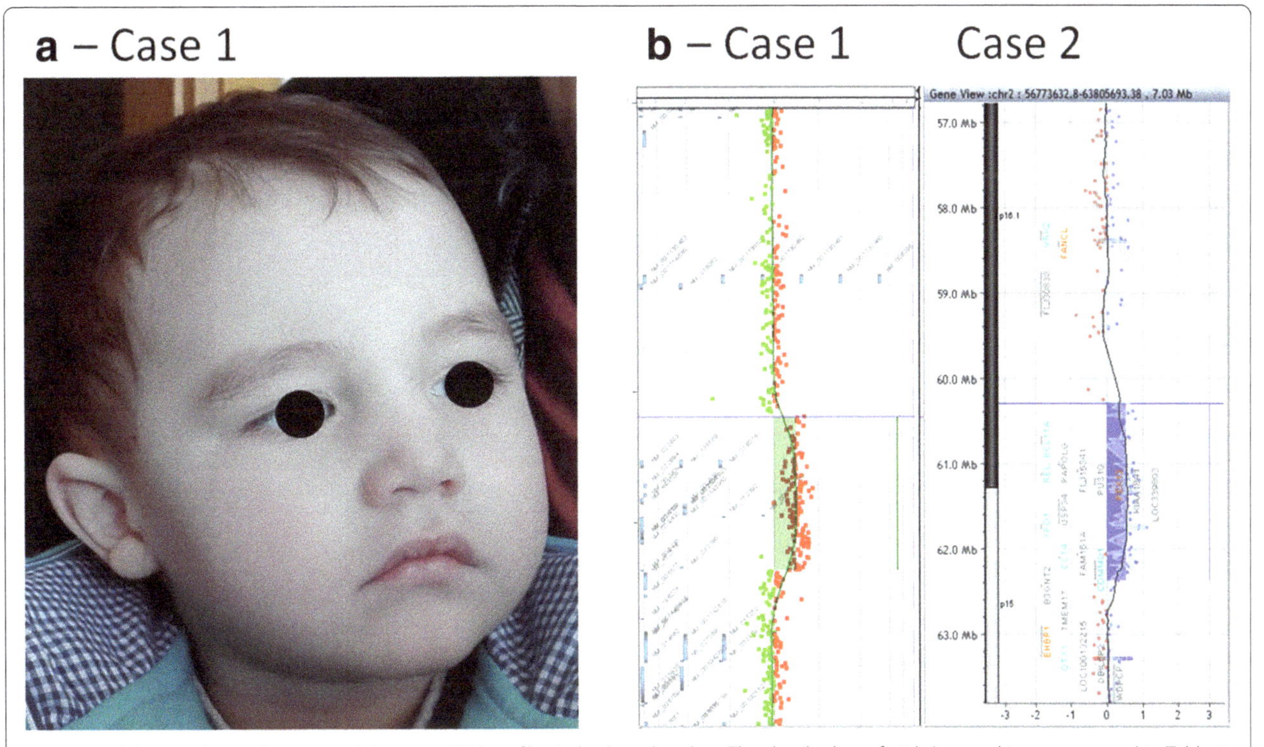

**Fig. 1** Facial dysmorphism of case 1 and the array CGH profiles in both probands. **a** The details about facial dysmorphis are presented in Table 1; **b** The array CGH results are presented for both Case 1 and Case 2. The reported duplications are almost the same. Case 1 - arr[GRCh37] 2p16.1p15(60113626_62111114)× 3 dn; Case 2 - arr[GRCh37] 2p16.1p15(60308869_62368583)× 3 dn

speech delay. Later, moderate intellectual disability was diagnosed. In the childhood, he had recurrent infections with neutropenia and thrombocytopenia. He has small ears and small hands. At 33 years his growth parameters were as follows: height 192 cm (95P), weight 95 kg (95P), head circumference 63.5 cm (>97P). Microarray analysis revealed a microduplication of 2.09 Mb in chromosome 2p16.1p15 region, confirmed by FISH (arr[GRCh37] 2p16.1p15(59938734–62,025,519)× 3 dn).

### Comparison with overlapping cases

The Database of Genomic Variants (DGV) [12] was checked for the presence of similar CNVs in control populations and none were revealed. A search through several databases, DECIPHER [13], ClinGen [14] and scientific literature indexed in PubMed (http://www.ncbi.nlm.nih.gov/pubmed) was performed.

According to all cases reported in the literature or deposited in databases with phenotype description (Table 1), there are 3 additional cases with overlapping duplications. One presented in detail as a case report [11] and 2 deposited in DECIPHER database. All were de novo. There are 4 additional cases, 1 in DECIPHER database with no phenotype data and 3 in ClinGen/ISCA database, listed under category "Developmental delay and additional significant developmental and morphological phenotypes referred for genetic testing". All CNVs are presented in Fig. 2.

The common features among the 7 patients with described phenotypic details are developmental delay, speech delay, mild to moderate intellectual disability, and unspecific dysmorphic features. Two patients have bilateral clinodactyly of the 5th finger and two have bilateral 2nd-3rd toes syndactyly. Interestingly, as opposed to the deletion phenotype, where microcephaly is reported in approximately 44% of patients [9], 2 out of 7 patients with duplication have macrocephaly. Such mirror phenotypes are often reported in the cases of microdeletion and microduplication syndromes of common region [15, 16].

The smallest region of overlap among reported cases encompasses 9 genes: *BCL11A, PAPOLG, REL, PUS10, PEX13,KIAA1841, C2orf74, ASHA2, USP34,* among them *BCL11A and PEX13* are OMIM Morbid genes. Gene PEX13 (OMIM*601789) is linked to the autosomal recessive Peroxisome biogenesis disorder 11A and 11B.

The second OMIM Morbid *BCL11A* has just recently been linked to new autosomal dominant Dias-Logan syndrome [17], with suggested clinical syndrome of at least mild dysmorphisms with intellectual disability and persistence of fetal haemoglobin. The type of mutation (missense mutations, truncating mutations, bigger deletions) partially defines the Dias-Logan phenotype, whereas the deletions of the neighbouring regions present as a 2p16.1p15 microdeletion syndrome with additional

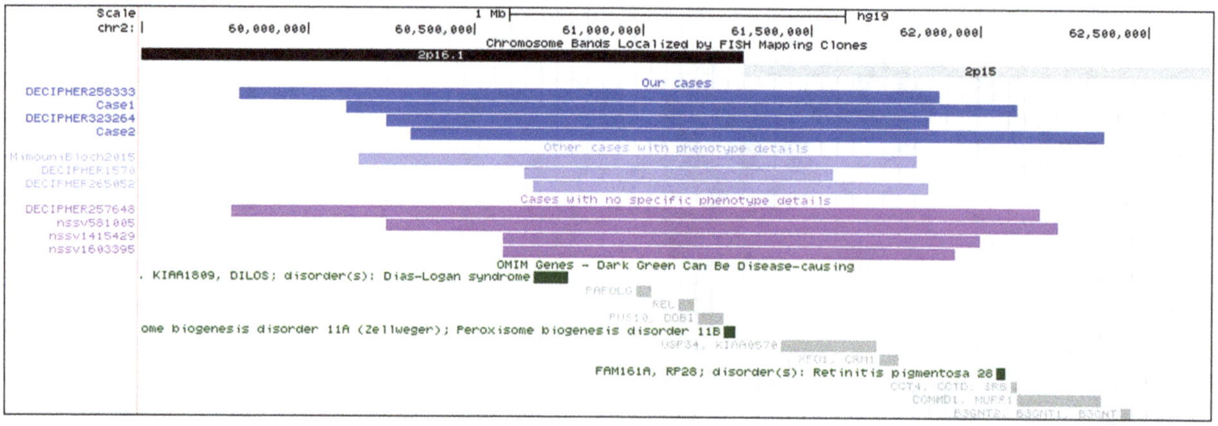

**Fig. 2** The duplication overlap with other reported/deposited casesSizes and locations of herein reported cases and other reported overlapping cases are shown. The UCSC Genome Browser is used. Gene content (OMIM genes) is presented under the reported cases

clinical features, as described above. The BCL11A is highly expressed in human cerebral cortex, hippocampus and cerebellum and the zebrafish knockdown models developed microcephaly and showed size reduction [18]. The 2p16.1p15 microdeletion syndrome patients have broad size range of deleted regions, and in addition to BCL11A, one more gene has shown potential link to the phenotype after extensive studies. Knockdown of REL in zebrafish resulted in specific structural brain anomalies, abnormal growth, and dysmorphisms. These findings are in accordance with known roles of REL in NF-kappaB pathway and memory formation [18].

When trying to decipher the meaning of duplications, search for copy number gain of selected genes was performed. There are currently no additional data (apart from the CNV sizes and some phenotype features of reported cases) available for the above mentioned genes in the literature. Telomeric borders of herein detailed duplications, including those from available databases with no specific phenotype data, do not differ by gene content (Fig. 2). On the centromeric border, there are 4 genes that are not uniformly duplicated in all cases, namely XPO1 (OMIM#602559), FAM16A1 (OMIM#613596), CCT4 (OMIM#605142) and COMMD1 (OMIM#607238). FAM16A1 is a known morbid gene, linked to autosomal recessive Retinitis pigmentosa 28. The other 3 genes have not been linked to human disease before and there are no individual phenotype features that could be linked to specific duplication sizes in the group of patients that are included in this report. Most likely explanation is that these genes do not cause significant additional clinical phenotype when present in 3 copies. Less likely, these might be increased gene dosage sensitive genes, but specific phenotype has not been sufficiently described in presented patients.

## Conclusion

Despite of almost two decades of molecular karyotyping in the group of individuals with developmental delay, intellectual disability, dysmorphic features and additional clinical characteristics, novel rare copy number variations are still identified. Their absence in the databases of normal copy number variation covering numerous populations renders further proof of potential significance or causality for specific phenotypes. Herein we report in detail 4 additional cases of 2p16.1p15 microduplication, which has been reported only once in the literature so far [11]. Each novel case of such a rare CNV provides important insights for clinicians, as well as for deciphering the human genome.

Together with previously reported data, our results suggest that the 2p16.1p15 microduplication might be linked to developmental delay, speech delay, mild to moderate intellectual disability, and unspecific dysmorphic features. Further cases are needed to decipher its clinical implications and decide if it represents a new clinical entity.


### Acknowledgements

We thank the families for their generous collaboration. We gratefully acknowledge the financial support of the University of Udine and Rotary Club Udine Nord for supporting FB.

This study makes use of data generated by the DECIPHER community. A full list of centres who contributed to the generation of the data is available from http://decipher.sanger.ac.uk and via email from decipher@sanger.ac.uk. Funding for the project was provided by the Wellcome Trust.

### Funding

This work is supported by funds of the Udine University to GD. We thank the Rotary Club Udine Nord for supporting FB.


### Authors' contributions

LL, CG, AF, SB, GD, and IB contributed to clinical evaluation. LL, CG, FB and BP performed genetic testing and interpretation. LL, GD and BP drafted the manuscript. All authors read and approved the final manuscript.

## Competing interests

The authors declare that they have no competing interests.

## Author details

[1]Clinical Institute of Medical Genetics, University Medical Center Ljubljana, Ljubljana, Slovenia. [2]Istituto di Genetica Medica, Azienda Ospedaliero-Universitaria di Udine, Udine, Italy. [3]Dipartimento di Medicina Interna e Specialità Mediche dell'Università Sapienza di Roma, Udine, Italy. [4]Department of Pediatric Endocrinology, Diabetes and Metabolic Diseases, University Children's Hospital, University Medical Center Ljubljana, Ljubljana, Slovenia. [5]Dipartimento di Area Medica, Università di Udine, Udine, Italy. [6]Service de génétique médicale, CHU de Nantes, Nantes, France.

## References

1. Miller DT, Adam MP, Aradhya S, et al. Consensus statement: chromosomal microarray is a first-tier clinical diagnostic test for individuals with developmental disabilities or congenital anomalies. Am J Hum Genet. 2010; 86(5):749–64.
2. Watson CT, Marques-Bonet T, Sharp AJ, Mefford HC. The genetics of microdeletion and microduplication syndromes: an update. Annu Rev Genomics Hum Genet. 2014;15:215–44.
3. Rajcan-Separovic E, Harvard C, Liu X, et al. Clinical and molecular cytogenetic characterisation of a newly recognised microdeletion syndrome involving 2p15-16.1. J Med Genet. 2007;44:269–76.
4. Chabchoub E, Vermeesch JR, de Ravel T, de Cock P, Fryns JP. The facial dysmorphy in the newly recognised microdeletion 2p15-p16.1 refined to a 570 kb region in 2p15. J Med Genet. 2008;45:189–92.
5. de Leeuw N, Pfundt R, Koolen DA, et al. A newly recognised microdeletion syndrome involving 2p15p16.1: narrowing down the critical region by adding another patient detected by genome wide tiling path array comparative genomic hybridisation analysis. J Med Genet. 2008;45:122–4.
6. Liang JS, Shimojima K, Ohno K, Sugiura C, Une Y, Yamamoto T. A newly recognised microdeletion syndrome of 2p15-16.1 manifesting moderate developmental delay, autistic behaviour, short stature, microcephaly, and dysmorphic features: a new patient with 3.2 Mb deletion. J Med Genet. 2009;46:645–7.
7. Felix TM, Petrin AL, Sanseverino MT, Murray JC. Further characterization of microdeletion syndrome involving 2p15-p16.1. Am J Med Genet A. 2010; 152A:2604–8.
8. Prontera P, Bernardini L, Stangoni G, et al. Deletion 2p15-16.1 syndrome: case report and review. Am J Med Genet A. 2011;155A:2473–8.
9. Piccione M, Piro E, Serraino F, et al. Interstitial deletion of chromosome 2p15-16.1: report of two patients and critical review of current genotype-phenotype correlation. Eur J Med Genet. 2012;55:238–44.
10. Hancarova M, Simandlova M, Drabova J, Mannik K, Kurg A, Sedlacek Z. A patient with de novo 0.45 Mb deletion of 2p16.1: the role of BCL11A, PAPOLG, REL, and FLJ16341 in the 2p15-p16.1 microdeletion syndrome. Am J Med Genet A. 2013;161A:865–70.
11. Mimouni-Bloch A, Yeshaya J, Kahana S, Maya I, Basel-Vanagaite L. A de-novo interstitial microduplication involving 2p16.1-p15 and mirroring 2p16.1-p15 microdeletion syndrome: clinical and molecular analysis. Eur J Paediatr Neurol. 2015;19:711–5.
12. DGV database, http://dgv.tcag.ca/, Accessed 20 Sept 2017.
13. Clinical Genome, ISCA Database, http://dbsearch.clinicalgenome.org/search/, Accessed 20 Sept 2017.
14. The Decipher Database, release version 9.10, http://decipher.sanger.ac.uk, Accessed 20 Sept 2017.
15. Shinawi M, Liu P, S-HL K, et al. Recurrent reciprocal 16p11.2 rearrangements associated with global developmental delay, bahavioural problems, dysmorphism, epilepsy, and abnormal head size. J Med Genet. 2010;47:332–41.
16. Jacquemont S, Reymond A, Zufferey F, et al. Mirror extreme BMI phenotypes associated with gene dosage at the chromosome 16p11.2 locus. Nature. 2011;478:97–102.
17. Peter B, Matsushita M, Oda K, Raskind W. De novo microdeletion of BCL11A is associated with severe speech sound disorder. Am J Med Genet A. 2014; 164A:2091–6.
18. Bagheri H, Badduke C, Qiao Y, et al. Identifying candidate genes for 2p15p16.1 microdeletion syndrome using clinical, genomic, and functional analysis. JCI Insight. 2016;1(3):e85461.

# A case of placental trisomy 18 mosaicism causing a false negative NIPT result

Jiexia Yang[1,2†], Yiming Qi[1,2†], Fangfang Guo[1,2], Yaping Hou[1,2], Haishan Peng[1,2], Dongmei Wang[1,2], Haoxin OY[1,2] and Aihua Yin[1,2*]

**Abstract**

**Background:** The non-invasive prenatal testing that evaluates circulating cell free DNA, and has been established as an additional pregnancy test for detecting the common fetal trisomies 21, 18 and 13 is rapidly revolutionizing prenatal screening as a result of its increased sensitivity and specificity. However, false positive and false negative results still exist.

**Case presentation:** We presented a case in which the non-invasive prenatal testing results were normal at 15 gestational age (GA), but an ultrasound examination at 30GA showed that the fetus had heart abnormalities, and the third trimester ultrasound at 33GA noted multiple anomalies including a 3.0 mm ventricular septal defect. Along with cordocentesis at 33GA, the cord blood sample cytogenetics analysis showed a mos 47,XN,+18[61]/46,XN[39] T18 karyotype. Six placental biopsies confirmed that the chromosome 18 placenta chimerism ratio had changed from 33% to 72%. Ultimately, the pregnancy was interrupted at 34GA.

**Conclusions:** We presented this case to highlight the need to clearly explain false positive or false negative results to patients. We believe that this information will also influence the development of future diagnostic test methodologies.

**Keywords:** The non-invasive prenatal testing (NIPT), Cell-free DNA (cfDNA), False negative, Placental mosaicism

## Background

Non-invasive prenatal testing (NIPT) which was established as an additional pregnancy test for detecting of the common fetal trisomies 21 (T21), 18 (T18) and 13 (T13), is rapidly becoming a common clinical practice [1]. It evaluates circulating cell-free DNA (cfDNA) as early as 9 gestational age (GA). These DNA fragments are derived from apoptotic placental cytotrophoblast cells [2]. Cell-free fetal DNA (cffDNA) can be described quantitatively as the fetal DNA fraction, and is determined by the ratio of the absolute concentration of cffDNA to the absolute concentration of total (maternal and fetal) cfDNA [3]. NIPT has used for several years as part of prenatal care to screen high-risk patients for fetal aneuploidy, and it has been used increasingly in clinical practice. The pooled sensitivities in the selected high-risk pregnant population were 0.998 (95% CI 0.981 to 0.999), 0.977 (95% CI 0.958 to 0.987) for T21 and T18, respectively. Pooled sensitivity for T13 sensitivity was closer to 0.900. The pooled specificity in the high-risk population for trisomies 21, 18, and 13 is 0.999 (95% 0.998 to 0.999) [4, 5]. However, false positive and false negative results till exist, as cffDNA comes from apoptotic placental trophoblast cells [6]. Therefore, the results may not always represent the actual fetal karyotype in all cases. In the vast majority of pregnancies, although the genetic component between the placental and fetal tissue is identical, false positive or false negative results still exist due to confined placental mosaicism (CPM) [7, 8]. Some positive NIPT results were finally confirmed to be false positive, and common reasons include placental mosaicism, vanishing twin or cotwin demise, fetal chromosome rearrangement, and maternal chromosome abnormalities or malignancy [9, 10]. In contrast, there is a small chance of a false negative result. The fact that cffDNA in the maternal plasma fraction originates from the cytotrophoblast explains a

* Correspondence: yinaiwa@126.com
†Equal contributors
1Prenatal Diagnosis Centre, Guangdong Women and Children Hospital, Guangzhou, Guangdong 511400, China
2Maternal and Children Metabolic-Genetic Key Laboratory, Guangdong Women and Children Hospital, Guangzhou, Guangdong 511400, China

part of the discrepancies between NIPT results and the actual fetal karyotype. A low level of cffDNA fraction in maternal plasma can also result a false negative NIPT result [11].

Herein, we presented one case of a patient whose fetus tested "negative" for T18 by NIPT but was diagnosed as mos 47,XN,+18[61]/46,XN[39]. Our report suggests that some pregnant women display regional placental mosaicism, which is sufficient to cause a discrepancy between the NIPT and karyotyping results.

## Methods

The NIPT test was performed at 15 and 34GA by sequencing cfDNA from the maternal peripheral blood. Blood collection, cfDNA extraction, library construction and sequencing were performed according to the instructions of JingXin Fetal Chromosome Aneuploidy (T21, T18, T13) Testing Kits (CFDA registration permit No. 0153400300) [12].

Based on our previous study, we developed a technique that uses the read length to estimate the concentration of fetal cfDNA in maternal plasma by sequencing [12]. The fetal DNA concentration was calculated as a quality control, as described in Yin's paper [12]. Combined GC-correction and Z-score testing methods were used to identify fetal autosomal aneuploidy for trisomy as described in Liao's paper [13]. Z score range from −3 to 3 was considered to indicate a low risk for a trisomy chromosome [14]. A cord blood sample was taken at 33GA. A cord blood sample and six placental biopsies (three from the maternal side and three from the fetal side) were taken for analysis. DNA sequencing, cfDNA extraction, library construction and sequencing were performed through bioconductor sequencing platform [12]. The speculated chimeric proportion of T18 was calculated from the ratio of the samples to the control. For example, for sample 1, the speculated chimeric proportion = 2*(1−3.327%/2.856%) =33%.

## Case presentation

A 32-year-old healthy pregnant woman was referred to the Medical Genetic Centre of Guangdong Women and Children Hospital. Maternal serum screening at 12GA combined nuchal translucency measurement (2.4 mm) showed a high risk of fetal T21 at 1 in 190. The NIPT at 15GA showed that the fetal DNA fraction in the maternal plasma sample was 7.8% (normal NIPT result) and the Chromosome18 Z scores were 1.889 (Table 1). NIPT provided at 15GA gave a low risk result.

As routine practice, ultrasound was conducted to monitor the developmental status of the fetus. The ultrasound examination at 24GA showed that the fetus displayed a defect in the ventricular compartment, which was confirmed by the ultrasound examination at 30 GA (Figure 1A). The ultrasound examination showed a 2.2 mm ventricular septal defect. At 33GA (Figure 1B), the patient was referred for further evaluation after a third trimester ultrasound revealed a 3.0 mm ventricular septal defect, and all four limbs were smaller than is observed at normal gestational weeks. For further counseling, the patient consented to have a cord blood sample taken by cordocentesis at 33GA. Cytogenetics analyses reported a karyotyping of mos 47,XN,+18[61]/46,XN[39] indicated that 61% of cells had trisomy 18 even though both parental karyotypes were normal. After genetic counseling and communicating with families, the pregnant woman opted to terminate her pregnancy at 34GA.

Maternal peripheral blood was collected for a confirmatory NIPT test before the pregnancy was interrupted at 34GA. Placental tissues were also retained. Six placental biopsies (three from the maternal side and three from the fetal side) were taken for sequencing. Placental biopsies confirmed that it was placental chimerism of chromosome18, with a chimeric ratio from 33% to 72% (Table 2). The chimeric ratios of the placental biopsies were consistently around 61%, which was the T18 mosaicism fetal umbilical cord blood type result. The NIPT reported Z-scores were −1.491, 5.500 and −0.016 for chromosome21, 18 and 13 respectily (Table 1), and the fetal fraction was 16.6%. These results confirmed that the fetus displayed T18 mosaicism, which indicated a false negative result for NIPT at 15GA.

## Discussion and conclusions

Increasing amounts of evidence have shown that the circulating fetal DNA in maternal blood during pregnancy mainly originates from placental trophoblastic cells, although there are still small contributions from fetal tissues [2]. Since cfDNA was identified, it has been widely promoted for the development of NIPT [15]. However, many factors can still affect NIPT results; for example, the maternal weight can significantly decrease the fetal DNA fraction [16], which usually leads to a false negative result. Otherwise, 0.8–1% of cases are confirmed as placental

**Table 1** NIPT results for the Case

| Gestational Weeks | Unique reads/ M | Fetal DNA Fraction | NIPT Z-scores | | | NIPT result |
|---|---|---|---|---|---|---|
| | | | Chromosome21 | Chromosome18 | Chromosome13 | |
| 15 | 3.25 | 7.80% | −0.466 | 1.889 | 1.369 | Low Risk |
| 34 | 3.36 | 16.6% | −1.491 | 5.500 | −0.016 | High Risk of T18 |

Z scores were calculated as previously described [12] with a normal range > −3 and <3

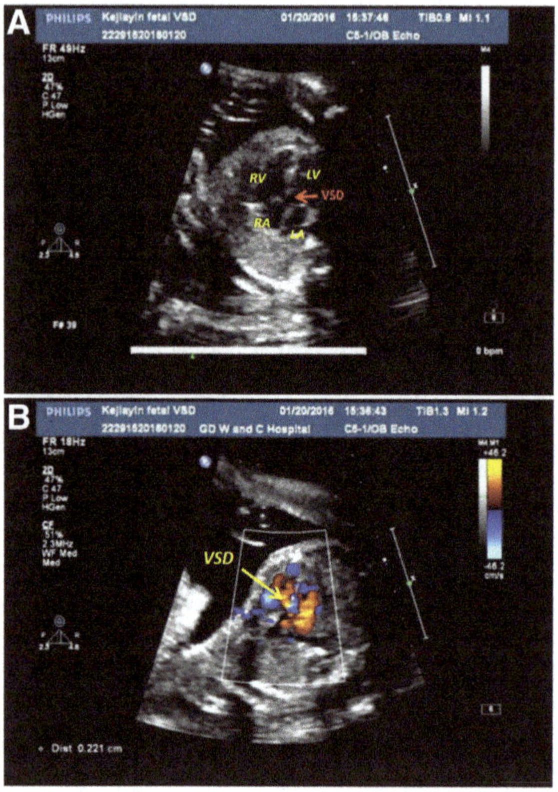

**Fig. 1** Ultrasound examination images. **a** Ultrasound examination result at 30wk. A ventricular septal defect for 2.2 mm was shown as the arrow in the image. Abbreviations: LA, left atrium; LV, left ventricle; RA, right atrium; RV, right ventricle; VSD, ventricular septal defect. **b** Ultrasound examination result at 33wk. A ventricular septal defect (VSD) for 3.0 mm was shown as the arrow in the image

mosaicism according to a large-scale evaluation of chorionic villi sampling (CVS) [17]. Placental mosaicism means that the cffDNA from cytotrophoblast cells has a different karyotype than that of the true fetal DNA [18]. Thus, in this study, we provided a false negative NIPT case caused by both fetal and placental mosaicism. Clinicians should be aware of this situation and patients should be informed of the possibility of discordant NIPT results.

**Table 2** Sequencing results for six placental biopsies

| Sample | | Chromosome 18 Z scores | Chromosome 18 ratio | Speculated chimeric proportion of T18 |
|---|---|---|---|---|
| maternal side | 1 | 40.279 | 3.327% | 33% |
| | 2 | 40.066 | 3.322% | 33% |
| | 3 | 49.474 | 3.427% | 40% |
| fetal side | 4 | 48.311 | 3.420% | 39% |
| | 5 | 89.007 | 3.884% | 72% |
| | 6 | 44.263 | 3.370% | 36% |
| Control | | −2.58944 | 2.856% | / |

Six placental biopsies (three from the maternal side, 1–3; three from the fetal side, 4–6) were taken for routine cytogenetics at 35GA

In this case, of placental mosaicism, the fetal DNA fraction in the maternal plasma sample at 15GA was 7.8% (normal NIPT result) with a chromosome18 Z-score of 1.889. Examination of the placental tissue at six sites showed that T18 mosaicism, as measured by the ratio of trisomy to disomy 18, averaged approximately 42%. Further, the chimeric ratio varied from 32% to 72% at different sites, which suggested that there were significant regional variations in the T18 mosaicism in this placenta. However, this was consistent with the fetal umbilical cord blood karyotype results, which showed a T18 mosaicism ratio of 61%. Furthermore, at 15GA, the fetal DNA percentage was 7.8% due to the mosaicism, and the effective/perceived fetal fraction observed by the algorithm on the trisomy chromosome was (100%−42%)*7.8% = 4.52%. However, a trisomy with an actual fetal fraction of 4.52% is mathematically insufficient to detect the 42% placental T18 when using our NIPT test. The fetal DNA concentration increases with gestational weeks [19]. At 35GA, the increased fetal DNA fraction was sufficient to detect the mosaicism. Similar patterns of mosaicism were also reported in cases with false negative cfDNA screening results [8, 9, 20].

This report describes a case of a false negative cell-free DNA result for trisomy 18 due to fetal and placental mosaicism. To date, few NIPT reports have demonstrated that placental mosaicism [14, 21, 22] manifests quite differently across individual pregnancies in pregnant women. The existence of false negatives due to mosaicism is not unique, and information pertaining to these cases is still limited. Multicenter studies have determined the frequency of mosaicism to be approximately 1% [23].In most situations, the mosaic cell line is only found in the placenta and will lead to a normal fetal outcome [24]. However the frequency of false negative fetal test results with maternal serum cffDNA testing due to placental mosaicism or other fetal-placental discrepancies is still unknown [7]. How should unexpected false negative NIPT results be handled in clinical practice? On the one hand, it is necessary that patients receive pretest counseling and informed consent prior to NIPT screening. Patients should be aware of the potential for false positive and false negative results as well as discordant results due to differences between the fetally and parentally derived analyzed samples [7]. We hope to give clinicians a reference with this case. Clinicians should be cognizant of false negative results when the fetal DNA concentrations are relatively low. In contrast, as the frequency and level of various types of mosaicism are still limited, new and accurate documents are valuable to the diagnostic and medical community. It is necessary for the NIPT field to improve its sensitivity and specificity and reduce the incidence of discordant results. This information can not only contribute to the development of future screening test methodologies and algorithms, but can also help optimize the counseling and medical decision applied by medical practitioners.

### Abbreviations
cfDNA: Cell free DNA; cffDNA: Cell-free fetal DNA; CPM: Confined placental mosaicism; CVS: Chorionic villi sampling; GA: Gestational age; NIPT: Non-invasive prenatal testing; T18: Trisomy 18


### Acknowledgements
Thanks to the CapitalBio Genomics Co., Ltd. and Wei Lei for data analysis and writing help.

### Funding
National Key Research and Development Program of China, 2016YFC1000700, 2016YFC1000703.


### Authors' contributions
All authors have materially participated in the study and manuscript preparation. Jiexia Yang and Yiming Qi carried out all the molecular genetic analysis, and paticipated in the design of the work; Fangfang Guo and Yaping Hou collected all clininal data and participated in conceiving the work; Dongmei Wang and Haoxin OY participated in conceiving the work, and revising the manuscript. Aihua Yin designed the work, drafted and revised the manuscript. All authors have approved the final article.

### Competing interests
The authors declare that they have no competing interests.

### References

1. Norwitz ER. Noninvasive prenatal testing: the future is now. Rev Obstet Gynecol. 2013;6(2):48–62.
2. Liao GJW, Gronowski AM, Zhao Z. Non-invasive prenatal testing using cell-free fetal DNA in maternal circulation. Clin Chim Acta. 2014;428:44–50. doi: 10.1016/j.cca.2013.10.007.
3. Bissell MG. Noninvasive prenatal diagnosis of fetal chromosomal Aneuploidies by maternal plasma nucleic acid analysis. Yearb Pathol Lab Med. 2009;2009:301–3. doi: 10.1016/s1077-9108(08)79012-1.
4. Kim S, Zhao C, Bombard AT, et al. Comment on "clinical application of massively parallel sequencing-based prenatal non-invasive fetal trisomy test for trisomies 21 and 18 in 11 105 pregnancies with mixed risk factors". Prenat Diagn. 2013;33(13):1310–3. doi: 10.1002/pd.4231.
5. Iwarsson E, Jacobsson B, Dagerhamn J, et al. Analysis of cell-free fetal DNA in maternal blood for detection of trisomy 21, 18 and 13 in a general pregnant population and in a high risk population - a systematic review and meta-analysis. Acta Obstet Gynecol Scand. 2017;96(1):7–18. doi: 10.1111/aogs.13047.
6. Chen EZ, Chiu RWK, Sun H, et al. Noninvasive prenatal diagnosis of fetal Trisomy 18 and Trisomy 13 by maternal plasma DNA sequencing. PLoS One. 2011;6(7):e21791. doi:10.1371/journal.pone.0021791.g001.
7. Hall AL, Drendel HM, Verbrugge JL, et al. Positive cell-free fetal DNA testing for trisomy 13 reveals confined placental mosaicism. Genet Med. 2013;15(9):729–32. doi: 10.1038/gim.2013.26.
8. Wang Y, Zhu J, Chen Y, et al. Two cases of placental T21 mosaicism: challenging the detection limits of non-invasive prenatal testing. Prenat Diagn. 2013;33(12):1207–10. doi: 10.1002/pd.4212.
9. Gao Y, Stejskal D, Jiang F, et al. False-negative trisomy 18 non-invasive prenatal test result due to 48,XXX,+18 placental mosaicism. Ultrasound Obstet Gynecol. 2014;43(4):477–8. doi: 10.1002/uog.13240.
10. Osborne CM, Hardisty E, Devers P, et al. Discordant noninvasive prenatal testing results in a patient subsequently diagnosed with metastatic disease. Prenat Diagn. 2013;33(6):609–11. doi: 10.1002/pd.4100.
11. Smith M, Lewis KM, Holmes A, et al. A case of false negative NIPT for down syndrome-lessons learned. Case Rep Genet. 2014;2014:1–3. doi: 10.1155/2014/823504.
12. A-h Y, C-f P, Zhao X, et al. Noninvasive detection of fetal subchromosomal abnormalities by semiconductor sequencing of maternal plasma DNA. Proc Natl Acad Sci. 2015;112(47):14670–5. doi: 10.1073/pnas.1518151112.
13. Liao C, Yin A, Cf P, et al. Noninvasive prenatal diagnosis of common aneuploidies by semiconductor sequencing. Proc Natl Acad Sci. 2014;111(20):7415 20. doi: 10.1073/pnas.1321997111.
14. Chiu RWK, Akolekar R, Zheng YWL, et al. Non-invasive prenatal assessment of trisomy 21 by multiplexed maternal plasma DNA sequencing: large scale validity study. BMJ. 2011;342(jan11 1):c7401. doi: 10.1136/bmj.c7401.
15. Langlois S, Brock J-A, Douglas Wilson R, et al. Current status in non-invasive prenatal detection of down syndrome, Trisomy 18, and Trisomy 13 using cell-free DNA in maternal plasma. J Obstet Gynaecol Can. 2013;35(2):177–81. doi: 10.1016/s1701-2163(15)31025-2.
16. Canick JA, Palomaki GE, Kloza EM, et al. The impact of maternal plasma DNA fetal fraction on next generation sequencing tests for common fetal aneuploidies. Prenat Diagn. 2013;33(7):667–74. doi: 10.1002/pd.4126.
17. Ledbetter DH, Zachary JM, Simpson JL, Golbus MS, Pergament E, Jackson L, Mahoney MJ, Desnick RJ, Schulman J, Copeland KL, et al. Cytogenetic results from the U.S. collaborative study on CVS. Prenat Diagn. 1992;12(5):317–45.
18. Flori E, Doray B, Gautier E, Kohler M, Ernault P, Flori J, Costa JM. Circulating cell-free fetal DNA in maternal serum appears to originate from cyto- and syncytio-trophoblastic cells. Case Rep Hum Reprod. 2004;19(3):723–4.
19. Hu H, Liu H, Peng C, Deng T, Fu X, Chung C, Zhang E, Lu C, Zhang K, Liang Z, Yang Y. Clinical experience of non-invasive prenatal chromosomal Aneuploidy testing in 190,277 patient samples. Curr Mol Med. 2016;16(8):759–66.
20. Pan Q, Sun B, Huang X, Jing X, Liu H, Jiang F, Zhou J, Lin M, Yue H, Hu P, Ning Y. A prenatal case with discrepant findings between non-invasive prenatal testing and fetal genetic testings. Mol Cytogenet. 2014;7(1):48.
21. Choi H, Lau TK, Jiang FM, et al. Fetal aneuploidy screening by maternal plasma DNA sequencing: 'false positive' due to confined placental mosaicism. Prenat Diagn. 2013;33(2):198–200. doi: 10.1002/pd.4024.
22. Pan M, Li FT, Li Y, et al. Discordant results between fetal karyotyping and non-invasive prenatal testing by maternal plasma sequencing in a case of uniparental disomy 21 due to trisomic rescue. Prenat Diagn. 2013;33(6):598–601. doi: 10.1002/pd.4069.
23. Lebo RV, Novak RW, Wolfe K, et al. Discordant circulating fetal DNA and subsequent cytogenetics reveal false negative, placental mosaic, and fetal mosaic cfDNA genotypes. J Transl Med. 2015;13(1). doi:10.1186/s12967-015-0569-y.
24. Mardy A, Wapner RJ. Confined placental mosaicism and its impact on confirmation of NIPT results. Am J Med Genet C: Semin Med Genet. 2016;172(2):118–22. doi: 10.1002/ajmg.c.31505.

# 23

# 18q22.1-qter deletion and 4p16.3 microduplication in a boy with speech delay and mental retardation

Chunjing Wang[1†], Huanhuan Ren[1†], Huaifu Dong[2], Meng Liang[1], Qi Wu[1] and Yaping Liao[1*]

**Abstract**

**Background:** Deletions involving the long arm of chromosome 18 have been associated with a highly variable phenotypic spectrum that is related to the extent of the deleted region. Duplications in chromosomal region 4p16.3 have also been shown to cause 4p16.3 microduplication syndrome. Most reported patients of trisomy 4p16.3 have more duplications, including the Wolf-Hirschhorn critical region (WHSCR). Here, we present a patient with speech delay and mental retardation caused by a deletion of 18q (18q22.1-qter) and terminal microduplication of 4p (4p16.3-pter) distal to WHSCR.

**Case presentation:** The patient was a 23-month-old boy with moderate growth retardation, severe speech delay, mental retardation, and dysmorphic features. Single nucleotide polymorphism (SNP) array analysis confirmed an 11.2-Mb terminal deletion at 18q22.1 and revealed a 1.8-Mb terminal duplication of 4p16.3. Our patient showed clinical overlap with these two syndromes, although his overall features were milder than what had been previously described. Some dosage-sensitive genes on the 18q terminal deleted region and 4p16.3 duplicated region of the present case may have contributed to his phenotype.

**Conclusions:** This is the first report of a patient with combined terminal deletion of 18q22.1 and duplication of 4p16.3. In this report, we provide clinical and molecular evidence supporting that the microduplication in 4p16.3, distal to WHSCR, is pathogenic. The coexistence of two chromosome aberrations complicates the clinical picture and creates a chimeric phenotype. This report provides further information on the genotype-phenotype correlation of 18q terminal deletion and 4p microduplication.

**Keywords:** 18q22.1 deletion, 4p16.3 duplication, Speech delay, Mental retardation, Facial dysmorphisms

## Background

Deletions of the long arm of chromosome 18 (18q deletion syndrome, OMIM #601808) are common abnormalities involving chromosome 18 [1]. Individuals with a terminal 18q deletion display variable phenotypes, including short stature, microcephaly, characteristic dysmorphic facial feature, cleft lip/palate, delayed myelination, foot deformities, hypotonia, congenital aural atresia (CAA), mental retardation (MR), and genitourinary malformations [2–5]. Some dosage-sensitive genes and critical regions on 18q that contribute to the clinical features have been identified, thereby providing a foundation for establishing the genotype-phenotype correlation for 18q deletions [1, 6].

Terminal deletions of chromosome 4p cause Wolf-Hirschhorn syndrome (WHS, OMIM #194190). Duplications involving 4p16.3 have also been reported in several individuals, giving rise to a proposed 4p16.3 microduplication syndrome [7, 8]. Larger imbalanced rearrangements on chromosome 4p in the form of deletions and duplications involving the Wolf–Hirschhorn critical region (WHSCR) have defined clinical features, such as developmental delay, delayed

* Correspondence: liaoyaping2003@sina.com
†Chunjing Wang and Huanhuan Ren contributed equally to this work.
[1]Department of Life Sciences, Bengbu Medical College, 2600 Donghai Avenue, Bengbu, Anhui 233030, People's Republic of China
Full list of author information is available at the end of the article

psychomotor development, intellectual disability, and craniofacial and skeletal malformations [9–12]. However, the significance and clinical presentation of patients with microduplication distal to WHSCR are not well understood. To the best of our knowledge, only two patients have been reported to date [8, 13].

Here, we report another case of a 23-month-old boy with a 1.8-Mb duplication at 4p16.3 distal to the WHSCR combined with an 11.2-Mb terminal deletion at the 18q22.1, who presents with similar and different symptoms previously seen in trisomy 4p and 18q deletion syndrome. This case provides further information regarding the clinical features and genotype-phenotype correlation of 18q deletion and 4p16.3 microduplication.

## Case presentation

The patient was a 23-month-old boy who was referred for cytogenetic studies because of speech delay and mental retardation. He was born at 38 weeks gestation following an unremarkable pregnancy by Caesarean section. His birth weight was 3.40 kg (<50th centile), and birth length was 52 cm (>75th centile). At birth, he had an umbilical hernia, which healed at 3 months of age.

The patient could sit at 8 months, and took his first steps at 18 months. At 23 months, his height was 90 cm (<75th centile), and his weight was 13 kg (<75th centile). He cannot speak meaningful words and walked with instability and large strides. Medical examination revealed developmental delay, sensory integration dysfunction, moderate MR, and reduced cognitive ability. Additional physical features included hypotonia, a moon face, midface hypoplasia, deep-set eyes, epicanthal folds, a wide nasal bridge, a flat nose, a protrusible mouth, short neck, and a longer fourth toe of the right foot. No significant defects such as cleft lip/palate, ears, heart, lung or genitourinary system were noted.

## Materials and methods

### Karyotyping

For chromosome analysis, metaphase chromosomes were obtained from peripheral blood lymphocytes after 72 h of incubation and were prepared for GTG banding according to standard protocols.

### Fish

According to standard protocols, the cultured blood lymphocytes of the patient were harvested to obtain metaphase chromosomes. FISH analysis was performed with six different chromosome 18 BAC probes; RP11-7H17, 185,880 bp, 18q23 (chr18:77,115,373-77,301,252); RP11-55 N14, 173,736 bp, 18p11.31 (chr18:2,744,753-2,918,488); RP11-53 N15, 678 bp, 18q22.3 (chr18:71,881,306-71,881,983); RP11-90 L7, 165,866 bp, 18q11.2 (chr18:23,355,089-23,520,954); RP11-79A24, 141,894 bp, 18q22.1 (chr18:66,593,997-66,735,890); and RP11-90E1, 182,823 bp, and 18q12.3 (chr18:41,350,363-41,533,185). Images were captured using a fluorescent microscope (Leica DM5000B), and signals were analyzed using Leica CW 4000 software.

### SNP array analysis

Infinium OmniZhongHua-8 SNP arrays (Illumina, San Diego, CA, USA) were utilized to analyze genome-wide copy number aberrations. DNA amplification, tagging, and hybridization were processed according to manufacturer's protocols. Illumina's iScan system was used to scan the beadchips. Image data was analyzed using Illumina's GenomeStudio.

## Results

The G-banding chromosomal analysis revealed a karyotype of 46, XY, del (18) (q22) (Figs. 1a and b). The karyotypes of his parents are normal. To investigate the deletion region of 18q, fluorescence in situ hybridization (FISH) analysis using chromosome 18 BAC probes was performed. Data showed hybridization signals in the region of 18q22.1 (chr18:66,593,997-66,735,890) (Fig. 1c) and no hybridization signal in the region of 18q23 (chr18:77,115,373-77,301,252) (Fig. 1d) and 18q22.3 (chr18:71,881,306-71,881,983) (Fig. 1e), indicating an 18q22 terminal deletion. To identify the size and position of the chromosomal aberrations, we performed SNP array analysis. The results showed a terminal deletion at 18q22.1 (Fig. 2a) and revealed the presence of a duplication at 4p16.3 (Fig. 2b). The terminal deletion 18q22.1 was approximately 11.2 Mb (66,794,478–78,015,180) in size and the 4p16.3 duplication was approximately 1.8 Mb (71,566–1,883,647) in size (UCSC genome browser, Human Assembly, GRCh37/hg19).

## Discussion

Using conventional karyotyping, FISH, and SNP array analyses, we report a case involving a terminal deletion of 18q22.1 and duplication of 4p16.3. Patients with terminal deletions of the long arm of chromosome 18 or microduplications of the short arm of chromosome 4 display diverse phenotypes. The clinical phenotypes of our patient show similarities and differences from previously reported cases.

The 18q22 deletion syndrome is characterized by mental retardation and development delay, as well as a range of physical anomalies, including microcephaly, short stature, hearing loss, CAA, cleft palate with or without cleft lip (CL/CP), white matter abnormalities of the brain, hand and foot malformations. Several reports have explored the genotype-phenotype correlations of 18q22 deletion syndrome. Recently, Cody et al. [6] viewed more than 350 individuals with 18q22 deletion syndrome and classified 133 of a total of 196 confirmed genes on 18q

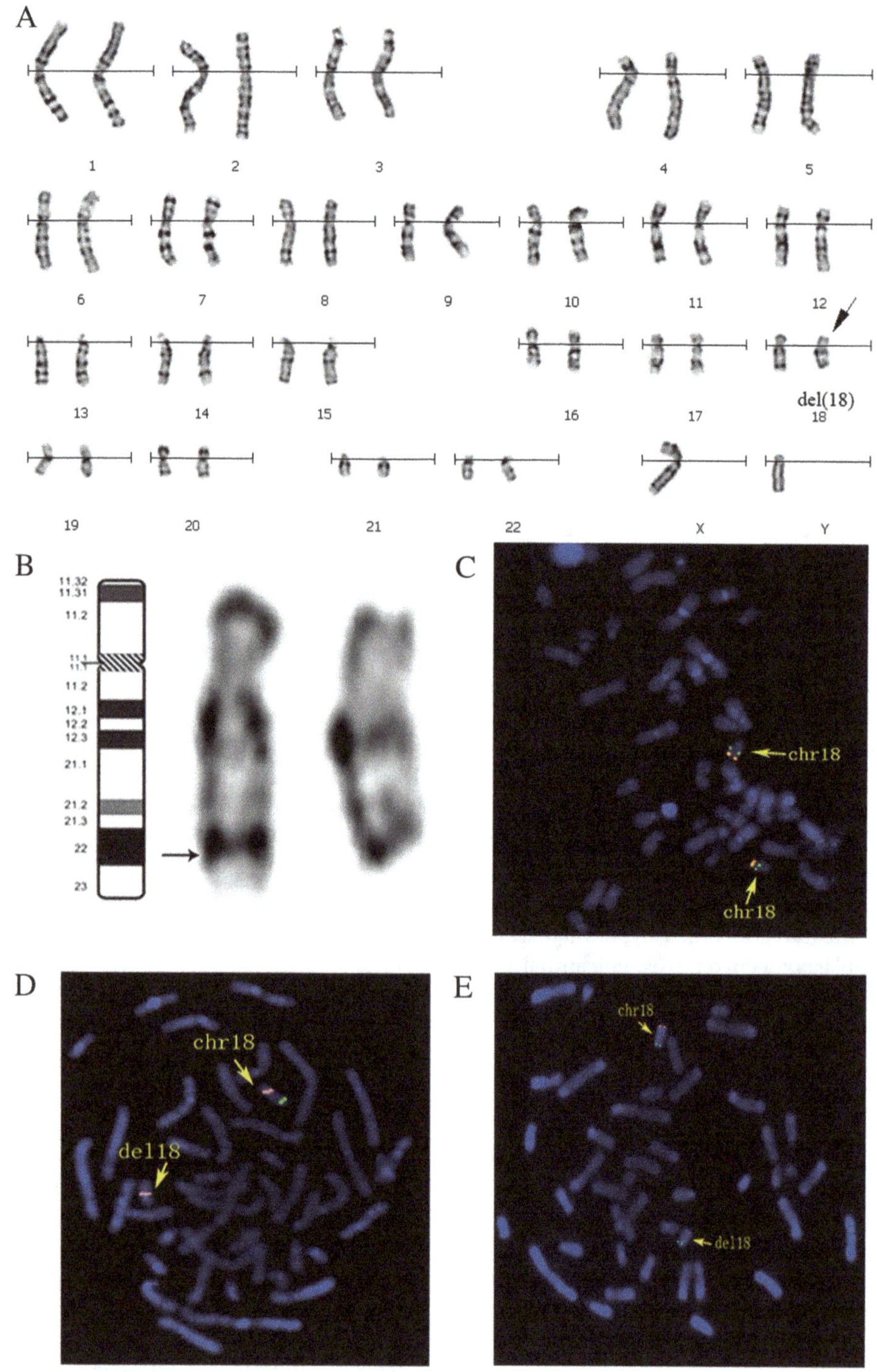


**Fig. 1** Identification of chromosome 18 terminal deletion. **a** GTG banded karyotype of the case showing an aberration at distal 18q indicated by an arrow. **b** G-banding of chromosome 18 showing the deletion of 18q. **c** BAC-probes RP11-79A24 (orange) (18q22.1) (chr18:66,593,997-66,735,890) and RP11-90E1 (green) (18q12.3) (chr18:41,350,363-41,533,185) showing no deletion at 18q22.1 (chr18:66,593,997-66,735,890). **d** BAC-probes (green) (18q22.3) (chr18:71,881,306-71,881,983) and RP11-90 L7 (orange) (18q11.2) (chr18:23,355,089-23,520,954) revealing the deletion of 18q22.3. **e** BAC-probes RP11-7H17 (orange) (18q23) (chr18:77,115,373-77,301,252) and RP11-55 N14 (green) (18p11.31) (chr18:2,744,753-2,918,488) revealing the deletion of 18q23

as dosage-insensitive and 15 (8%) as dosage-sensitive leading to haploinsufficiency, whereas another 10 (5%) have effects that are conditionally haploinsufficient and dependent on another factor, such as genetic or environmental, to cause an abnormal phenotype. Our patient's deletion region includes 5 of the 15 genes. Those genes

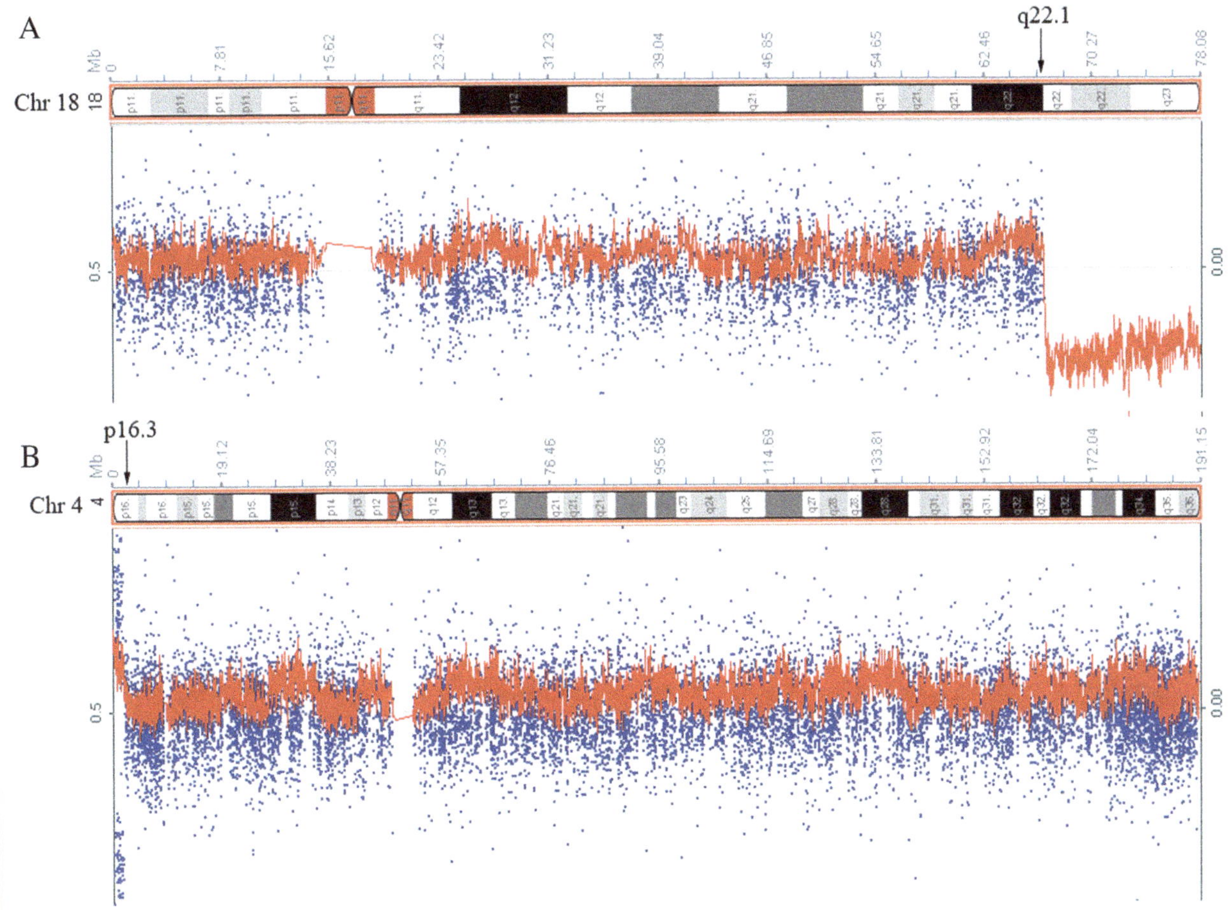

**Fig. 2** SNP array-based chromosome analysis. **a** Identification of the deletion in chromosome 18 revealed an 11.2-Mb deletion at 18q22.1 (chr18:66,794,478–78,015,180). **b** Revealing a 1.8-Mb duplication at 4p16.3 (chr4:71,566–1,883,647)

are *NETO1* (chr18:70,409,549-70,534,810), *CYB5A* (chr18: 71,983,110-72,026,422), *TSHZ1* (chr18:72,997,498-73,000, 596), *MBP* (chr18:74,690,789-74,844,774), and *NFATC1* (chr18:77,160,326-77,289,323).

Although the terminal deletion involving 18q was approximately 11.2 Mb in size and included five dosage-sensitive genes, our patient's clinical features were relatively mild and distinct from those described in 18q- syndrome. Abnormal phenotypes in our case were only associated with *NETO1* and *MBP* genes. In terms of *NETO1* (chr18:70,409,549-70,534,810), patients who are hemizygous for this gene represent executive function difficulties [14]. Haploinsufficiency of this gene has been associated with impaired spatial learning and memory. The *MBP* gene lies within the 18q23 CNS dysmyelination critical region (chr18:72,980,819-75,485,284), and hemizygosity of the *MBP* gene can cause dysmyelination of the brain for people with distal 18q- [14, 15]. Our patient presents MR, walking instability, and large strides, which may be attributed to CNS dysmyelination. However, high-frequency sensorineural hearing loss, which has been associated with the *MBP* gene, was not observed in our patient. In addition, defects in the *TSHZ1* gene would cause cleft soft palate and CAA [16], but our patient does not exhibit both symptoms, although the deletion region of this case included this gene. The other case with a larger deletion of 18q21.3-qter that we previously reported also did not present sensorineural hearing loss, CAA, and CL/CP [17]. Some cases presenting with a mild phenotype suggest that features associated with this deletion is highly heteregeneous. It seems that hemizygosity of some dosage-sensitive genes, such as *TSHZ1* and *MBP*, may not lead to an abnormal phenotype. We infer that variable phenotypes may be attributed to potential gene-gene interactions and gene-environmental interactions.

Interestingly, our patient presents severe speech delay, although the deleted region in 18q does not include the dosage-sensitive gene *SETBP1* (chr18:42,260,863-42,648, 475), which is associated with severe delay in expressive speech with intact receptive language [6, 18, 19]. It may be due to a 1.8-Mb duplication involving 4p16.3 that was also observed in this case. Two critical regions within 4p16.3-WHSCR1 and WHSCR2 for WHS were identified [20, 21]. Most patients with trisomy 4p16.3 have more duplications, which include WHSCR1 and WHSCR2. In contrast, smaller duplications in 4p16.3 distal to WHSCR1 and WHSCR2 are rare. To the best of our knowledge, only two patients have been reported to have this defect [8, 13]. In addition, the duplication involving chromosome 4p16.3 in our patient does not involve WHSCR2 and the coding region of WHSCR1. His clinical features also overlap with the two previously reported cases, including developmental delay, dysmorphic facial features, and speech and cognitive delay. Clinical features of the three patients are discussed in detail and summarized in Table 1.

Some dosage-sensitive genes, such as *LETM1*, *WHSC1*, and *WHSC2*, can be responsible for the duplication 4p phenotype [22]. However, the phenotypic spectrum of patients without the involvement of the WHS critical region is not well understood [13]. The 1.8-Mb microduplication in the present case includes at least 34 RefSeq genes, and some of the genes in this region may have a role in the 4p trisomy phenotype, which include *TACC3*, *FAM53A*, *FGFR3*,

**Table 1** Clinical features of the duplication 4p16.3 cases

| Clinical features | Present case | Cyr et al. [13] | Palumbo et al. [8] |
|---|---|---|---|
| Duplication positions | 71,566–1,883,647 | 1,326,373-1,832,617 | 1,405,662-1,798,461 |
| Other chromosome anomalies | Terminal deletion of 18q22.1 | – | – |
| Gestational age (weeks) | 39 | 38–4/7 | Unknown |
| Sex and age at diagnosis | M, 23 months | M, 9 months | M, 13 years |
| Weight | < 50th centile | 30th centile | > 97th centile |
| Height | > 75th centile | 30th centile | 90-97th centile |
| Head circumference | > 75th centile | > 95th centile | 25-50th centile |
| Neurologic | | | |
| Speech delay | Yes (severe) | Yes | Yes |
| Developmental delay | Yes | Yes | Yes |
| seizure | No | Yes | No |
| Sensory Integration | Dysfunction (squinting while running) | Unknown | Dysfunction (ADHD) |
| Short stature/failure to thrive | No | Yes | No |
| MRI | Unknown | Dilatation of the lateral ventricles | Normal |
| Craniofacial | | | |
| Macro/microcephaly | No | Yes (Macrocephaly) | No |
| Frontal bossing | Yes | Yes | Yes |
| Hypertelorism | Yes | Yes | Yes |
| Epicanthal folds | Yes | Yes | Yes |
| palpebral fissures | Normal | Narrow and long | Downslanted |
| Eyes | Normal | Iris heterochromia; hyperopia | Hyperopia |
| Ears | Low-set and dysmorphic | Low-set and posteriorly rotated | Normal |
| Nose | Broad nasal root and short nasal bridge | Broad nasal root and short nasal bridge | Normal |
| Palate | Normal | Normal | High arched |
| Retrognathia/micrognathia | No | No | Yes |
| Neck | Short | Short | Short |
| Musculoskeletal | | | |
| Hypotonia/ Hypertonia | Yes (Hypotonia) | No | No |
| Balance difficulty | Yes | No | Unknown |
| Upper/Lower extremity | Longer fourth toe of the right foot | Bridged palmar crease, syndactyly, | Bilateral flatfoot |
| Others | Umbilical hernia | Prominent fetal pads; slightly more hair in the lumbosacral region | Scoliosis, dental abnormalities, gynecomastia |

*ADHD* Attention deficit hyperactivity disorder

*LETM1, SLBP,* and *CRIPAK.* TACC3 (transforming acidic coiled-coil containing protein 3) is involved in microtubule dynamic regulation during cell division. Microtubule dynamics are essential to mitotic spindle assembly for appropriate neurogenesis in the cerebral cortex [23, 24]. Peset and Vernos [25] showed that the overexpression of *TACC3* cause defects in chromosome alignment and eventually mitotic arrest. Piekorz et al. [26] reported that TACC3 is a critical component of the centrosome/mitotic spindle apparatus, and its absence triggers p53-mediated apoptosis. Based on this evidence, we hypothesize that the overexpression of *TACC3* influences early embryonic neural development by interfering with neuronal apoptosis and/or cell cycle. Another gene, *FAM53A*, is also known as a candidate gene for neurodevelopmental features because it is highly expressed in the early embryonic central nervous system, suggesting that it plays critical roles in neuronal development [8, 13]. In summary, neurodevelopmental delay, which we have described in this case study and in other patients, [13, 22] may be caused by an increased dosage of the *TACC3* and *FAM53A* genes.

Another key gene of the 4p16.3 duplication may be *LETM1.* It encodes a leucine zipper EF hand-containing transmembrane protein 1 that is involved in mitochondrial morphology, protein transport, and mitochondrial $K^+/H^+$ exchange [27, 28]. It has been suggested that the overexpression of *LETM1* can cause seizures [8, 13, 22, 29], but our patient did not exhibit this symptom. No duplication carriers of a three-generation family described by Schönewolf-Greulich's group [12] experienced seizures either. Data from these patients with 4p16 duplications suggest variable penetrance of epilepsy [8, 13, 22, 29]. It is not clear how duplication of the *FGFR3, CRIPAK,* and *SLBP* genes could affect the phenotype expressed in our patient. Evaluation of additional patients with well-characterized 4p16.3 duplication and/or point mutations in this region will be useful to illuminate the role of individual genes in these clinical features.

In addition, severe speech delay is the outstanding clinical symptom of our patient, which has also been observed in the other two individuals. As of writing, the patient is nearly 4 years old. We followed the patient and found that he could not speak complete sentences. Hannes et al. [22] suggested that speech development may be impaired by the aberration involving the WHSCR, whereas the duplicated region of the three individuals does not include WHSCR. Although these evidences suggest there may be a candidate region or genes, such as *TACC3, FAM53A,* and *LETM1,* shared by all three patients associated with speech delay on 4p16.3 distal to WHSCR, additional experimental and clinical data are needed to support our hypothesis.

## Conclusions

We describe a 23-month-old male with a combined terminal deletion of 18q22.1 and duplication of 4p16.3. Compared to other individuals with 18q22.1 deletions, our patient presents a relatively mild phenotype. The coexistence of two chromosomal rearrangements complicates the clinical symptoms and creates a chimeric disorder marked by characteristics of both chromosomal abnormalities. Additionally, our case report provides clinical and molecular evidence supporting the existence of a novel 4p16.3 microduplication syndrome. The *TACC3* and *LETM1* genes apparently play a key role in the etiology of the clinical phenotype of 4p16.3 microduplication.

### Abbreviations

FISH: Fluorescence in situ hybridization; SNP array: Single nucleotide polymorphism array; WHS: Wolf–Hirschhorn syndrome; WHSCR: Wolf-Hirschhorn critical region


### Acknowledgments

We thank the patient and his family for participating in this study.

### Funding

The Natural Science Foundation of the Higher Education Institutions of Anhui Province, China (Nos. KJ2015A263 and KJ2016A473), and The National Undergraduate Innovative Training Program (201510367042) supported this study. These funding agencies had no role in this study.


### Authors' contributions

LP designed the study. WJ and RH drafted the paper and interpreted the SNP-array data. WQ conducted conventional and molecular cytogenetic analysis. LM and DF performed SNP arrays. All of the authors have read and approved the final manuscript.

### Competing interests

The authors have no competing interests to declare.


### Author details

[1]Department of Life Sciences, Bengbu Medical College, 2600 Donghai Avenue, Bengbu, Anhui 233030, People's Republic of China. [2]Department of Paediatrics, The First Affiliated Hospital of Bengbu Medical College, 2600 Donghai Avenue, Bengbu, Anhui, China.


### References


1. Feenstra I, Vissers LE, Orsel M, et al. Genotype-phenotype mapping of chromosome 18q deletions by high-resolution array CGH: an update of the phenotypic map. Am J Med Genet A. 2007;143(16):1858–67.
2. Cody JD, Heard PL, Crandall AC, et al. Narrowing critical regions and determining penetrance for selected 18q- phenotypes. Am J Med Genet A. 2009;149(7):1421–30.
3. Cody JD, Semrud-Clikeman M, Hardies LJ, et al. Growth hormone benefits children with 18q deletions. Am J Med Genet A. 2005;137(1):9–15.
4. Cody JD, Ghidoni PD, DuPont BR, et al. Congenital anomalies and anthropometry of 42 individuals with deletions of chromosome 18q. Am J Med Genet. 1999; 85(5):455–62.
5. Kulikowski LD, Yoshimoto M, da Silva Bellucco FT, et al. Cytogenetic molecular delineation of a terminal 18q deletion suggesting neo-telomere formation. Eur J Med Genet. 2010;53(6):404–7.
6. Cody JD, Sebold C, Heard P, et al. Consequences of chromsome18q deletions. Am J Med Genet C Semin Med Genet. 2015;169(3):265–80.
7. Bi W, Cheung SW, Breman AM, et al. 4p16.3 microdeletions and microduplications detected by chromosomal microarray analysis: new insights into mechanisms and critical regions. Am J Med Genet A. 2016;170(10):2540–50.

8. Palumbo O, Palumbo P, Ferri E, et al. Report of a patient and further clinical and molecular characterization of interstitial 4p16.3 microduplication. Mol Cytogenet. 2015;8:15.
9. Dai Y, Yang J, Chen Y, et al. Microarray analysis of unbalanced translocation in wolf-Hirschhorn syndrome. Pediatr Int. 2013;55(3):368–70.
10. Partington MW, Fagan K, Soubjaki V, et al. Translocations involving 4p16.3 in three families: deletion causing the Pitt-Rogers-Danks syndrome and duplication resulting in a new overgrowth syndrome. J Med Genet. 1997;34(9):719–28.
11. Patel SV, Dagnew H, Parekh AJ, et al. Clinical manifestations of trisomy 4p syndrome. Eur J Pediatr. 1995;154(6):425–31.
12. Schonewolf-Greulich B, Ravn K, Hamborg-Petersen B, et al. Segregation of a 4p16.3 duplication with a characteristic appearance, macrocephaly, speech delay and mild intellectual disability in a 3-generation family. Am J Med Genet A. 2013;161(9):2358–62.
13. Cyr AB, Nimmakayalu M, Longmuir SQ, et al. A novel 4p16.3 microduplication distal to WHSC1 and WHSC2 characterized by oligonucleotide array with new phenotypic features. Am J Med Genet A. 2011;155(9):2224–8.
14. Miller G, Mowrey PN, Hopper KD, et al. Neurologic manifestation in 18q- syndrome. Am J Med Genet. 1990;37(1):128–32.
15. Gay CT, Hardies LJ, Rauch RA, et al. Magnetic resonance imaging demonstrates incomplete myelination in 18q- syndrome: evidence for myelin basic protein haploinsufficiency. Am J Med Genet. 1997;74(4):422–31.
16. Feenstra I, Vissers LE, Pennings RJ, et al. Disruption of teashirt zinc finger homeobox 1 is associated with congenital aural atresia in humans. Am J Hum Genet. 2011;89(6):813–9.
17. Liao YP, Liang YH, Dong HF, et al. 18q terminal deletion identified by high resolution chromosome and fluorescence in situ hybridization. Fudan Univ J Med Sci. 2010;37(4):479–82.
18. Filges I, Shimojima K, Okamoto N, et al. Reduced expression by SETBP1 haploinsufficiency causes developmental and expressive language delay indicating a phenotype distinct from Schinzel–Giedion syndrome. J Med Genet. 2011;48(2):117–22.
19. Marseglia G, Scordo MR, Pescucci C, et al. 372 kb microdeletion in 18q12.3 causing SETBP1 haploinsufficiency associated with mild mental retardation and expressive speech impairment. Eur J Med Genet. 2012; 55(3):216–21.
20. Wright TJ, Ricke DO, Denison K, et al. A transcript map of the newly defined 165 kb wolf-Hirschhorn syndrome critical region. Hum Mol Genet. 1997;6(2): 317–24.
21. Zollino M, Lecce R, Fischetto R, et al. Mapping the wolf-Hirschhorn syndrome phenotype outside the currently accepted WHS critical region and defining a new critical region, WHSCR-2. Am J Hum Genet. 2003;72(3):590–7.
22. Hannes F, Drozniewska M, Vermeesch JR, et al. Duplication of the wolf-Hirschhorn syndrome critical region causes neurodevelopmental delay. Eur J Med Genet. 2010;53(3):136–40.
23. Buchman JJ, Tsai LH. Spindle regulation in neural precursors of flies and mammals. Nat Rev Neurosci. 2007;8(2):89–100.
24. Yang YT, Wang CL, Van Aelst L. DOCK7 interacts with TACC3 to regulate interkinetic nuclear migration and cortical neurogenesis. Nat Neurosci. 2012; 15(9):1201–10.
25. Peset I, Vernos I. The TACC proteins: TACC-ling microtubule dynamics and centrosome function. Trends Cell Biol. 2008;18(8):379–88.
26. Piekorz RP, Hoffmeyer A, Duntsch CD, et al. The centrosomal protein TACC3 is essential for hematopoietic stem cell function and genetically interfaces with p53-regulated apoptosis. EMBO J. 2002;21(4):653–64.
27. Frazier AE, Kiu C, Stojanovski D, et al. Mitochondrial morphology and distribution in mammalian cells. Biol Chem. 2006;387(12):1551–8.
28. Nowikovsky K, Froschauer EM, Zsurka G, et al. The LETM1/YOL027 gene family encodes a factor of the mitochondrial K+ homeostasis with a potential role in the wolf-Hirschhorn syndrome. J Biol Chem. 2004;279(29):30307–15.
29. McQuibban AG, Joza N, Megighian A, et al. A Drosophila mutant of LETM1, a candidate gene for seizures in wolf-Hirschhorn syndrome. Hum Mol Genet. 2010;19(6):987–1000.

# A boy with developmental delay and mosaic supernumerary inv dup(5)(p15.33p15.1) leading to distal 5p tetrasomy

Pavel Tesner[1*], Jana Drabova[1], Miroslav Stolfa[1], Martin Kudr[2], Martin Kyncl[3], Veronika Moslerova[1], Drahuse Novotna[1], Radka Kremlikova Pourova[1], Eduard Kocarek[1], Tereza Rasplickova[1], Zdenek Sedlacek[1] and Marketa Vlckova[1]

**Abstract**

**Background:** With only 11 patients reported, 5p tetrasomy belongs to rare postnatal findings. Most cases are due to small supernumerary marker chromosomes (sSMCs) or isochromosomes. The patients share common but unspecific symptoms such as developmental delay, seizures, ventriculomegaly, hypotonia, and fifth finger clinodactyly. Simple interstitial duplications leading to trisomies of parts of 5p are much more frequent and better described. Duplications encompassing 5p13.2 cause a defined syndrome with macrocephaly, distinct facial phenotype, heart defects, talipes equinovarus, feeding difficulties, respiratory distress and anomalies of the central nervous system, developmental delay and hypotonia.

**Case presentation:** We present a boy with dysmorphic features, developmental delay, intellectual disability and congenital anomalies, and a mosaic sSMC inv dup(5)(p15.33p15.1). He is the fourth and the oldest reported patient with distal 5p tetrasomy. His level of mosaicism was significantly different in lymphocytes (13.2%) and buccal cells (64.7%). The amplification in our patient is smaller than that in the three previously published patients but the only phenotype difference is the absence of seizures in our patient.

**Conclusions:** Our observations indicate that for the assessment of prognosis, especially with respect to intellectual functioning, the level of mosaicism could be more important than the extent of amplification and the number of extra copies. Evaluation of the phenotypical effect of rare chromosomal aberrations is challenging and each additional case is valuable for refinement of the genotype-phenotype correlation. Moreover, our patient demonstrates that if the phenotype is severe and if the level of sSMC mosaicism is low in lymphocytes, other tissues should be tested.

**Keywords:** 5p tetrasomy, Marker chromosome, Mosaicism, Intellectual disability

* Correspondence: pavel.tesner@lfmotol.cuni.cz
[1]Department of Biology and Medical Genetics, Charles University 2nd Faculty of Medicine and University Hospital Motol, V Uvalu 84, 15006 Prague 5, Czech Republic
Full list of author information is available at the end of the article

## Background

Tetrasomies of a part or the whole 5p belong to rare postnatal findings and can be the result of a small supernumerary marker chromosome (sSMC) with inverted duplication (inv dup) or an isochromosome. Clinical outcomes of sSMCs vary from an unaffected to a severely affected status with major anomalies and intellectual disability (ID). sSMCs are often present in mosaics and can even be absent in some tissues. The clinical manifestation is frequently influenced by the level of mosaicism in specific tissues [1].

Only 11 postnatal patients of 5p tetrasomy have been reported, seven with supernumerary i(5)(p10) [2–8], three with amplification of the distal part of 5p – one interstitial triplication [9] and two supernumerary inv dup [10, 11], and one patient had proximal 5p tetrasomy but his phenotype description and sSMC characterization were rather incomplete [12]. The features of 5p tetrasomy are developmental delay, seizures, ventriculomegaly, hypotonia, short stature or growth delay, and fifth finger clinodactyly [11]. A single transverse palmar crease, recurrent infections, abnormalities of the diaphragm, abnormalities of the pinna, microretrognathia, abnormalities of the philtrum and thin upper lip vermilion are also frequently observed. Interestingly, the phenotype seems to be rather similar irrespective of whether the whole 5p or just its distal part is amplified.

In contrast to 5p tetrasomies, partial or complete 5p trisomies are much more frequent. Proximal 5p trisomies are associated with a specific phenotype with macrocephaly, facial anomalies (upslanted palpebral fissures, hypertelorism, epicanthus, depressed nasal bridge, midface retrusion, micrognathia, and abnormality of the pinna), short neck, hypoplasia of the abdominal wall musculature, congenital heart defects, talipes equinovarus, feeding difficulties, respiratory distress, recurrent respiratory infections, and anomalies of the central nervous system (CNS), especially ventriculomegaly. Generalized hypotonia, seizures and ID are also common [13]. The critical region for this phenotype was primarily placed to 5p11-p13 by Chia et al. [14] and later refined to 5p13.1-p13.3 by Loscalzo et al. [15]. The 5p13.2 duplication syndrome was finally defined by Yan et al. [16], and *NIPBL* was suggested as its critical gene [17].

We present a 5-year-old boy with dysmorphic features, feeding difficulties, hypotonia, developmental delay, ID, autistic features, and mosaic sSMC inv dup(5)(p15.33p15.1) resulting in tetrasomy of distal 5p not involving the 5p13.2 region. We compared the genotype and phenotype of our patient with previously described patients of 5p tetrasomy and reviewed the literature for clinical effects of tetrasomy and trisomy of distinct parts of 5p. We found just slight and non-specific differences among the phenotypes of the patients compared. Our observations indicate that for the assessment of prognosis, especially with respect to intellectual functioning, the level of mosaicism could be more important than the extent of the region amplified and the number of extra copies.

## Case presentation

### Clinical report

The boy was born via spontaneous delivery from the second uneventful pregnancy to healthy unrelated Caucasian parents. The age of the mother and the father was 31 and 32 years, respectively. Birth weight was 3650 g (82nd centile) and birth length was 53 cm (87th centile). No congenital anomalies were observed in the newborn, and the neonatal period was unremarkable. During the infant period the boy suffered from feeding difficulties and recurrent upper airways infections. His psychomotor development was delayed. Pyelectasia, foramen ovale apertum and hiatal hernia were detected at the age of 14 months, and brain MRI revealed a cyst in posterior cranial fossa.

He was examined again at the age of 3 years and 5 months due to global developmental delay. He was not able to walk but he started to stand with support. The speech was absent and he used only vocalizations. He had problems with chewing and he could eat only mashed food. His parents described frequent aggressive behavior with biting. Hypotonia (central hypotonic syndrome), hypermobility of joints and pedes planovalgi were also present. His height was 96 cm (11th centile), weight was 13.5 kg (7th centile) and head circumference was 52.5 cm (96th centile). Dysmorphic features included dolichocephaly, frontal bossing, low set ears, abnormality of the pinna, hypotelorism, downslanted palpebral fissures, epicanthus, depressed nasal bridge, low hanging columella, long philtrum, thin upper lip vermilion, short chin, slight midface retrusion, single transverse palmar crease on the right hand, pectus excavatum, and kyphosis (Fig. 1a, b).

At the last examination at the age of 5 years and 1 month his height was 110 cm (18th centile; however, according to growth prediction from the mid parent height, the height of the boy would be expected to be around 97th centile, and thus the actual observation might rather indicate a more significant growth delay), weight was 15.5 kg (2th centile) and head circumference was 54 cm (95th centile). Speech was still absent and feeding and chewing difficulties persisted, but the boy was able to walk independently. He showed symptoms of an autism spectrum disorder such as stereotypical hand movements, frequent bruxism and a very sporadic eye contact. Macrocephaly, dolichocephaly, central hypotonic syndrome and hypermobility of the joints persisted. Pedes planovalgi were accompanied by valgus

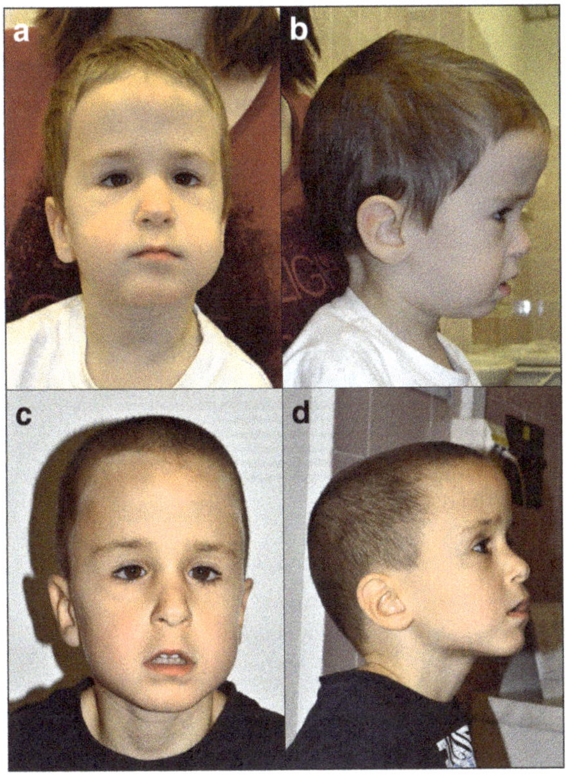


**Fig. 1** The patient at the age of 3 years and 5 months (**a**, **b**) and 5 years and 1 month (**c**, **d**). Apparent features include low set ears, hypotelorism, downslanted palpebral fissures, epicanthus, depressed nasal bridge, low hanging columella, long philtrum, and thin upper lip vermilion. While short chin is present only at younger age, frontal bossing is more remarkable at older age

deformity of the knees. In addition, a small umbilical hernia was present. Midface retrusion and short chin observed previously were not present, but the forehead was even more prominent (Fig. 1c, d).

### Laboratory analysis

The research was prospectively reviewed and approved by a duly constituted ethics committee. Informed consent was obtained from the parents of the patient. Examination of G-banded chromosomes from peripheral blood lymphocytes was performed using standard protocols. For fluorescence in situ hybridization (FISH) analysis of blood lymphocytes and buccal cells, Cytocell Aquarius Cri-du-chat and SOTOS Probe Combination (LPU 013) (Oxford Gene Technology, UK) was used. High-resolution array comparative genomic hybridization (aCGH) and single nucleotide polymorphism (SNP) analysis of the lymphocyte genomic DNA isolated using AutoGen Flex STAR (Autogen, USA) employed the SurePrint G3 ISCA V2 CGH 8x60K Microarray and the SurePrint G3 ISCA CGH + SNP 4x180K Microarray, respectively, according to the protocol of the manufacturer (Agilent Genomics, USA).

### Results

The patient had a mosaic sSMC and karyotype mos 47,XY,+mar[10]/46,XY[28] (Fig. 2a). Parental karyotypes were normal and the sSMC occurred de novo. aCGH analysis of the patient revealed gain of material in 5p15.33p15.1, in the region chr5:22149_15009591 (hg19) (Fig. 2b). FISH analysis confirmed the origin of the sSMC from 5p15.33p15.1 and revealed its inv dup structure (Fig. 2c), with the final karyotype mos 47,XY,+dup(5)(pter→p15.1::p15.1→pter)dn[10]/46,XY[28]. The region of tetrasomy was 15 Mb long and encompassed 137 genes including 54 protein-coding genes, of which 14 are known disease-causing genes (Additional file 1). Considering the tetrasomic nature of the aberration, the mean $\log_2$ratio of 0.176 observed in aCGH indicated a mosaic of 13.0% according to the formula by Valli et al. [18]. FISH analysis of 409 cell nuclei of peripheral lymphocytes showed the sSMC in 13.2% of cells. In contrast, interphase FISH analysis of 312 nuclei of buccal mucosa cells showed the sSMC in 64.7% of cells. SNP array CGH analysis identified 71 at least partly informative SNPs in the interval of the 5p tetrasomy allowing to deduce the parental origin of the sSMC. The analysis was complicated by the low level of mosaicism of the sSMC in lymphocytes, and the almost 1% error rate of the array as indicated by genome-wide discrepancies with Mendelian inheritance. Nevertheless, 18 informative SNPs clearly indicated the paternal origin of the sSMC, and 51 additional SNPs were not at odds with this scenario. Of the SNPs which could discriminate between the paternal alleles, 10 clearly indicated that both SNP alleles on the sSMC were identical to the allele present on the normal chromosome 5 inherited by the patient from the father, and 8 additional SNPs were not at odds with this scenario (showing that the sSMC alleles could originate either from the paternal chromosome 5 inherited by the patient, or from the other paternal chromosome 5). Of the 51 SNPs which were not at odds with the paternal origin, 20 showed alleles identical to the sSMC and the normal paternal chromosome 5, and 29 could not discriminate between the two scenarios.

## Discussion and conclusions

According to literature reports, isochromosomes of the whole 5p (i(5)(p10)) [2–8] are more frequent than inv dups of distal 5p [9–11]. Our patient is the fourth and the oldest case with tetrasomy of distal 5p. He is the only patient old enough to allow proper evaluation of his intellectual functioning, not only developmental delay, but also of all other features.

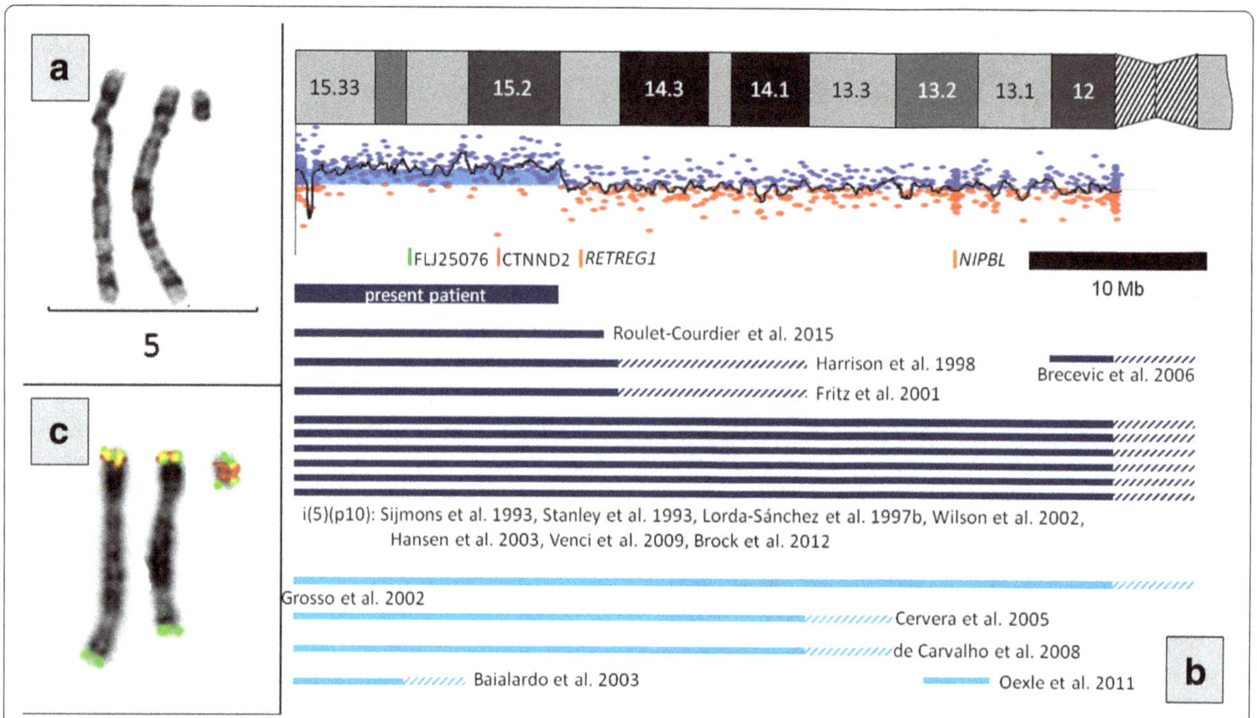


**Fig. 2** **a** Partial G-banded karyotype of normal chromosomes 5 and the sSMC. **b** Scheme showing the banding pattern of 5p, the result of array CGH in the present patient, FISH probes for the cri-du-chat region employed in our study (5p15.31 (FLJ25076) in green, 5p15.2 (CTNND2) in red), disease-causing genes discussed (orange), the extent of 5p amplification in the present patient (thick dark blue bar) and previously published tetrasomies (inv dups, isochromosomes, an interstitial triplication; thin dark blue bars) and trisomies (terminal and interstitial duplications, unbalanced translocations; thin light blue bars). Uncertain ranges in published patients are hatched. A megabase scale bar is also shown. **c** FISH examination of normal chromosomes 5 and the sSMC. See (**b**) for 5p probe colors. The 5q35 (NSD1) probe is in green. The pattern of signals on the sSMC indicates its structure of inv dup of distal 5p

Phenotypes of the tetrasomic patients are similar and only few unspecific differences can be observed (Additional file 2). Recurrent respiratory infections were observed in our patient and in two other patients with distal 5p tetrasomy [10, 11], and another patient died at the age of 35 days because of bronchopneumonia [9]. Respiratory infections were also described in a patient with mos i(5)(p10) [4]. A possible explanation for this feature was proposed in a patient with trisomy of the whole 5p by Grosso et al. [19], who found low level of secretory immunoglobulins A (IgA). Nevertheless, detailed immunological examination was not performed and the finding could be coincidental. Patients with 5p tetrasomy published in the literature were not tested for IgA and in our patient it was within the normal range. More detailed immunological examination of patients with 5p amplifications is needed to elucidate the cause of recurrent infections.

Compared to the other patients with distal 5p tetrasomy [9–11], the tetrasomy in our patient does not encompass six of their amplified genes. The previous patients manifested seizures in infancy but our patient did not, and thus one of these genes could cause the seizures. Inactivating *RETREG1* mutations cause autosomal recessive hereditary sensory and autonomic neuropathy IIB (OMIM #613115), but our patient does not show this phenotype. No diseases are associated with the other genes. While the *FBXL7* [20], *MARCH11* [21], *ZNF622* [22], and *BASP1* [23] genes are expressed in brain and could possibly contribute to seizures, no data exist on *MYO10* expression in CNS.

The comparison of phenotypes associated with 5p tetrasomy and 5p trisomy is summarized in Additional file 3. The common features of all 5p amplifications are anomalies of CNS, hypotonia, seizures, and ID. Although the critical region of the 5p13.2 duplication syndrome is involved neither in the tetrasomic region of our patient nor in the distal 5p tetrasomy regions of the previous patients [9–11], many of their traits are similar to those of patients with the 5p13.2 duplication syndrome, including congenital heart defects and seizures (in two and three of the four distal 5p tetrasomy patients, respectively). The presence of these symptoms in patients with tetrasomies not involving *NIPBL* indicates that other gene(s) for these conditions may exist in 5p14 and 5p15. Phenotypic overlap among carriers of amplifications of non-overlapping regions of 5p was noted by Cervera et al. [24]. Their patient with dup(5)(p13.3p15.3) had severe

ID, seizures, macrocephaly, upslanted palpebral fissures, epicanthal folds, depressed nasal bridge, and abnormal pinna, which are also characteristic for the 5p13.2 duplication syndrome. Also de Carvalho et al. [25] reported t(5;15)(p13.3;p12) leading to distal 5p trisomy in five individuals with features resembling the 5p13.2 duplication syndrome. This reopens the question if the 5p trisomy phenotype is caused solely by trisomy of 5p13.2 with *NIPBL* as the possible candidate gene [26]. Conversely, also a normal individual with a terminal 5p trisomy resulting from der(15)t(5;15)(p15.1;p13) was reported [27].

The tetrasomy in our patient affected a total of 137 genes. Extensive data collected on their disease involvement, expression and sensitivity to variation are in Additional file 1. The majority of the protein-coding genes are expressed in all tissues including the brain, and some of them show lack of tolerance to loss-of-function variation. Evidence for sensitivity to increased copy number is generally sparser, and the ClinGen Dosage Sensitivity Map (https://www.ncbi.nlm.nih.gov/projects/dbvar/clingen/) indicates triplosensitivity in none of these genes. Evidence exists for haploinsufficiency of *TERT* and *CTNND2*, but neither the phenotype caused by the loss of these genes nor a "mirror" phenotype could be observed in our patient. The *TRIO* gene has the strongest evidence for haploinsufficiency and causes autosomal dominant mental retardation 44 (MRD44, OMIM #617061). Our patient and also other patients with 5p tetrasomy showed some features of this disorder such as downslanting palpebral fissures, short nose, micrognathia, facial asymmetry, large ears, clinodactyly, feeding difficulties, developmental delay, ID, poor speech, autistic features and recurrent infections, while microcephaly and seizures are present only in some of them [9–11].

Moreover, according to the STRING database (https://string-db.org/), the TRIO protein activates RAC1, and the *RAC1* gene causes autosomal dominant mental retardation 48 (MRD48, OMIM #617751) with a very variable phenotype. Other possibly interesting protein interactions may exist. For example, the *NDUFS6* gene amplified in our patient encodes the NADH:ubiquinone oxidoreductase subunit S6 of the mitochondrial complex I (MCI). Biallelic *NDUFS6* mutations cause MCI deficiency (OMIM #252010) but no evidence exists for the sensitivity of this gene to amplification. A duplication of *NDUFS4*, an interaction partner of *NDUFS6*, in case 331431 from DECIPHER was considered to be possibly pathogenic. The phenotype and severity of MCI deficiency is highly variable and it is difficult to decide if the phenotype of our patient could fit at least partly this condition because of his rather unspecific symptoms; his phenotype is definitely not discordant with mild MCI deficiency. Similarly, the product of *MED10* is a component of the Mediator complex, a coactivator for DNA-binding factors activating transcription by RNA polymerase II [28]. Mutations in a possible interacting partner of *MED10*, *MED12*, cause X-linked ID (OMIM #309520, #300895, #305450). Another highly interconnected protein encoded by the sSMC is CCT5, a subunit of the chaperonin containing TCP1 complex involved in folding of cytoskeletal proteins. Multiple subunits of this complex have been associated with various neurodevelopmental disorders [29, 30]. It must be noted that it is unclear from in silico analysis how much the levels of proteins encoded by genes in the amplified interval are changed, if these changes cause any disturbances of stechiometric ratios in the protein complexes, and if these disturbances impair the functions of these complexes.

As the sSMC does not contain the normal chromosome 5 centromere, it is likely to carry a neocentromere (reviewed in [31]). A variable postzygotic mitotic stability of the sSMC in individual tissues (possibly due to the differences in the time of neocentromere activation [32]) or a different proliferation disadvantage of different cell types with the sSMC could cause the different level of mosaicism observed in lymphocytes and buccal cells of our patient. The SNP array CGH analysis revealed the paternal origin of the sSMC and showed that the two copies of distal 5p present on the sSMC are identical with the corresponding part of the normal paternal chromosome 5 present in the patient. This could point to the paternal meiotic origin of the sSMC from an acentric fragment via hairpin formation, reduplication and neocentromere acquisition described by Murmann et al. [32]. In contrast to usually non-mosaic 5p trisomies, the phenotype of 5p tetrasomy due to a sSMC can be influenced by the level of mosaicism. Three patients with mosaic i(5)(p10) in fibroblasts but a normal karyotype in lymphocytes were reported. A girl had a 62% mosaic of i(5)(p10) in fibroblasts and developmental delay, seizures, mild ID and hypotonia [3]. Another girl with a milder phenotype (borderline intelligence and psychomotor skills, but with complex partial seizures) had only 10% mosaic in fibroblasts [6]. Finally, a boy having in addition ventriculomegaly, short stature, and macrocephaly, had a 14% mosaic in fibroblasts [8]. All three children exhibited mosaic hyperpigmentation of skin, and therefore the biopsy should target the hypo- or hyperpigmented lesions generally following the lines of Blaschko [33]. Skin biopsy can be replaced by buccal smear but if the examination is negative and the suspicion for mosaicism persists, invasive sampling is necessary to reach the diagnosis. Because aCGH cannot distinguish trisomy from 50% mosaic of tetrasomy, FISH should be used to elucidate the type of aberration. However, in contrast to i(5)(p10) cases, skin signs of mosaicism have not been observed in patients with mosaic distal 5p tetrasomy. The pitfalls of mosaicism are illustrated also by an infertile man with no dysmorphic features, ID nor congenital defects who carried mos i(5)(p10) in 16% of lymphocytes, but no such sSMC in skin fibroblasts and urothelial cells [7]. The similarly low level of mosaicism in lymphocytes of our patient initially also shed doubts on its causality, until the buccal analysis was performed which showed a much higher percentage of cells carrying the sSMC. Similarly to Pallister-Killian syndrome with supernumerary isochromosome 12p in skin fibroblasts (and other tissues), but with no or insignificant representation in lymphocytes [34], our case showed that the examination of another tissue is essential, and the easily accessible buccal cells could serve this aim. The decision if the sSMC is causal or if it is just a coincidental finding not explaining the phenotype is very important as it is crucial for planning of possible additional examinations.

#### Abbreviations

aCGH: Array comparative genomic hybridization; CNS: Central nervous system; FISH: Fluorescence in situ hybridization; inv dup: Inverted duplication; SNP: Single nucleotide polymorphism; sSMC: Small supernumerary marker chromosome

#### Acknowledgements

We thank the patient and the parents for their cooperation.

#### Funding

The work was supported by grants 17-29423A, 15-33041A, 00064203 (project IP6003) by Czech Ministry of Health and TA01010931 by Technology Agency of the Czech Republic.

#### Authors' contributions

All authors have actively participated in the study and manuscript preparation. Clinical analysis: MKu, MKy, RKP, MV. Anthropological analysis: VM. Laboratory analysis: MS, JD, TR. Manuscript writing and revision: PT, RKP, JD, DN, EK, ZS, MV. All authors read and approved the final manuscript.

#### Competing interests

The authors declare that they have no competing interests.

#### Author details

[1]Department of Biology and Medical Genetics, Charles University 2nd Faculty of Medicine and University Hospital Motol, V Uvalu 84, 15006 Prague 5, Czech Republic. [2]Department of Paediatric Neurology, Charles University 2nd Faculty of Medicine and University Hospital Motol, V Uvalu 84, 15006 Prague 5, Czech Republic. [3]Department of Radiology, Charles University 2nd Faculty of Medicine and University Hospital Motol, V Uvalu 84, 15006 Prague 5, Czech Republic.

#### References

1. Liehr T, Klein E, Mrasek K, Kosyakova N, Guilherme RS, Aust N, et al. Clinical impact of somatic mosaicism in cases with small supernumerary marker chromosomes. Cytogenet Genome Res. 2013;139:158–63.
2. Sijmons RH, Leegte B, van Lingen RA, de Pater JM, van der Veen AY, del Canho H, et al. Tetrasomy 5p mosaicism in a boy with delayed growth, hypotonia, minor anomalies, and an additional isochromosome 5p [46,XY/47,XY, + i(5p)]. Am J Med Genet. 1993;47:559–62.
3. Stanley WS, Powell CM, Devine GC, Ellingham T, Samango-Sprouse CA, Vaught DR, et al. Mosaic 5p tetrasomy. Am J Med Genet. 1993;45:774–6.
4. Lorda-Sánchez I, Villa A, Urioste M, Bernal E, Jaso E, García A, Martínez-Frías ML. Tetrasomy 5p mosaicism due to an extra i(5p) in a severely affected girl. Am J Med Genet. 1997;68:481–4.
5. Wilson SC, Susman M, Bain S, Wohlferd M, Van Dyke D, Daniel A, et al. Isochromosome 5p mosaicism at prenatal diagnosis: observations and outcomes in six cases at chorionic villus sampling and one at amniocentesis. Prenat Diagn. 2002;22:681–5.
6. Hansen LK, Brandrup F, Rasmussen K. Pigmentary mosaicism with mosaic chromosome 5p tetrasomy. Br J Dermatol. 2003;149:414–6.
7. Venci A, Bettio D. Tetrasomy 5p mosaicism due to an additional isochromosome 5p in a man with normal phenotype. Am J Med Genet A. 2009;149A:2889–91.
8. Brock JA, Dyack S, Ludman M, Dumas N, Gaudet M, Morash B. Mosaic tetrasomy 5p resulting from an isochromosome 5p marker chromosome: case report and review of literature. Am J Med Genet A. 2012;158A:406–11.
9. Harrison KJ, Teshima IE, Silver MM, Jay V, Unger S, Robinson WP, et al. Partial tetrasomy with triplication of chromosome (5) (p14-p15.33) in a patient with severe multiple congenital anomalies. Am J Med Genet. 1998;79:103–7.
10. Fritz B, Dietze I, Wandall A, Aslan M, Schmidt A, Kattner E, et al. A supernumerary marker chromosome with a neocentromere derived from 5p14->pter. J Med Genet. 2001;38:559–65.
11. Roulet-Coudrier F, Rouibi A, Thuillier C, Bourthoumieu S, Lebbar A, Dupont JM, Yardin C. Unusual isochromosome 5p marker chromosome. Am J Med Genet A. 2015;167A:455–9.
12. Brecevic L, Michel S, Starke H, Müller K, Kosyakova N, Mrasek K, et al. Multicolor FISH used for the characterization of small supernumerary marker chromosomes (sSMC) in commercially available immortalized cell lines. Cytogenet Genome Res. 2006;114:319–24.
13. Lorda-Sánchez I, Urioste M, Villa A, Carrascosa MC, Vázquez MS, Martínez A, Martínez-Frías ML. Proximal partial 5p trisomy resulting from a maternal (19; 5) insertion. Am J Med Genet. 1997;68:476–80.
14. Chia NL, Bousfield LR, Johnson BH. A case report of a de novo tandem duplication (5p) (p14——pter). Clin Genet. 1987;31:65–9.
15. Loscalzo ML, Becker TA, Sutcliffe M. A patient with an interstitial duplication of chromosome 5p11-p13.3 further confirming a critical region for 5p duplication syndrome. Eur J Med Genet. 2008;51:54–60.
16. Yan J, Zhang F, Brundage E, Scheuerle A, Lanpher B, Erickson RP, et al. Genomic duplication resulting in increased copy number of genes encoding the sister chromatid cohesion complex conveys clinical consequences distinct from Cornelia de Lange. J Med Genet. 2009;46:626–34.
17. Novara F, Alfei E, D'Arrigo S, Pantaleoni C, Beri S, Achille V, et al. 5p13 microduplication syndrome: a new case and better clinical definition of the syndrome. Eur J Med Genet. 2013;56:54–8.
18. Valli R, Maserati E, Marletta C, Pressato B, Lo Curto F, Pasquali F. Evaluating chromosomal mosaicism by array comparative genomic hybridization in hematological malignancies: the proposal of a formula. Cancer Genet. 2011;204:216–8.
19. Grosso S, Cioni M, Garibaldi G, Pucci L, Galluzzi P, Canapicchi R, et al. De novo complete trisomy 5p: clinical and neuroradiological findings. Am J Med Genet. 2002;112:56–60.
20. Nagase T, Ishikawa K, Suyama M, Kikuno R, Hirosawa M, Miyajima N, et al. Prediction of the coding sequences of unidentified human genes. XII. The complete sequences of 100 new cDNA clones from brain which code for large proteins in vitro. DNA Res. 1998;5:355–64.
21. Morokuma Y, Nakamura N, Kato A, Notoya M, Yamamoto Y, Sakai Y, et al. MARCH-XI, a novel transmembrane ubiquitin ligase implicated in ubiquitin-dependent protein sorting in developing spermatids. J Biol Chem. 2007;282:24806–15.

22. Seong HA, Gil M, Kim KT, Kim SJ, Ha H. Phosphorylation of a novel zinc-finger-like protein, ZPR9, by murine protein serine/threonine kinase 38 (MPK38). Biochem J. 2002;361:597–604.
23. Park S, Kim YI, Kim B, Seong C, Oh Y, Baek K, Yoon J. Characterization of bovine and human cDNAs encoding NAP-22 (22 kDa neuronal tissue-enriched acidic protein) homologs. Mol Cells. 1998;8:471–7.
24. Cervera M, Sánchez S, Molina B, Alcántara MA, Del Castillo V, Carnevale A, et al. Trisomy of the short arm of chromosome 5 due to a de novo inversion and duplication (5)(p15.3 p13.3). Am J Med Genet A. 2005;136A:381–5.
25. de Carvalho AF, da Silva Bellucco FT, Kulikowski LD, Toralles MB, Melaragno MI. Partial 5p monosomy or trisomy in 11 patients from a family with a t(5; 15)(p13.3;p12) translocation. Hum Genet. 2008;124:387–92.
26. Oexle K, Hempel M, Jauch A, Meitinger T, Rivera-Brugués N, Stengel-Rutkowski S, Strom T. 3.7 Mb tandem microduplication in chromosome 5p13.1-p13.2 associated with developmental delay, macrocephaly, obesity, and lymphedema. Further characterization of the dup(5p13) syndrome. Eur J Med Genet. 2011;54:225–30.
27. Baialardo EM, Torrado Mdel V, Barreiro CZ, Gallego MS. Partial distal 5p trisomy resulting from paternal translocation (5;15)(p15.1;p13) in a boy with no mental retardation. Clin Dysmorphol. 2003;12:257–9.
28. Sato S, Tomomori-Sato C, Banks CAS, Sorokina I, Parmely TJ, Kong SE, et al. Identification of mammalian mediator subunits with similarities to yeast mediator subunits Srb5, Srb6, Med11, and Rox3. J Biol Chem. 2003;278: 15123–7.
29. Iossifov I, Levy D, Allen J, Ye K, Ronemus M, Lee YH, et al. Low load for disruptive mutations in autism genes and their biased transmission. Proc Natl Acad Sci U S A. 2015;112:E5600–7.
30. Krishnan A, Zhang R, Yao V, Theesfeld CL, Wong AK, Tadych A, et al. Genome-wide prediction and functional characterization of the genetic basis of autism spectrum disorder. Nat Neurosci. 2016;19:1454–62.
31. Scott KC, Sullivan BA. Neocentromeres: a place for everything and everything in its place. Trends Genet. 2014;30:66–74.
32. Murmann AE, Conrad DF, Mashek H, Curtis CA, Nicolae RI, Ober C, Schwartz S. Inverted duplications on acentric markers: mechanism of formation. Hum Mol Genet. 2009;18:2241–56.
33. Thomas IT, Frias JL, Cantu ES, Lafer CZ, Flannery DB, Graham JG Jr. Association of pigmentary anomalies with chromosomal and genetic mosaicism and chimerism. Am J Hum Genet. 1989;45:193–205.
34. Peltomaki P, Knuutila S, Ritvanen A, Kaitila I, de la Chapelle A. Pallister-Killian syndrome: cytogenetic and molecular studies. Clin Genet. 1987;31:399–405.

25

# Chromosomal abnormalities and copy number variations in fetal ventricular septal defects

Meiying Cai, Hailong Huang, Linjuan Su, Na Lin, Xiaoqing Wu, Xiaorui Xie, Gang An, Ying Li, Yuan Lin, Liangpu Xu* and Hua Cao*

**Abstract**

**Background:** This study aimed to evaluate the applicability of chromosomal microarray analysis (CMA), rather than traditional chromosome analysis, in prenatal diagnosis of ventricular septal defects (VSDs) for superior prenatal genetic counseling and to reveal a potential correlation between submicroscopic chromosomal aberrations and VSDs.

**Results:** Among the 151 VSD cases, 79 (52.3%) had isolated defects and 72 (47.7%) had additional ultrasound anomalies. Karyotype analysis identified 16 chromosomal abnormalities. Besides the 14 cases of chromosome abnormalities consistent with karyotype analysis, CMA identified an additional 20 cases (13.2%) of abnormal copy number variations (CNVs), of which 13 were pathogenetic CNVs, 5 were variations of uncertain clinical significance (VOUS) and 2 were benign CNVs. The detection rate of pathogenic CNVs in non-isolated-VSDs was significantly higher than that in isolated-VSDs (36.1% (26/72) vs. 1.3% (1/79), $p = 0.001$). We also found that CMA results indicating pathogenic abnormalities affected the rate of pregnancy termination.

**Conclusions:** This study showed that CMA combined with cytogenetic analysis is particularly effective in identifying CNVs in fetuses with VSDs and can have an effect on obstetrical outcomes. The elucidation of the etiology of VSDs suggested that gene mutations or other factors may be implicated.

**Keywords:** Ventricular septal defects, Chromosomal microarray analysis, Chromosomal abnormality, Prenatal diagnosis

## Background

Congenital heart disease (CHDs) is one of the most common types of birth defects, affecting up to 8 in every 1000 babies born in the China [1]. Ventricular septal defects (VSDs) are the most common cardiac defects seen postnatally, accounting for 30–35% of all CHDs detected after birth and 10% of all fetal cases [2, 3]. Recent studies have shown that approximately 20–40% of VSDs are attributable to chromosomal aneuploidies or Mendelian diseases, while the remaining are attributable to non-Mendelian causes that are poorly understood [4–7]. Prenatal ultrasonography suggested that 33–47% percent of fetuses with VSD had chromosomal abnormalities, among which trisomy 18, trisomy 21, and DiGeorge syndrome were the most common [5, 8].

Genomic microarrays include micro-array based comparative genomic hybridization (aCGH) and single nucleotide polymorphism (SNP) arrays, both of which can detect micro-deletions and micro-duplications in the genome. Aside from the detection of CNVs, SNP arrays can detect uniparental disomy and chimeric DNA. In this study, we performed whole-genome scanning using SNP arrays as well as karyotyping of 151 fetuses that were diagnosed as having VSD by ultrasonic cardiography. We tried to elucidate genetic factors that cause fetal VSD and explore the clinical value of the application of CMA in the diagnosis of VSD in fetuses.

* Correspondence: xiliangpu@fjmu.edu.cn; caohua69@hotmail.com
Department of the Prenatal Diagnosis Center, Fujian Provincial Maternity and Children's Hospital, affiliated hospital of Fujian Medical University, Fujian Key Laboratory for Prenatal Diagnosis and Birth Defect, Fuzhou, China

## Methods

### Patient data

We conducted a retrospective study on VSD cases diagnosed prenatally with ultrasound in the Prenatal Diagnosis Center of the Fujian Provincial Maternal and Children Health Hospital, from January 2017 to April 2018. Fetal samples were collected by amniocentesis ($n = 85$) or cord blood sampling ($n = 66$) depending on the gestation period. Amniotic fluid was collected by amniocentesis at the gestational age of 16–24 weeks and fetal blood was collected by cord blood sampling at a gestational age over 24 weeks. The fetuses underwent a routine ultrasonic scan, and fetal biometry was performed at a median gestational age of 25 + 5 (range, 18 + 3 to 33 + 4) weeks. This study was approved by the ethics committee at the Fujian Provincial Maternal and Child Health Hospital, and informed consent was obtained from the parents for invasive prenatal diagnosis. Once fetal pathogenic CNVs were confirmed, approximately 2.0 mL of peripheral venous blood was collected from their parents. DNA was extracted using the Gentra Puregene blood kit (QIAGEN, Santa Clara, CA, USA).

The cases were classified as isolated or non-isolated-VSD, the latter comprising cases with other cardiac anomalies, extracardiac structural anomalies, or sonographic soft markers. A total of 151 VSD cases were included, of which 79 (52.3%) cases were isolated-VSD and 72 (47.7%) cases were non-isolated-VSD (detailed information in Table 1).

### Cytogenetic analysis

Cultured amniocytes or lymphocytes were analyzed by regular karyotype analysis using the Giemsa banding technique at a resolution of 450–550 bands.

### CMA

Genomic DNA was directly extracted from uncultured amniotic fluid and cord blood samples using the QIAamp DNA Blood Mini kits (Qiagen, Germany). DNA was quantified using a NanoDrop spectrophotometer (Thermo Fisher Scientific, Waltham, MA, USA), according to the manufacturer's instructions. The DNA quality was assessed by agarose gel electrophoresis. The genome-wide high-resolution SNP array CytoScan HD (Affymetrix Genome CytoScan 750 K, Affymetrix, Santa Clara, CA, USA) including both SNPs and oligonucleotide probes was used in this study. DNA (250 ng) was amplified, labeled, and hybridized according to the manufacturer's protocol. Procedures for DNA digestion, ligation, polymerase chain reaction (PCR), fragmentation, labeling, and hybridization to the arrays were performed according to the manufacturer's protocols. The CNV reporting filter was set at > 100 kb in size with a minimum set of 50 marker counts. The results obtained from the CytoScan arrays were analyzed with Chromosome Analysis Suite software (Affymetrix), using annotations of the genome version GRCH37 (hg19). The detected copy number gains or losses were systematically evaluated by comparing them with values available in the literature and the publicly available databases, including database of genomic variants (DGV, http://projects.tcag.ca/variation/), DECIPHER database (http://decipher.sanger.ac.uk/), the International Standards for Cytogenomic Arrays (ISCA, https://www.iscaconsortium.org/), and Online Mendelian Inheritance in Man (OMIM, http://www.omim.org). The CNVs were classified as benign, pathogenic, or variants of uncertain significance (VOUS) according to the American College of Medical Genetics (ACMG) guidelines [9]. Microarray analysis of DNA from maternal and paternal blood samples was used to determine whether CNVs detected in the fetal samples were inherited or de novo. All de novo CNVs were experimentally validated by fluorescence in situ hybridization (FISH).

### Statistical analysis

IBM SPSS Statistics 20 (IBM, Armonk, NY, USA) was used for statistical analysis. The detection rate of pathogenic variants in the isolated and non-isolated-VSD fetuses was compared between cytogenetic analysis and CMA. A value of $p < 0.05$ was considered statistically significant.

## Results

### Cytogenetic analysis of VSD fetuses

In the 151 VSD cases analyzed, karyotyping identified 16 chromosomal abnormalities. Among the 79 isolated-VSD fetuses, karyotyping identified only one chromosomal abnormality associated with 13p+, which was not found with CMA. However, of the 72 non-isolated-VSD fetuses,

**Table 1** Phenotypic characteristics of 151 VSD fetuses

| Classification | Number of fetuses | Number of Karyotype abnormality | Number of CHA | | |
|---|---|---|---|---|---|
| | | | Pathogenic CNVs | VOUS | Benign CNVs |
| Isolated- VSD | 79 | 1 | 1 | 1 | 1 |
| Non-isolated-VSD | 72 | 15 | 12 | 4 | 1 |
| Total | 151 | 16 | 13 | 5 | 2 |

*CMA* chromosomal microarray analysis, *CNVs* copy number variations, *VOUS* variation of uncertain clinical significance, *VSD* ventricular septal defect

karyotyping identified 15 clinically significant chromosomal abnormalities, involving trisomy 18 ($n = 5$), trisomy 21 ($n = 2$), trisomy 13 ($n = 1$), Klinefelter syndrome ($n = 1$), deletions of 4q25q28 ($n = 1$), and duplications of 16p13.3 ($n = 1$), 22q11.2 ($n = 1$), and 8q21 ($n = 1$), and an unusual partial aneuploidy- monosomy 18 and trisomy 18 with one chromosome exhibiting a 18p11.32p11.31 microdeletion and 18p11.31p11.21 duplication. Additionally, we found one pericentric (9)(p12q13) inversion, which was not found with CMA (Table 2).

### Detection rates of CMA with karyotyping

CMA was performed in 151 VSD fetuses, with 22.5% (34/151) of the cases showing chromosomal abnormalities. Fourteen of these cases were also identified with the karyotype analysis, but the other 20 were identified only with CMA, of which 13 were pathogenetic CNVs, 5 were VOUS, and 2 were benign CNVs. Among the 13 fetuses with pathogenic CNVs, only one fetus had isolated-VSD. These 13 CNVs involved deletions of 3q24q25.1, 15q24.1q24.2, and 22q11.21; duplications of 3q29, 7q11.23, 17p11.2, 22q11.21, 22q11.1q11.21, and Xp28; and loss of heterozygosity of 16q23.2q24.3 and 16p13.3p12.3. There were 7 cases with pathogenic CNVs related to known chromosomal disorder syndromes-DiGeorge syndrome ($n = 4$), Schmid-Fraccaro syndrome ($n = 2$), and Potocki-Lupski syndrome ($n = 1$) (Table 3).

### Comparison of pathogenic CNV detection rates

Overall, the detection rate of pathogenic CNVs with CMA was significantly higher than that with karyotype analysis (17.9% vs. 10.6%, $p < 0.05$). The detection rate of CNVs in non-isolated-VSDs was significantly higher than that in isolated-VSDs (36.1% (26/72) vs. 1.3% (1/79), $p = 0.001$).

### Inheritance analysis and obstetrical outcomes

We screened the hereditary information of 27 families in which karyotyping showed chromosomal abnormalities (9 cases of chromosome aneuploidies were exempted) and abnormal CNVs. Parental analysis showed that that in 5 fetuses the abnormalities were inherited from unaffected parents (Table 4), and in 18 cases, the CNVs occurred de novo. The reasons for termination of pregnancies in the 28 women analyzed were chromosome abnormalities ($n = 14$), pathogenic CNVs ($n = 13$), and VOUS CNVs ($n = 1$). We also found that in 2.5% (2/79) of isolated-VSD cases and 44.4% (32/72) of non-isolated-VSD cases, pregnancy was terminated.

## Discussion

The development of CMA technology, including aCGH and SNP arrays, in the early 2000s provided a new research tool for chromosomal analysis. Since then, a number of studies have used CMA to locate novel candidate genes involved in heterotaxy [10], isolated tetralogy of

**Table 2** Abnormal karyotyping results of VSD fetuses

| Case | Karyotype | CMA results | Prenatal ultrasound | Postnatal outcome |
|---|---|---|---|---|
| 1 | 47,XX,+ 18 | arr[hg19](18) × 3 | VSD; Posterior fossa widening; Single umbilical artery | TP |
| 2 | 47,XX,+ 18 | arr[hg19](18) × 3 | VSD; TS; FGR | TP |
| 3 | 47,XX,+ 18 | arr[hg19](18) × 3 | VSD; ARA; TS; Absence of nasal bone | TP |
| 4 | 47,XY,+ 18 | arr[hg19](18) × 3 | VSD; Single umbilical artery; FGR | TP |
| 5 | 47,XY,+ 18 | arr[hg19](18) × 3 | VSD; FGR; Absence of nasal bone; Overriding fingers | TP |
| 6 | 47,XY,+ 21 | arr[hg19](21) × 3 | VSD; ARA; PVS; Absence of nasal bone | TP |
| 7 | 47,XY,+ 21 | arr[hg19](21) × 3 | VSD; TGA | TP |
| 8 | 47,XY,+ 13 | arr[hg19](13) × 3 | VSD; COA; LSVC; Single umbilical artery | TP |
| 9 | 47,XXY | arr[hg19](1–22) × 2,(XXY) × 1 | VSD; FGR | TP |
| 10 | 46,XX,-18,+mar | arr[hg19]18p11.32p11.31(136,227-3,348,254) × 1,18p11.31p11.21(3,350,736-13,083,388) × 3 | VSD; COA; PVS; AOO | TP |
| 11 | 46,XY,del,(4)(q25q28) | arr[hg19]4q25q28.1(112,192,577-127,874,789) × 1 | VSD; widening of left lateral ventricle | TP |
| 12 | 46,XY,add(16)(p13.3) | arr[hg19]16P13.3(85,880-536,631) × 1,17q24.2q25.3 (64,966,574-81,041,823) × 3 | VSD; LSVC; widening of left lateral ventricle | TP |
| 13 | 47,XY,add(22)(q11.1) | arr[hg19]22q11.1q11.21(16,888,899-18,649,190) × 4 | VSD; HA; Single umbilical artery | TP |
| 14 | 46,XX,add(8)(q21) | arr[hg19]8q21.2q23.3(86,553,128-114,877,447) × 3 | VSD; PTA | TP |
| 15 | 46,XX,inv.(9)(p12q13) | arr[hg19](1–22) × 2,(XX) × 1 | VSD; choroid plexus cysts | TD |
| 16 | 46,XY,13p+ | arr[hg19](1–22) × 2,(XY) × 1 | VSD | TD |

*AOO* augmentation of oval, *ARA* aortic ride across, *COA* coarctation of the aorta, *CMA* chromosomal microarray analysis, *FGR* fetal growth restriction, *HA* hypoplastic aorta, *HLHS* hypoplastic left heart syndrome, *LSVC* left superior vena cava, *PTA* persistent truncus arteriosis, *PVS* pulmonary valve stenosis, *SV* single ventricle, *TD* term delivery, *TGA* transposition of the great arteries, *TP* termination of pregnancy, *TS* tricuspid stenosis, *VSD* ventricular septal defect

**Table 3** Chromosomal microarray analysis of VSD fetuses with normal karyotyping results

| Case | CMA results | Size (Mb) | Prenatal ultrasound | Pathogenicity classification | Obstetrical outcomes | Inheritance |
|---|---|---|---|---|---|---|
| 1 | arr[hg19]22q11.21(18,648,855-21,800,471) × 1 | 3.1 | VSD; RAA; vascular circle; ALSA | P (DiGeorge syndrome) | TP | de novo |
| 2 | arr[hg19]22q11.21(18,648,855-21,800,471) × 1 | 3.1 | VSD; ARA; PA; thymic hypoplasia | P (DiGeorge syndrome) | TP | de novo |
| 3 | arr[hg19]22q11.21(18,631,364-20,729,389) × 1 | 2.0 | VSD; thymic hypoplasia | P (DiGeorge syndrome) | TP | de novo |
| 4 | arr[hg19]22q11.21(18,648,855-21,800,471) × 1 | 3.1 | VSD; RAA | P (DiGeorge syndrome) | TP | de novo |
| 5 | arr[hg19]22q11.21(18,648,855-21,800,471) × 1 | 3.1 | VSD; ARSA; TR; LSVC; Single umbilical artery | P (Cat Eye Syndrome) | TP | de novo |
| 6 | arr[hg19]22q11.1q11.21(16,888,899-18,649,190) × 4 | 1.7 | VSD; ARSA; TR; LSVC; Single umbilical artery | P (Cat Eye Syndrome) | TP | de novo |
| 7 | arr[hg19]17p11.2(16,567,623-18,743,354) × 3 | 2.1 | VSD; PA; FGR | P (Potocki-Lupski Syndrome) | TP | de novo |
| 8 | arr[hg19]Xp28(152,713,658-153,421,838) × 3 | 0.69 | VSD; TR | P | TP | de novo |
| 9 | arr[hg19]3q24q25.1(143,476,996-151,222,561) × 1 | 7.7 | VSD; ocular hypertelorism; widening of lateral ventricle | P | TP | de novo |
| 10 | arr[hg19]15q24.1q24.2(72,965,465-75,567,135) × 1 | 2.6 | VSD; PA; FGR; Absence of nasal bone | P | TP | de novo |
| 11 | arr[hg19]3q29(195,743,957-197,386,180) × 3 | 1.6 | VSD | P | TP | de novo |
| 12 | arr[hg19]7q11.23(72,701,098-74,069,645) × 3 | 1.3 | VSD; Left kidney dysplasia | P | TP | de novo |
| 13 | arr[hg19]16q23.2q24.3(79,800,878-90,146,366)hmz,16p13.3p12.3(94,807-19,302,326)hmz | 10.3 | VSD; PVS; Left kidney dysplasia; FGR | P | TP | UPD |
| 14 | arr[hg19]11P15.1P14.3(20,745,930-21,780,075) × 3 | 1.0 | VSD; Right hydronephrosis; widening of left lateral ventricle | VOUS | TP | De novo |
| 15 | arr[hg19]4q24(106,284,925-107,545,257) × 3 | 1.2 | VSD; ARSA; FGR | VOUS | TD | De novo |
| 16 | arr[hg19]9q21.33q22.1(89,868,507-90,975,015) × 3 | 1.1 | VSD | VOUS | TD | De novo |
| 17 | arr[hg19]16p13.11(14,897,401-16,534,031) × 1 | 0.5 | VSD; Left ventricular hyperechoic | VOUS | TD | De novo |
| 18 | arr[hg19]2q31.2q31.3(180,558,684-181,901,189) × 3 | 0.5 | VSD; OFB | VOUS | TD | De novo |
| 19 | arr[hg19]5q14.1(76,983,283-77,512,158) × 3 | 0.5 | VSD | B | TD | Maternal |
| 20 | arr[hg19]10q21.1(59,095,330-60,684,488) × 1 | 1.5 | VSD; TR | B | TD | Maternal |

*ALSA* aberrant left subclavian artery, *ARA* aortic ride across, *ARSA* aberrant right subclavian artery, *B* benign, *CMA* chromosomal microarray analysis, *CNVs* copy number variations, *FGR* fetal growth restriction, *LSVC* left superior vena cava, *OFB* oval flaps bulging, *P* Pathogenic, *PA* pulmonary atresia, *PVS* pulmonary valve stenosis, *RAA* right aortic arch, *TR* tricuspid regurgitation, *TD* term delivery, *TP* termination of pregnancy, *UPD* uniparental disomy, *VOUS* variation of uncertain clinical significance, *VSD* ventricular septal defect, *VC* vascular circle

**Table 4** Chromosomal abnormalities inherited from unaffected parents in VSD fetuses

| Case | Prenatal ultrasound | Abnormal fetal chromosomes | Pathogenicity classification | Inheritance | Postnatal outcome |
|---|---|---|---|---|---|
| 1 | VSD | 46,XX,inv.(9)(p12q13) | B | Maternal | TD |
| 2 | VSD | 46,XY,13pstk+ | B | Maternal | TD |
| 3 | VSD, TR | arr[hg19]5q14.1(76,983,283-77,512,158) × 3 | B | Maternal | TD |
| 4 | VSD, single umbilical artery | arr[hg19]10q21.1(59,095,330-60,684,488) × 1 | B | Maternal | TD |
| 5 | VSD, RAA, left kidney dysplasia | arr[hg19]16q23.2q24.3(79,800,878-90,146,366)hmz,16p13.3p12.3(94,807-19,302,326)hmz | P (LOH) | Maternal Normal phenotype | TP |

*B* benign, *P* pathogenic, *RAA* right aortic arch, *TD* term delivery, *TP* termination of pregnancy, *TR* tricuspid regurgitation, *VSD* ventricular septal defect, *LOH* loss of heterozygosity

Fallot (TOF) [11], and left-sided CHD [12], as well as novel genomic regions of interest [13]. However, little is known about the involvement of CNVs in either isolated or non-isolated-VSDs. Therefore, we used CMA combined with cytogenetic analysis to identify chromosomal abnormalities and CNVs in fetuses with VSDs, for superior prenatal genetic counseling and revealed a potential correlation between submicroscopic chromosomal aberrations and VSDs.

VSDs are attributable to both Mendelian diseases or chromosomal aneuploidies, as well as to non-Mendelian causes [2]. In our study, karyotype analysis identified 16 chromosomal abnormalities in 151 VSD cases. Among the isolated-VSD fetuses, karyotyping only identified one chromosomal abnormality associated with 13p+, a type of heterochromatin polymorphism, which was not found with CMA. Heterochromatin is regarded as a morphological manifestation of genetic silencing [14]. However, in the non-isolated-VSD fetuses, karyotyping identified clinically significant chromosomal abnormalities involving trisomy 18, trisomy 21, trisomy 13, Klinefelter syndrome, 22q11.2 deletion, and trisomy 18 with one chromosome exhibiting a 18p11.32p11.31 microdeletion and 18p11.31p11.21 duplication. A previous study has reported the association between VSD and major aneuploidies (trisomy 21, trisomy 18, trisomy 13, and Klinefelter syndrome), as well as 22q11.2 deletion syndrome [15], confirming our findings. Karyotype analysis also identified deletion of 4q25q28, and duplications of 16p13.3 and 8q21. These three chromosomal abnormalities are associated with abnormal cardiac development, according to the DECIPHER database. Additionally, we found one pericentric (9)(p12q13) inversion, which was not found with CMA. Some reports have predicted that the genes responsible for normal heart development could be present on chromosome 9, around the p11-q13 region, which might be rendered defective during the process of inversion and thereby resulted in CHD; however, this theory needs further study.

According to the study [16], CMA is unable to replace karyotype analysis due to its failure in detecting chromosome translocations or inversions. But CMA is superior to karyotype analysis because of its high accuracy and resolution in detecting and identifying CNVs, without the need for amniotic fluid cell culture. We observed that the detection rate of pathogenic abnormalities with CMA was significantly higher than with karyotype analysis. According to some reported studies, the yield of CMA in prenatal evaluation ranges from 6.6 to 19.2% [17–20]. The actual rates of clinical detection in our cohort are consistent with the reported studies.

In this study, the most frequently detected CNVs in VSD cases were 22q11.2 deletions. CHDs are known to be associated with 22q11.2 microdeletion [21]. According to the DECIPHER database, *TBX1* is the key causative gene for CHD phenotypes resulting from the 22q11.2 deletion. Besides 22q11.2 deletions, we identified two CNVs associated with Cat Eye Syndrome [22] and Potocki-Lupski Syndrome [23]. Patients with these syndromes display a range of physical and mental disabilities as well as CHDs, including VSDs. Although there is no reported correlation between Xq28 duplication and VSDs, this fragment is important for intellectual development and has been confirmed as a pathogenic CNV [24]. It is well accepted that when VSD is detected in the presence of other structural anomalies, it is more likely related to genetic disorders [25]. We identified a diverse set of four CNVs associated with rare chromosomal syndromes- 3q24q25.1 and 15q24.1q24.2 and the two microduplications, 3q29 and 7q11.23. These syndromes display a range of physical and mental disabilities as well as congenital organ malformations, including VSD. Syndromic VSDs are related to a variety of etiologies such as microscopic and sub-microscopic chromosomal abnormalities, monogenic syndromes, as well as epigenetic and environmental factors [26]. We also found one VSD case with loss of heterozygosity in 16q23.2q24.3 and 16p13.3p12.3. CMA on the parents showed that it was a result of maternal uniparental disomy, which was a classified pathogenic variation.

We observed five cases of VOUS. The result is consistent with the frequency reported in other studies using similar CMA [6, 18]. One case had a 1.0 Mb duplication in chromosome 11p15.1p14.3 that involved an OMIM gene, NELL1, which is associated with the differentiation of brain cells and the growth, differentiation, and mineralization of osteoblasts. The parents' CMA results were normal. Thus, the fetal CNV was de novo, but its clinical significance is uncertain. Due to the non-isolated-VSDs with other severe ultrasound anomalies, the parents opted to terminate the pregnancy.We checked the reference genes involved in the other four cases of VOUS, and none of them are known to be associated with embryonic heart development.The parents opted to delivery the pregnancy. As the use of CMA for genetic disorders expands, increasing data on CNVs is expected to decrease the number of VOUS remarkably in the future.

In this study, the detection rate of CNVs in non-isolated-VSDs was significantly higher than that in isolated-VSDs. In contrast, An et al. [27] showed that there was no significant difference in the detection rate between isolated-VSD and not-isolated-VSD. One reason for the varying detection rates might be due to different prenatal ultrasound equipment and array probe scales. We found that 2.5% (2/79) of isolated-VSD cases and 44.4% (32/72) resulted with termination of pregnancy, with the reasons being chromosome abnormalities, pathogenic CNVs, and other severe ultrasound anomalies. We also found that pregnant women were more likely to continue pregnancy when known chromosomal abnormalities were excluded. This highlights the importance of improving genetic counseling, providing psychological support, and raising awareness of VSDs in parents to reduce unnecessary termination of pregnancies.

## Conclusion

The accuracy of CMA testing is significant in cases of prenatally detected CHD, for both isolated- and non-isolated-VSD cases. In conclusion, CMA combined with cytogenetic analysis is particularly effective in identifying chromosomal abnormalities and CNVs in fetuses with VSDs, which could aid parental counselling. Based on this study and others [28], a majority of the cases still remain elusive, suggesting that different gene mutations or other factors may be implicated in the etiology of VSDs.

#### Abbreviations

CHD: Congenital heart disease; CMA: Chromosomal microarray analysis; CNV: Copy number variation; FISH: Fluorescence in situ hybridization; LOH: Loss of heterozygosity; PCR: Polymerase chain reaction; SNP: Single nucleotide polymorphism; VOUS: Variation of uncertain clinical significance; VSD: Ventricular septal defects

#### Acknowledgments

We thank the patients that participated in this study.

#### Funding

This work was supported by the Key Special Projects of Fujian Provincial Department of Science and Technology [no. 2013YZ0002–1], the Key Clinical Specialty Discipline Construction Program of Fujian [no. 20121589], and the Fujian Provincial Natural Science Foundation [no. 2017 J01238].

#### Authors' contributions

Study concepts: LX, HC; Study design: MC; CMA analysis: HH, GA; Karyotyping: XW, YL; FISH analysis: HH; Data analysis and interpretation: NL; Statistical analysis: XX, LS; Manuscript preparation: MC, LX. All authors read and approved the final manuscript.

#### Competing interests

The authors declare that they have no competing interest.

#### References

1. Lin KY, D'Alessandro LC, Goldmuntz E. Genetic testing in congenital heart disease: ethical considerations. World J Pediatr Congenit Heart Surg. 2013;4(1):53–7.
2. Li G, Yang N, Xie M, Xu Y, Han N, Chen Q, et al. Perinatal and follow-up outcome study of fetal anomalies with multidisciplinary consultation. Ther Clin Risk Manag. 2017;13:1303–7.
3. Mosimann B, Zidere V, Simpson JM, Allan LD. Outcome and requirement for surgical repair following prenatal diagnosis of ventricular septal defect. Ultrasound Obstet Gynecol. 2014;44(1):76–81.
4. Paladini D, Palmieri S, Lamberti A, Teodoro A, Martinelli P, Nappi C. Characterization and natural history of ventricular septal defects in the fetus. Ultrasound Obstet Gynecol. 2000;16(2):118–22.
5. Axt-Fliedner R, Schwarze A, Smrcek J, Germer U, Krapp M, Gembruch U. Isolated ventricular septal defects detected by color Doppler imaging: evolution during fetal and first year of postnatal life. Ultrasound Obstet Gynecol. 2006;27(3):266–73.
6. Du L, Xie HN, Huang LH, Xie YJ, Wu LH. Prenatal diagnosis of submicroscopic chromosomal aberrations in fetuses with ventricular septal defects by chromosomal microarray-based analysis. Prenat Diagn. 2016; 36(13):1178–84.
7. Goldmuntz E. DiGeorge Syndrome: New Insights. Clin Perinatol. 2005;32(4): 963–78.
8. Paladini D, Russo M, Teodoro A, Pacileo G, Capozzi G, Martinelli P, et al. Prenatal diagnosis of congenital heart disease in the Naples area during the years 1994-1999 -- the experience of a joint fetal-pediatric cardiology unit. Prenat Diagn. 2002;22(7):545–52.
9. Hanemaaijer NM, Sikkema-Raddatz B, van der Vries G, Dijkhuizen T, Hordijk R, van Essen AJ, et al. Practical guidelines for interpreting copy number gains detected by high-resolution array in routine diagnostics. Eur J Hum Genet. 2012;20(2):161–5.
10. Thienpont B, Mertens L, de Ravel T, Eyskens B, Boshoff D, Maas N, et al. Submicroscopic chromosomal imbalances detected by array-CGH are a frequent cause of congenital heart defects in selected patients. Eur Heart J. 2007;28(22):2778–84.
11. Breckpot J, Tranchevent LC, Thienpont B, Bauters M, Troost E, Gewillig M, et al. BMPR1A is a candidate gene for congenital heart defects associated with the recurrent 10q22q23 deletion syndrome. Eur J Med Genet. 2012; 55(1):12–6.
12. Hitz MP, Lemieux-Perreault LP, Marshall C, Feroz-Zada Y, Davies R, Yang SW, et al. Rare copy number variants contribute to congenital left-sided heart disease. PLoS Genet. 2012;8(9):e1002903.
13. Geng J, Picker J, Zheng Z, Zhang X, Wang J, Hisama F, et al. Chromosome microarray testing for patients with congenital heart defects reveals novel disease causing loci and high diagnostic yield. BMC Genomics. 2014;15: 1127.
14. Elgin SC, Reuter G. Position-effect variegation, heterochromatin formation, and gene silencing in drosophila. Cold Spring Harb Perspect Biol. 2013;5(8): a017780.
15. Costain G, Silversides CK, Bassett AS. The importance of copy number variation in congenital heart disease. Npj Genom Med. 2016;1:16031.
16. Wapner RJ, Martin CL, Levy B, Ballif BC, Eng CM, Zachary JM, et al. Chromosomal microarray versus karyotyping for prenatal diagnosis. N Engl J Med. 2012;367(23):2175–84.
17. Mademont-Soler I, Morales C, Soler A, Martínez-Crespo JM, Shen Y, Margarit E, et al. Prenatal diagnosis of chromosomal abnormalities in fetuses with abnormal cardiac ultrasound findings: evaluation of chromosomal microarray-based analysis. Ultrasound Obstet Gynecol. 2013;41(4):375–82.
18. Liao C, Li R, Fu F, Xie G, Zhang Y, Pan M, et al. Prenatal diagnosis of congenital heart defect by genome-wide high-resolution SNP array. Prenat Diagn. 2014;34(9):858–63.
19. Yan Y, Wu Q, Zhang L, Wang X, Dan S, Deng D, et al. Detection of submicroscopic chromosomal aberrations by array-based comparative genomic hybridization in fetuses with congenital heart disease. Ultrasound Obstet Gynecol. 2014;43(4):363.
20. Zhu X, Li J, Ru T, Wang Y, Xu Y, Yang Y, et al. Identification of copy number variations associated with congenital heart disease by chromosomal microarray analysis and next-generation sequencing. Prenat Diagn. 2016; 36(4):321–7.
21. Ferencz C, Neill CA, Boughman JA, Rubin JD, Brenner JI, Perry LW. Congenital cardiovascular malformations associated with chromosome abnormalities: an epidemiologic study. J Pediatr. 1989;114(1):79–86.
22. Johnson A, Minoshima S, Asakawa S, Shimizu N, Shizuya H, Roe BA, et al. A 1.5-Mb Contig within the cat eye syndrome critical region at human chromosome 22q11.2. Genomics. 1999;57(2):306–9.
23. Potocki L, Bi W, Treadwell-Deering D, Carvalho CM, Eifert A, Friedman EM, et al. Characterization of Potocki-Lupski syndrome (dup(17)(p11.2p11.2)) and delineation of a dosage-sensitive critical interval that can convey an autism phenotype. Am J Hum Genet. 2007;80(4):633–49.
24. Amir RE, Van den Veyver IB, Wan M, Tran CQ, Francke U, Zoghbi HY. Rett syndrome is caused by mutations in X-linked MECP2, encodingmethyl-CpG-binding protein 2. Nat Genet. 1999;23(2):185–8.
25. Donnelly JC, Platt LD, Rebarber A, Zachary J, Grobman WA, Wapner RJ. Association of copy number variants with specific ultrasonographically detected fetal anomalies. Obstet Gynecol. 2014;124(1):83–90.
26. Sukenik-Halevy R, Sukenik S, Koifman A, Alpert Y, Hershkovitz R, Levi A, et al. Clinical aspects of prenatally detected congenital heart malformations and the yield of chromosomal microarray analysis. Prenat Diagn. 2016;36(13): 1185–91.

26

# Rare partial octosomy and hexasomy of 15q11-q13 associated with intellectual impairment and development delay

Haiyu Li[1], Juan Du[1,2], Wen Li[1,2], Dehua Cheng[1,2], Wenbin He[1,2], Duo Yi[2], Bo Xiong[2], Shimin Yuan[2], Chaofeng Tu[1], Lanlan Meng[2], Aixiang Luo[1], Ge Lin[1,2], Guangxiu Lu[1,2] and Yue-Qiu Tan[1,2*]

**Abstract**

**Background:** Small supernumerary marker chromosomes (sSMCs) are common structurally abnormal chromosomes that occur in 0.288% of cases of mental retardation. Isodicentric 15 (idic(15)) is common in sSMCs and usually leads to a rare chromosome disorder with distinctive clinical phenotypes, including early central hypotonia, developmental delay, epilepsy, and autistic behavior. It was previously shown that the partial tetrasomy 15q and partial hexasomy 15q syndromes are usually caused by one and two extra idic(15), respectively. Karyotypes containing a mosaic partial octosomy 15q resulting from three extra idic(15) have rarely been reported.

**Case presentation:** Two patients with profound intellectual impairment, development delay and hyperpigmentation were recruited for this study. The phenotype was relatively more severe in patient 1 than in patient 2. Conventional cytogenetic analysis of peripheral blood obtained from patients 1 and 2 revealed rare mosaic karyotypes containing sSMCs, i.e., mos 49,XX,+mar × 3[83]/48,XX,+mar × 2[7]/46,XX[10] and mos 48,XX,+mar × 2[72]/47,XX,+mar[28], respectively. The results of analyses of copy number variation (CNV) and fluorescence in situ hybridization (FISH) analyses, showed that the sSMCs were found to be idic(15) involving the Prader-Willi/Angelman Syndrome Critical Region (PWACR) genes and the *P* gene, with duplication sizes of 6.3 Mb and 9.7 Mb, respectively. DNA fingerprinting analysis of patient 1 showed a maternal origin for the idic(15). Both patients had mosaic idic(15) karyotypes: patient 1 had cells with a 15q partial octosomy (83%), and patient 2 had cells with a 15q partial hexasomy (72%).

**Conclusions:** We detected two rare mosaic idic(15) karyotypes that were associated with congenital abnormalities, including a rare mosaic octosomy of 15q11-q13. Our cases further validate the notion that the phenotypic severity is correlated with the level of mosaicism and the dosage effect of related genes in the proximal 15q.

**Keywords:** Isodicentric 15, Partial octosomy of 15q, Mental retardation, Developmental delay, Hyperpigmentation, *P* gene

* Correspondence: tanyueqiu@csu.edu.cn
[1]Institute of Reproduction and Stem Cell Engineering, Central South University, Changsha, Hunan 410078, People's Republic of China
[2]Reproductive and Genetic Hospital of CITIC-Xiangya, Changsha, Hunan 410078, People's Republic of China

## Background

Small supernumerary marker chromosomes (sSMCs) can be defined as small structurally abnormal chromosomes that occur in addition to the normal 46 chromosomes [1]. Usually, an sSMC is smaller than chromosome 20 and cannot be unambiguously identified or characterized using only conventional chromosome banding techniques [2]. These chromosomes occur in 0.04% of newborns and 0.288% of cases with mental retardation [3]. Individuals who carry sSMCs present with a broad spectrum of clinical characteristics, and ranging from a normal presentation to severe birth defects [4]. The effects of sSMCs on a patient's features are associated with their size, the presence of euchromatic material and the level of mosaicism [5].

The sSMCs that originate from chromosome 15, i.e. sSMC(15), are common and can usually be identified using molecular cytogenetic techniques. Chromosome 15 contains many low copy repeats which is prone to unequal crossover, and can form inverted duplication 15 (inv dup(15)) or special sSMC(15) named isodicentric 15 (idic(15)) which includes a chromosome fragment that is duplicated from end-to-end as a mirror image. The phenotypes of patients with idic(15) appear to be highly dependent on the breakpoint. For example, almost no clinical signs were detectable in a case with idic(15)(pter→q12), whereas clinical signs were presented in a patient with the karyotype 47,+idic(15)(pter→q13) [6]. Some researchers have proposed that an idic(15) without the PWS/AS critical region (PWACR) is clinically neutral, while an idic(15) containing the PWACR might result in severe clinical phenotypes, such as intellectual disability, development delay, autism, seizures, and behavioral problems [7–9]. Furthermore, paternally inherited idic(15) might be associated with a normal phenotype, whereas maternally inherited idic(15) is likely to result in development impairments [10].

The number of idic(15) reported across different cases has varied. Partial tetrasomy 15q, which is caused by one idic(15), is relatively common (approximately 80% of cases) [7, 8, 11–19], and partial hexasomy 15q, which is caused by one or two idic(15) or tricentric der(15), has also been occasionally described [9, 20–23]. However, individuals who carry more than two idic(15) have rarely been reported. In this study, we described two children with congenital abnormalities who carried rare types of idic(15) in mosaic forms that were identified by molecular cytogenetic techniques, including single-nucleotide polymorphism (SNP) arrays and fluorescence in situ hybridization (FISH). To improve the value of genetic counseling in affected cases, we explored the relationship between the phenotypes and karyotypes of these patients.

## Case presentation

Patient 1 was a 3-year-old Chinese girl who was born after 38 weeks of uneventful gestation to non-consanguineous healthy parents. She was the first pregnancy and first child of the parents. Her birth weight, length and head circumference were normal, but she exhibited obvious birth defects. She had a cleft palate and extensive skin hyperpigmentation at birth. Her Apgar scores were 7 and 5 at one and five minutes after birth, respectively.

Her growth was nearly normal, but she was slow to reach her developmental motor milestones. Her height, weight, and head circumference were 55.6 cm (25$^{th}$ percentile), 3900 g (< 3$^{rd}$ percentile) and 34.2 cm (< 3$^{rd}$ percentile), respectively, at 2 months. She began to stably raise her head at 20 months. Although she is currently 3 years old, she cannot sit, crawl, or walk independently. With the help of her parents, she can stand for a short time but tires easily. Her daily needs are completely taken care of by her family. She was severely delayed in intelligence with a development quotient (DQ) score of 20 at 20 months. She has exhibited extensive skin hyperpigmentation over her whole body, particularly in the trunk, limbs and perineum, since birth. A darker color is distributed diffusely on her back and buttocks and linearly on her arms. The light coloration on her face, neck, hands, a part of the abdominal skin and the left leg are the only areas of normal coloration on her whole body. The percentage of her body covered with hyperpigmentation is estimated to exceed 85% (Fig. 1). Other tests, such as brain magnetic resonance imaging (MRI), hearing tests, and biochemical tests, were normal.

Patient 2 was an eight-month-old girl. She was born after 39 weeks of uneventful gestation. She was the second pregnancy and second child of the parents, and all other members of her family were healthy. Her birth weight was 4450 g (> 97$^{th}$percentile). Even though she is currently eight months old, she cannot turn over, sit or crawl and can only raise her head unsteadily. She was seriously delayed for 5 months in motor and intelligence with a DQ score of 29.7. The clinical phenotype of patient 2 was similar to that of patient 1, but patient 2 only had slight hyperpigmentation and no cleft palate (Fig. 2). Her brain computed tomography (CT) scan and electroencephalography (EEG) were abnormal. Her skin hyperpigmentation was also found on her neck and limbs; notably, a hemangioma (2 cm × 4 cm) on her left leg broadened the phenotypic spectrum of the 15q duplication (Fig. 2).

### Cytogenetic and molecular cytogenetic analyses

Chromosome analysis was performed by G-banded and/not C-banded metaphases in cultured peripheral blood

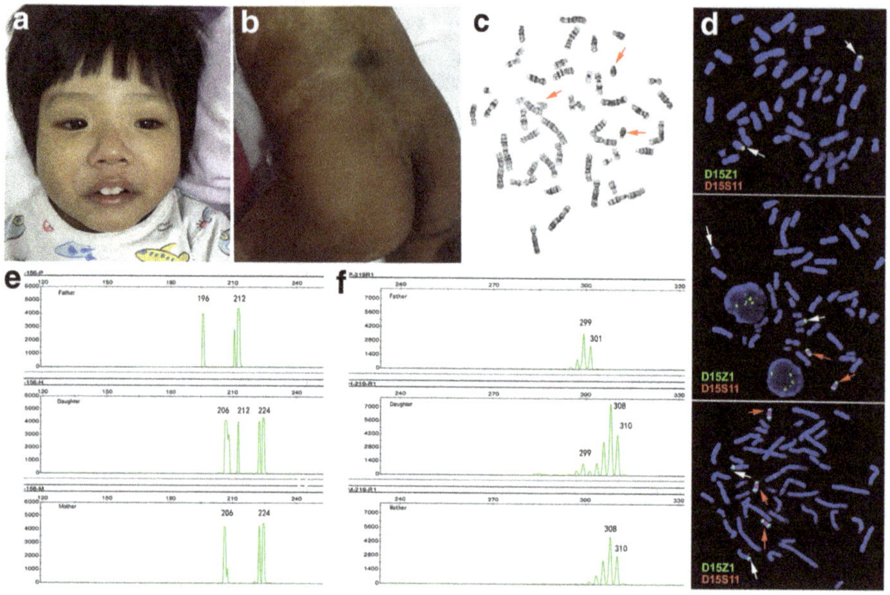

**Fig. 1** The appearance, karyotyping, FISH and DNA fingerprinting results for patient 1. **a** Frontal view of patient 1 displays some facial dysmorphism, including ocular hypertelorism, nystagmus and uneven pigmentation. **b** Deeper pigmentation on the buttocks and back. **c** Partial karyotype by G-banding showing three extra idic(15) regions (red arrow) **d** FISH analysis using D15Z1 (green arrow) and D15S11 (red arrow) showing that each idic(15) has two green hybridization signals and two red hybridization signals. A normal chromosome 15 has one green and one red hybridization signal. **e** and **f** Electropherograms of the markers D15S156 (**e**) and D15S219 (**f**) in the father, children and mother (top to bottom). The children have three different alleles of D15S156 and D15S219. **e** The informative marker of D15S156 shows two different maternal alleles (206 and 224) and one paternal allele (212), indicating that the duplicated region of patient 1 was maternal. **f** The informative marker of D15S219 shows two different maternal alleles (308 and 310) and one paternal allele (299), again illustrating that the duplicated region was maternal

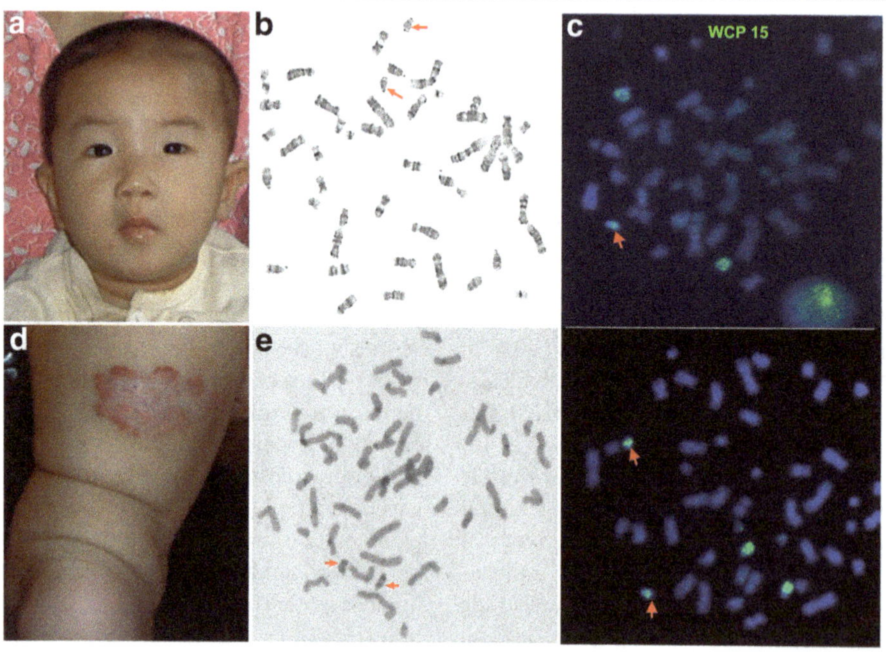

**Fig. 2** The appearance, karyotyping and FISH results for patient 2. **a** The proband has mild facial dysmorphism with low-set ears, a depressed nasal bridge and ocular hypertelorism. **b** Partial karyotype by G-banding showing two extra idic(15) regions (red arrow) **c** FISH analysis of patient 2 using whole-chromosome painting (WCP) probes showing one and two idic(15) regions **d** The patient 2 had a hemangioma (2 cm × 4 cm) on her left leg. **e** Partial karyotype by C-banding showing that each SMC(15) had two centromeres, indicating that the SMC(15) was idic(15)

lymphocytes. FISH analysis was performed on metaphase chromosomes in peripheral blood lymphocytes and oral mucosal cells with D15Z1 (15p11, green signal)/D15S11 (15q11.2, red signal) probes, which covered the critical region of the PWS/AS syndrome (PWACR) in the patient 1, and whole-chromosome painting (WCP) probes were used in patient 2 according to the manufacturer's instruction. All probes were purchased from Abbott-Vysis (Downers Grove, IL, USA). Single hybridization patterns were analyzed using VideoTesT-FISH 2.1 software (Version number 5.0.74.4803, VideoTesT, Ltd., Russia). SNP microarrays were used to analyze genomic DNA that were extracted from the peripheral blood of patients using QIAamp® DNA Midi Kit (QIAGEN, Hilden, Germany). DNA concentration was measured using NanoDrop spectrophotometer (ND-1000, Thermo Fisher Scientific, USA) and DNA quality was determined by agarose gel electrophoresis (1%). For each sample, 2.0 μg of genomic DNA was used for testing which was performed according to the protocol of CytoScan750K reagent kit (Affymetrix, USA). Image scanning and data analyses were performed on Chromosome Analysis Suite (CHAS, Affymetrix, USA). The base pair positions of detected genomic imbalances were designated according to the February 2009 (GRCh37/hg19) Assembly in the UCSC Human Genome browser (http://genome.ucsc.edu).

### DNA fingerprinting analysis

Genomic DNA was extracted using the methods described above. Markers were chosen from previous studies based on the breakpoint in patient 1 [24, 25]. These markers included D15S219, D15S156, D15S1048, D15S1019, D15S1043, D15S165, and D15S184 (Table 1).

## Results

Conventional G-banding showed that the karyotypes of the patients were mos 49,XX,+mar × 3[83]/48,XX,+mar × 2[7]/46,XX[10] and mos 48,XX,+mar × 2[72]/47,XX,+mar[28] (Figs. 1 and 2), respectively. Chromosome microarray analysis performed using Cytoscan 750 k SNP array revealed an abnormal female array profile with a copy number gain in the regions 15q11.2–13.1(22,770,421–29,073,540, 6.3 Mb) and 15q11.2–13.3 (22,770,421–32,444,043, 9.7 Mb) (Fig. 3). The results of FISH analyses confirmed that the sSMC was derived from chromosome 15 and was an idic(15) chromosome because each sSMC had two hybridization signals (Fig. 1). Therefore, patient 1 had a mosaic partial octosomy karyotype, 49,XX,+idic(15) × 3(pter→q13::q13 → pter)[83]/48,XX,+idic(15) × 2(pter→q13::q13 → pter)[7]/46,XX[10].ish idic(15)(q13.1)(D15Z1++,D15S11++).arr 15q11.2q13.1(22,770,421–29,073,540) × 4 dn (reaching the maximum of the software design), while patient 2 had a mosaic partial hexasomy karyotype, 48,XX,+idic(15) × 2(pter→q13::q13 → pter)[72]/47,XX,+idic(15)(pter→q13::q13 → pter)[28].arr 15q11.2q13.3 (22,770,421–32,444,043] × 4 dn (reaching the maximum of the software design). Similar FISH results were obtained using oral

**Table 1** DNA fingerprinting results for 7 STR loci in patient 1

| | Size of the fragment | | |
|---|---|---|---|
| Locus | Father | Patient 1 | Mother |
| D15S219 | (299, 301) | (299, 308/310) | (308, 310) |
| D15S156 | (196, 212) | (212, 206/224) | (206, 224) |
| D15S1048 | (197, 216) | (197, 220) | (220, 220) |
| D15S1019 | (198, 201) | (199, 201) | (199, 201) |
| D15S1043 | (87, 95) | (81, 87) | (81, 87) |
| D15S165 | (165, 178) | (165, 178) | (165, 178) |
| D15S184 | (223, 278) | (223, 278) | (223, 278) |

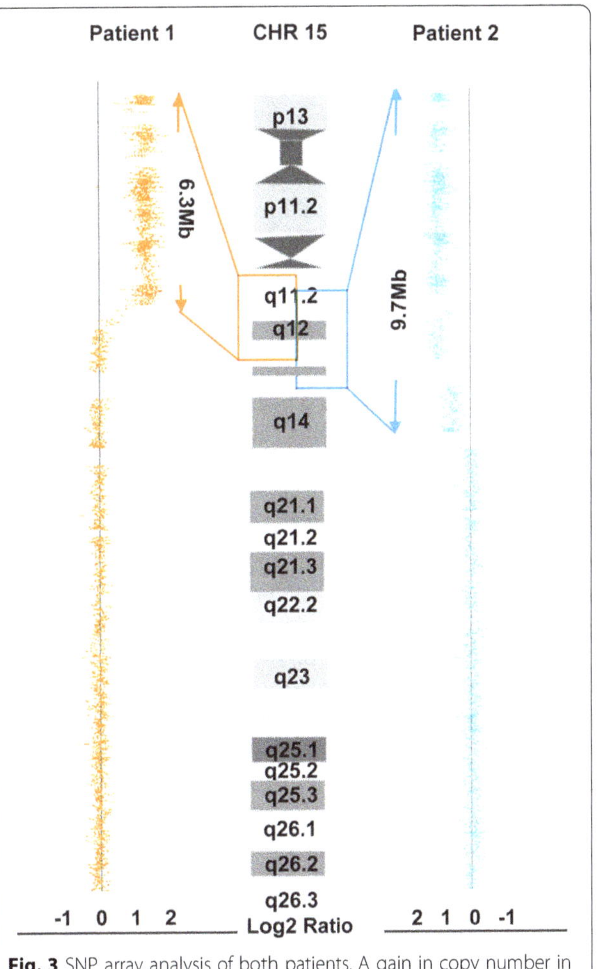


**Fig. 3** SNP array analysis of both patients. A gain in copy number in the 15q11q13 region of patient 1 (left) and patient 2 (right). The orange box shows the location of the copy number gain on chromosome 15 in patient 1, and the blue box shows the location of the copy number gain on chromosome 15 in patient 2. The copy number was beyond the maximum limit of the software (4×). The values on the X-axis represent the log2 ratios for the patients

mucosal cells from patient 1, in whom the ratio of octosomy 15q cells was 85% (180/210). In addition, DNA fingerprinting analysis of patient 1 showed that the child had three different alleles at D15S156 and D15S219, respectively (Fig. 1). These informative markers revealed that one allele was of paternal origin and the remaining two distinct alleles were of maternal origin. These results suggested that in patient 1, biparental inheritance of two normal chromosome 15 s and maternal inheritance of the idic(15) had occurred, which eliminated the possibility of uniparental disomy (UPD).

## Discussion

In this study, we report two patients with serious intellectual impairment and development delay who carried high ratios of mosaic sSMCs. The sSMCs were confirmed by karyotyping, FISH and SNP arrays to be idic(15) and derived from 15pter-15q13.

The chromosome region 15q11-q13 is a potential hot spot for chromosomal duplication and deletion due to numerous interspersed and tandem segmental duplications in this region [26, 27]. Small duplications without the PWACR are usually believed to be clinically neutral [8, 28], but larger genomic rearrangements that cover the PWACR can result in three distinct neurodevelopmental disorders, namely, Prader-Willi syndrome (PWS), Angelman syndrome (AS), and 15q duplication syndrome (Dup15q syndrome) [29]. The two patients presented in this study had severe phenotypes, including cognitive disabilities, psychomotor delays, and speech and behavioral problems. They also had segment gains of 6.3 Mb and 9.7 Mb in 15q, respectively, which is consistent with previously reported cases of Dup15q syndrome [29].

Dup15q syndrome could be caused by interstitial duplication or idic(15), and patients with an interstitial duplication exhibited a milder phenotype than those with idic(15) [19]. An interstitial duplication usually comprises one extra copy of 15q11-q13, which results in trisomy of 15q11-q13. And an idic(15) typically adds two extra copies of 15q11-q13, leading to tetrasomy of 15q11-q13. Nevertheless, a single idic(15) that included four extra copies of 15q11-q13 resulting in hexasomy of 15q, has also been reported [22]. To date, different copy number variations (CNVs) of the 15q11-q13 fragment have been observed to range from 3 to 6 copies, resulting in triplication [15, 30], tetrasomy [11, 12, 16–18], pentasomy [14] and hexasomy [9, 21–23]. Tetrasomy 15q, containing one extra idic(15), is relatively common.

Battaglia reviewed the phenotypes of patients with 15q duplication and showed that tetrasomy of 15q causes a more serious phenotype than 15q triplication [31]. Therefore, more repeats are likely to result in more serious phenotypes. In our study, the symptoms of patient 1, who carried mosaic partial octosomy and hexasomy of 15q, were more severe than those observed in patient 2, who carried a mosaic partial hexasomy and tetrasomy of 15q. Compared with patient 2, patient 1 had a lower DQ and more delayed developmental milestone events. For example, patient 1 could not hold her head up at 8 months, while patient 2 could do so. The data in our study further support the above mentioned hypothesis regarding the relationship between the 15q copy number and the phenotypic severity.

In the present study, the karyotype of patient 1 was mos 49,XX,+idic(15) × 3(pter→q13::q13 → pter)[83]/48,XX,+idic(15) × 2(pter→q13::q13 → pter)[7]/46,XX[10]. To the best of our knowledge, only two similar cases have previously been reported [32, 33]. Cockwell et al. described a patient with dynamic mosaicism of inv. dup(15) [32]. Chromosome and FISH analyses showed that 35 of 50 GTG-banded metaphases had morphologically distinct sSMCs dervied from chromosome 15. Furthermore, 3 of 35 cells had 3 sSMCs, including inv. dup(15), a ring chromosome and a minute chromosome. The other case was a girl with mental retardation, who carried the mosaic karyotype, 49,XX,+mar × 3[1]/47,XX,+mar[9]/46,XX[10], as described on the sSMC database (No.15-W-q14/7–1) [33]. In these two cases, the proportions of cells with 49 chromosomes were only 6% and 5%, respectively. However, this proportion was as high as 83% in the patient 1 of our study. A comparison of the phenotypes observed between our cases and the two previously reported individuals described above revealed that patient 1 in our study not only exhibited mental retardation but also cleft palate and hyperpigmentation. Thus, we speculated that the phenotypic severity is related to the level of mosaicism.

Idic(15) syndrome has a distinctive clinical phenotypes consisting of early central hypotonia, developmental delay, epilepsy, and autistic behavior (Table 2). Furthermore, partial idic(15) patients exhibit increased pigmentation, and the most affected individuals have subtle facial features, including a small button nose, downslanting palpebral fissures, and low-set and/or posteriorly rotated ears [29]. Our patients possessed nearly all of the known phenotypes, except for epilepsy. The age of onset of epilepsy is usually between 6 months and 9 years old [31]. Therefore, these two patients could potentially develop epilepsy in the future.

A few of patients with Dup15q syndrome had presented hyperpigmentation [33]. In our study, both patients presented with skin hyperpigmentation, which was especially prominent in patient 1. The *P* gene, which is located in 15q(27,754,875–28,099,358), encodes a melanosomal transmembrane protein. Homozygous loss-of-function mutations in the *P* gene could cause hypopigmentation [OMIM#611409], while copy number increases in the *P* gene could cause hyperpigmentation

**Table 2** Overview of the clinical presentation of different numbers of idic(15) as reported in the literature

| Clinical phenotype | Tetrasomy (*N* = 44) [7, 11–18] | Hexasomy (*N* = 8) [9, 20–23] | Octosomy (*N* = 3)[a] [32, 33] |
|---|---|---|---|
| Mental retardation | 33/44(75%) | 6/8(75%) | 3/3 |
| Autism | 10/44(22.7%) | 2/8(25%) | _ |
| Seizures | 17/44(38.6%) | 7/8(87.5%) | 1/3 |
| Aggressiveness | 18/44(40.9%) | 6/8(75%) | 1/3 |
| Sleep problems | 4/44(9.1%) | _ | 1 |
| Short stature | 10/44(22.7%) | _ | 2/3 |
| Language delay | 17/44(38.6%) | 6/8(75%) | 1/3 |
| Abnormal EEG | 10/44(22.7%) | 5/8(62.5%) | _ |
| Abnormal MRI | 6/44(13.6%) | 2/8(25%) | normal |
| Dizziness | _ | 1/8(12.5%) | _ |
| Mild facial anomalies | 26/44(59.1%) | 7/8(87.5%) | 2/3 |
| Strabismus | 7/44(15.9%) | _ | _ |
| Nystagmus | 1/44(2.3%) | _ | 1/3 |
| Tympanitis/nervous deafness | 16/44(36.4%) | 2/8(25%) | normal |
| Cleft palate | _ | 1/8(12.5%) | 1/3 |
| Short neck | _ | 1/8(12.5%) | _ |
| Low muscle tension | 27/44(61.3%) | 6/8(75%) | 1/3 |
| Hyperpigmentation | 6/44(13.6%) | 3/8(37.5%) | 1/3 |
| Bone disorders | 4/44(9.1%) | 1/8(12.5%) | _ |
| Cryptorchidism | 1/44(2.3%) | 1/8(12.5%) | _ |
| Joint abnormality | 6/44(13.6%) | 5/8(62.5%) | _ |
| Exaggerated tendon reflex | 1/44(2.3%) | 1/8(12.5%) | Normal or _ |
| Cannot walk | 3/44(6.8%) | 2/8(25%) | 1/3 |

*N* the total number of patients, _ not available or no phenotype, *EEG* electroencephalography, *MRI* magnetic resonance imaging
[a]the data were obtained from patients in our study, in the literature and in databases

[9, 12, 15, 16, 29]. Both patients were hyperpigmented, which is consistent with an increase in the *P* gene copy number. In patient 1, most of the body presented hyperpigmented, while patient 2 exhibited only partial hyperpigmentation, Additionally, the color in patient 1 was much deeper than that observed in patient 2, indicating that the phenotype associated with the *P* gene is dosage-sensitive. Furthermore, our patients displayed pigmentary mosaicism, which is consistent with a mosaic karyotype. Patient 2 presented with a hemangioma on her left leg while patient 1 had none. Nietzel et al. reported a girl with 48,XX,+mar × 2 who also presented with a hemangioma(5 × 5 cm) on her back [6]. However, we found no conclusive evidence indicating a correlation between idic(15) and hemangioma. The results of SNP analyses revealed that the duplication segment in patient 2 (9.7 Mb) was larger than in patient 1 (6.3 Mb). Therefore, we hypothesized that the reason for the hemangioma observed in patient 2 might be associated with the patient's larger repeat segment.

Cook et al. firstly demonstrated that maternally inherited idic(15) is more likely than paternally inherited idic(15) to result in development impairments [10]. Idic(15) covers the PWACR area, which contains many imprinted genes. The genes that are maternally preferentially expressed in the PWACR area are specifically expressed in the brain, such as *UBE3A* and *ATP10A*. This area also contains bi-allelically expressed genes, such as $GABA_A$ receptor subunit genes (*GABRB3, GABRA5,* and *GABRG3*), which may be overexpressed in patients with idic(15) in whom they can cause clinical effects [34, 35], including intellectual disabilities, autism and epilepsy [10, 13, 31, 35, 36]. In our study, we used DNA fingerprinting analysis to verify that the idic(15) of patient 1 was maternal. Thus, we think that the phenotype of patient 1 was associated with an increases in the maternal genes copy number.

A few of patients with Dup15q syndrome presented with cleft palate [9, 37]. In the present study, this symptom was also observed in patient 1. Erdogan et al. reported that candidate genes for cleft palate were located on chromosome 15 and included *GREM1* (32,717,974-32,745,107), *CX36* (34,751,032-34,754,965), and *MEIS2* (36,889,204-37,101,299) [38]. As these genes are outside of the range of the duplicated segment detected in patient 1, the cleft palate observed in patient 1 may be caused by another unknown gene.

## Conclusion

In summary, we report two cases with profound intellectual impairment, development delay and hyperpigmentation and identify a rare mosaic octosomy of 15q11-q13. We explored the relationship between phenotypes and karyotypes in these patients and verified that phenotypic severity was correlated with the level of mosaicism and the dosage effect of related genes in the proximal 15q region.

### Abbreviations

AS: Angelman syndrome; CNV: Copy number variation; FISH: Fluorescence in situ hybridization; PWACR: PWS/AS critical region; PWS: Prader-Willi syndrome (PWS); SMC: Supernumerary marker chromosome; SNP: Single-nucleotide polymorphism

### Acknowledgements

We thank American Journal Experts for providing language editing service in our manuscript. We are grateful to the patients and their family members for participating in this study.

### Funding

This study was supported by grants from the National Natural Science Foundation of China (No.81771645 and No. 81471432).

### Authors' contributions

LH collected patient data, performed the DNA fingerprinting analysis and drafted the initial manuscript. DJ and LW carried out instruments and approved the final manuscript as submitted. HW analyzed the data of DNA fingerprinting analysis. CD and YD performed the FISH experiments and interpreted the results. XB performed the SNP experiments and interpreted the results. YS helped draft the initial manuscript. TC, ML and LA reviewed all laboratory results. LG and LG carried out instruments, critically reviewed the manuscript, and approved the final manuscript as submitted. TY conceived the study, participated in its design and coordination, and helped draft the initial manuscript and write the manuscript. All authors read and approved the final manuscript.

### Competing interests

The authors declare that they have no competing interests.

### References

1. Crolla JA, Howard P, Mitchell C, Long FL, Dennis NR. A molecular and FISH approach to determining karyotype and phenotype correlations in six patients with supernumerary marker(22) chromosomes. Am J Med Genet. 1997;72(4):440–7.
2. Liehr T, Claussen U, Starke H. Small supernumerary marker chromosomes (sSMC) in humans. Cytogenet Genome Res. 2004;107(1–2):55–67.
3. Liehr T, Weise A. Frequency of small supernumerary marker chromosomes in prenatal, newborn, developmentally retarded and infertility diagnostics. Int J Mol Med. 2007;19(5):719–31.
4. Stavber L, Bertok S, Kovac J, Volk M, Lovrecic L, Battelino T, et al. Characterization of a de novo sSMC 17 detected in a girl with developmental delay and dysmorphic features. Mol Cytogenet. 2017;10:10.
5. Starke H, Nietzel A, Weise A, Heller A, Mrasek K, Belitz B, et al. Small supernumerary marker chromosomes (SMCs): genotype-phenotype correlation and classification. Hum Genet. 2003;114(1):51–67.
6. Nietzel A, Albrecht B, Starke H, Heller A, Gillessen-Kaesbach G, Claussen U, et al. Partial hexasomy 15pter–>15q13 including SNRPN and D15S10: first molecular cytogenetically proven case report. J Med Genet. 2003;40(3):e28.
7. Kleefstra T, de Leeuw N, Wolf R, Nillesen WM, Schobers G, Mieloo H, et al. Phenotypic spectrum of 20 novel patients with molecularly defined supernumerary marker chromosomes 15 and a review of the literature. Am J Med Genet A. 2010;152A(9):2221–9.
8. Cheng SD, Spinner NB, Zackai EH, Knoll JH. Cytogenetic and molecular characterization of inverted duplicated chromosomes 15 from 11 patients. Am J Hum Genet. 1994;55(4):753–9.
9. Qumsiyeh MB, Rafi SK, Sarri C, Grigoriadou M, Gyftodimou J, Pandelia E, et al. Double supernumerary isodicentric chromosomes derived from 15 resulting in partial hexasomy. Am J Med Genet A. 2003;116A(4):356–9.
10. Cook EH Jr, Lindgren V, Leventhal BL, Courchesne R, Lincoln A, Shulman C, et al. Autism or atypical autism in maternally but not paternally derived proximal 15q duplication. Am J Hum Genet. 1997;60(4):928–34.
11. Galizia EC, Palmer R, Waters JJ, Koepp MJ, Hennekam RC, Sisodiya SM. The idic(15) syndrome: expanding the phenotype. Am J Med Genet A. 2012; 158A(6):1505–8.
12. Al Ageeli E, Drunat S, Delanoe C, Perrin L, Baumann C, Capri Y, et al. Duplication of the 15q11-q13 region: clinical and genetic study of 30 new cases. Eur J Med Genet. 2014;57(1):5–14.
13. Park DH, Lim S, Park ES, Sim EG. A nine-month-old boy with isodicentric chromosome 15: a case report. Ann Rehabil Med. 2013;37(2):291–4.
14. Yang J, Yang Y, Huang Y, Hu Y, Chen X, Sun H, et al. A study of two Chinese patients with tetrasomy and pentasomy 15q11q13 including Prader-Willi/Angelman syndrome critical region present with developmental delays and mental impairment. BMC Med Genet. 2013;14:9.
15. Tan ES, Yong MH, Lim EC, Li ZH, Brett MS, Tan EC. Chromosome 15q11-q13 copy number gain detected by array-CGH in two cases with a maternal methylation pattern. Mol Cytogenet. 2014;7:32.
16. Akahoshi K, Spritz RA, Fukai K, Mitsui N, Matsushima K, Ohashi H. Mosaic supernumerary inv dup(15) chromosome with four copies of the P gene in a boy with pigmentary dysplasia. Am J Med Genet A. 2004;126A(3):290–2.
17. Wang Q, Wu W, Xu Z, Luo F, Zhou Q, Li P, et al. Copy number changes and methylation patterns in an isodicentric and a ring chromosome of 15q11-q13: report of two cases and review of literature. Mol Cytogenet. 2015;8:97.
18. Szabo A, Czako M, Hadzsiev K, Duga B, Komlosi K, Melegh B. Partial tetrasomy of the proximal long arm of chromosome 15 in two patients: the significance of the gene dosage in terms of phenotype. Mol Cytogenet. 2015;8:41.
19. Finucane BM, Lusk L, Arkilo D, Chamberlain S, Devinsky O, Dindot S, et al. 15q duplication syndrome and related disorders. In: Adam MP, Ardinger HH, Pagon RA et al., editors. GeneReviews® [Innternet]. Seattle: University of Washington; 2016.
20. Conant KD, Finucane B, Cleary N, Martin A, Muss C, Delany M, et al. A survey of seizures and current treatments in 15q duplication syndrome. Epilepsia. 2014;55(3):396–402.
21. Maggouta F, Roberts SE, Dennis NR, Veltman MW, Crolla JA. A supernumerary marker chromosome 15 tetrasomic for the Prader-Willi/ Angelman syndrome critical region in a patient with a severe phenotype. J Med Genet. 2003;40(7):e84.
22. Kraoua L, Chaabouni M, Ewers E, Chelly I, Ouertani I, Ben Jemaa L, et al. Hexasomy of the Prader-Willi/Angelman critical region, including the OCA2 gene, in a patient with pigmentary dysplasia: case report. Eur J Med Genet. 2011;54(4):e446–50.
23. Mann SM, Wang NJ, Liu DH, Wang L, Schultz RA, Dorrani N, et al. Supernumerary tricentric derivative chromosome 15 in two boys with intractable epilepsy: another mechanism for partial hexasomy. Hum Genet. 2004;115(2):104–11.
24. Wolpert CM, Menold MM, Bass MP, Qumsiyeh MB, Donnelly SL, Ravan SA, et al. Three probands with autistic disorder and isodicentric chromosome 15. Am J Med Genet. 2000;96(3):365–72.
25. Wu DJ, Wang NJ, Driscoll J, Dorrani N, Liu D, Sigman M, et al. Autistic disorder associated with a paternally derived unbalanced translocation leading to duplication of chromosome 15pter-q13.2: a case report. Mol Cytogenet. 2009;2:27.
26. Bailey JA, Gu Z, Clark RA, Reinert K, Samonte RV, Schwartz S, et al. Recent segmental duplications in the human genome. Science. 2002;297(5583):1003–7.

27. Zody MC, Garber M, Sharpe T, Young SK, Rowen L, O'Neill K, et al. Analysis of the DNA sequence and duplication history of human chromosome 15. Nature. 2006;440(7084):671–5.
28. Browne CE, Dennis NR, Maher E, Long FL, Nicholson JC, Sillibourne J, et al. Inherited interstitial duplications of proximal 15q: genotype-phenotype correlations. Am J Hum Genet. 1997;61(6):1342–52.
29. Kalsner L, Chamberlain SJ. Prader-Willi, Angelman, and 15q11-q13 duplication syndromes. Pediatr Clin N Am. 2015;62(3):587–606.
30. Akahoshi K, Fukai K, Kato A, Kimiya S, Kubota T, Duplication SRA. Of 15q11.2-q14, including the P gene, in a woman with generalized skin hyperpigmentation. Am J Med Genet. 2001;104(4):299–302.
31. Battaglia A. The inv dup(15) or idic(15) syndrome: a clinically recognisable neurogenetic disorder. Brain and Development. 2005;27(5):365–9.
32. Cockwell AE, Davalos IP, Rivera HR, Crolla JA. FISH characterisation of dynamic mosaicism involving an inv dup(15) in a patient with mental retardation. Am J Med Genet. 2001;103(4):289–94.
33. Liehr T. Small supernumerary marker chromosomes. http://ssmc-tl.com/chromosome-15-abnormal.html. Accessed 8 Dec 2017.
34. Chamberlain SJ, Lalande M. Neurodevelopmental disorders involving genomic imprinting at human chromosome 15q11-q13. Neurobiol Dis. 2010;39(1):13–20.
35. Chamberlain SJ, Lalande M. Angelman syndrome, a genomic imprinting disorder of the brain. J Neurosci. 2010;30(30):9958–63.
36. Battaglia A, Bernardini L, Torrente I, Novelli A, Scarselli G. Spectrum of epilepsy and electroencephalogram patterns in idic (15) syndrome. Am J Med Genet A. 2016;170(10):2531–9.
37. Hou JW, Wang TR. Unusual features in children with inv dup(15) supernumerary marker: a study of genotype-phenotype correlation in Taiwan. Eur J Pediatr. 1998;157(2):122–7.
38. Erdogan F, Ullmann R, Chen W, Schubert M, Adolph S, Hultschig C, et al. Characterization of a 5.3 Mb deletion in 15q14 by comparative genomic hybridization using a whole genome "tiling path" BAC array in a girl with heart defect, cleft palate, and developmental delay. Am J Med Genet A. 2007;143A(2):172–8.

# Unique amplification of BCR-ABL1 gene fusion in a case of T-cell acute lymphoblastic leukemia

Rima Koka[1,3*], Najeebah A. Bade[2,3], Edward A. Sausville[2,3], Yi Ning[4] and Ying Zou[1,3]

**Abstract**

**Background:** ABL1 gene translocations can be seen in precursor T-acute lymphoblastic leukemia (T-ALL). The typical translocation partner is the NUP214 gene. BCR-ABL translocations are relatively rare in this entity. Furthermore, while there have been unique patterns of amplification noted among the NUP214-ABL fusion genes, there have been few such reports among cases with BCR-ABL fusion genes.

**Case presentation:** Here we report a unique case of a 44-year old patient with T-ALL in which the blasts demonstrated a derivative chromosome 9 involving a 9;22 translocation and a dicentric Philadelphia chromosome 22 with a homogeneously staining region at the interface of the 9;22 translocation, leading to BCR-ABL1 gene amplification. Fluorescence in-situ hybridization (FISH) showed abnormal BCR/ABL1 fusions with the BCR-ABL1 gene amplification in 48% of the interphase cells analyzed. The translocation was confirmed by SNP array.

**Conclusions:** We present a novel derivative chromosome 9 that shows BCR-ABL gene fusion along with a dicentric Philadelphia chromosome 22 with BCR-ABL1 gene amplification. This is a unique pattern of BCR-ABL fusion which has never been described in T-ALL. It is significant that the patient responded to standard treatment with the CALGB 10403 protocol and supplementation with a tyrosine kinase inhibitor. Identification of additional patients with this pattern of BCR-ABL fusion will allow for enhanced risk assessment and prognostication.

**Keywords:** T-lymphoblastic leukemia, BCR/ABL, Gene amplification, Isodicentric chromosome 22, Derivative chromosome 9

## Background

Precursor T-lymphoblastic lymphoma/leukemia is a malignancy derived from T-cell precursors. It can manifest as a mass-forming lesion, designated as lymphoma, of the thymus and/or lymph nodes or as leukemia, with involvement of the peripheral blood and bone marrow. The distinction between lymphoma and leukemia is somewhat arbitrary, particularly since all cases have some involvement of the bone marrow; however, the presence of greater than 25% lymphoblasts in the bone marrow should be classified as leukemia [1]. The lymphoblasts are characterized by small to medium-sized cells with moderately condensed to dispersed chromatin, indistinct nucleoli and scant basophilic cytoplasm. Cytoplasmic vacuoles may also be seen. There is no morphologic distinction between T-lymphoblasts from the B-lymphoblasts seen in precursor B-lymphoblastic lymphoma/leukemia (B-ALL). In order to distinguish T-lymphoblasts from B-lymphoblasts, ancillary testing using flow cytometry and/or immunohistochemistry is necessary. The most lineage specific marker is cytoplasmic CD3 although other T-cell markers CD2, CD4, CD8, CD5, CD7 and CD8 can be expressed, often in a pattern that reflects the stage of intrathymic differentiation. In order to distinguish from a mature T cell malignancy, expression of one or more immature markers CD1a, CD34 or TdT is needed. Approximately 19–32% of cases aberrantly express myeloid markers CD13 and CD33 while CD117 may be expressed in cases with activating FLT-3 mutations [2–4]. Precursor T-lymphoblastic lymphoma (T-LBL) constitutes 85–90% of all lymphoblastic lymphomas while precursor

* Correspondence: mkoka@som.umaryland.edu
[1]Department of Pathology, University of Maryland School of Medicine Baltimore, 22 S. Greene St NBW53, Baltimore, MD 21201, USA
[3]University of Maryland Marlene and Stewart Greenebaum Cancer Center, Baltimore, MD, USA
Full list of author information is available at the end of the article

T-lymphoblastic leukemia (T-ALL) accounts for approximately 15% and 25% of childhood and adult lymphoblastic leukemias respectively [1]. Both T-LBL and T-ALL demonstrate slight male predominance.

An abnormal karyotype is found in approximately 50% of T-ALL/LBL cases with a significant proportion involving T-cell receptor (TCR) genes; the alpha and delta loci at 14q11.2, the beta locus at 7q35 and the gamma locus at 7p14–15 partner with a variety of genes [5–8]. These translocations often lead to transcriptional dysregulation of the partner gene. Translocations not involving the TCR genes are rare in T-ALL/LBL. One of these unusual translocations involves the balanced translocation of the Abelson (ABL1) oncogene at chromosome 9q34 to BCR on chromosome 22q11 to produce what is known as the Philadelphia chromosome. In this report, we present a unique case of T-ALL/LBL with amplification of BCR-ABL1 fusion gene in an isodicentric derivative Philadelphia chromosome 22 (idic der (22) t (9;22) (q34;q11.2) hsr (9;22)) with a homogeneously staining region at the interface of the 9;22 translocation.

## Case presentation

A 44 year old Caucasian female with a history of hypertension, obstructive sleep apnea, and morbid obesity, presented to the hospital with severe bony pains, worsening fatigue, and shortness of breath. She had a 25 pound weight loss over the past 1 month as well as drenching night sweats. She did not smoke cigarettes, drink alcohol or use illicit drugs. She had not started any new medications recently.

She was found to have a white blood cell count of 109,500/mcL (differential: 31% segmented neutrophils, 25% myelocytes, 21% lymphocytes, 2% monocytes, 7% eosinophils, 14% blasts), hemoglobin 8.5 g/dL, and platelet count of 111,000/mcL. Her creatinine was 1.6 mg/dL, serum calcium 14.8 mg/dL, LDH 581 units/L, and uric acid was 18.6 mg/dL. Peripheral blood smear showed marked leukocytosis with several immature myeloid precursors and blasts. The blasts were intermediate in size with loosely clumped chromatin, inconspicuous nucleoli and scant basophilic cytoplasm. The bone marrow biopsy and clot section demonstrated a hypercellular (90%) marrow for the age of the patient. Maturing granulopoiesis and erythropoiesis were scant secondary to replacement by a monotonous population of immature cells. Flow cytometric analysis confirmed the presence of an abnormal T-cell population expressing cytoplasmic CD3, CD2, CD4, CD5, CD7, CD8, CD45, and CD1a. Surface CD3 and TdT expression levels were dim to negative.

Twenty metaphase cells from three cultures were analyzed by GTG banding at the 450 band level. 11 cells had a normal karyotype. Nine cells (45%) were abnormal with a derivative chromosome 9 involving a 9;22 translocation and a dicentric derivative chromosome 22 involving a 9;22 translocation and a homogeneously staining region at the interface of the 9;22 translocation, which was associated BCR-ABL1 gene amplification (Fig. 1a-b).

Fluorescence in-situ hybridization (FISH) was performed using a BCR/ABL1 dual color dual fusion probe set to rule out a 9;22 translocation. 200 interphase cells were examined. Abnormal BCR/ABL1 fusions with the BCR-ABL1 gene amplification were found in 48% of the interphase cells analyzed (Fig. 1c-e). Single nucleotide polymorphism (SNP) microarray analysis was performed and demonstrated gain of 9q34 from genomic position (hg19) 133,624,374–139,394,573 (5.8 Mb) including the ABL1 gene, and gain of 22q11 from 16,114,244–23,648,478 (7.5 Mb) including the BCR gene (Fig. 2). Additional findings included loss of heterozygosity at 22q12 (5 Mb), 4q, 5q, 6q, and 22q; all of these were noted in 100% of cells and thus, likely represent constitutional changes. Small changes of uncertain significance were also noted in 7q and 16p, but in less than 1 Mb.

Following diagnosis, hydroxyurea was used for cytoreduction to which the white blood cell count quickly responded. The patient was initially treated for tumor lysis syndrome with hydration and rasburicase, but eventually required continuous venovenous hemofiltration (CVVH) for acute renal failure. She also developed respiratory failure and required intubation.

Treatment was initiated with CALGB 10403 protocol which included Prednisone 60 mg/m2/day for days 1–28, vincristine 1.5 mg/m2 on days 1, 8, 15, and 22, daunorubicin 25 mg/m2 on days 1, 8, 15, and 22, and peg-asparaginase of 2500 units/m2 on day 4. She was also started on Imatinib at a dose of 400 mg by mouth daily on day 3 following initiation of chemotherapy. This dose was continued throughout her treatment. She also received intrathecal chemotherapy with cytarabine and methotrexate. Her course was complicated by septic shock which eventually led to initiation of pressor support. Throughout the hospitalization, the patient remained on CVVH. She also had chronic respiratory failure and required tracheostomy and continued ventilator support. A repeat bone marrow biopsy after count recovery showed no morphologic or immunophenotypic evidence of acute leukemia, was 40% cellular and had trilineage hematopoiesis; however, there was persistent neutropenia based on peripheral counts. Karyotype was 46XX and BCR-ABL PCR was negative.

Unfortunately, she eventually developed sacral decubitus ulcers that resulted in multiple infectious complications including persistent bacteremia and fungemia. Ultimately, the decision was made for comfort care. The patient passed away 86 days after admission although her leukemia was in complete remission.

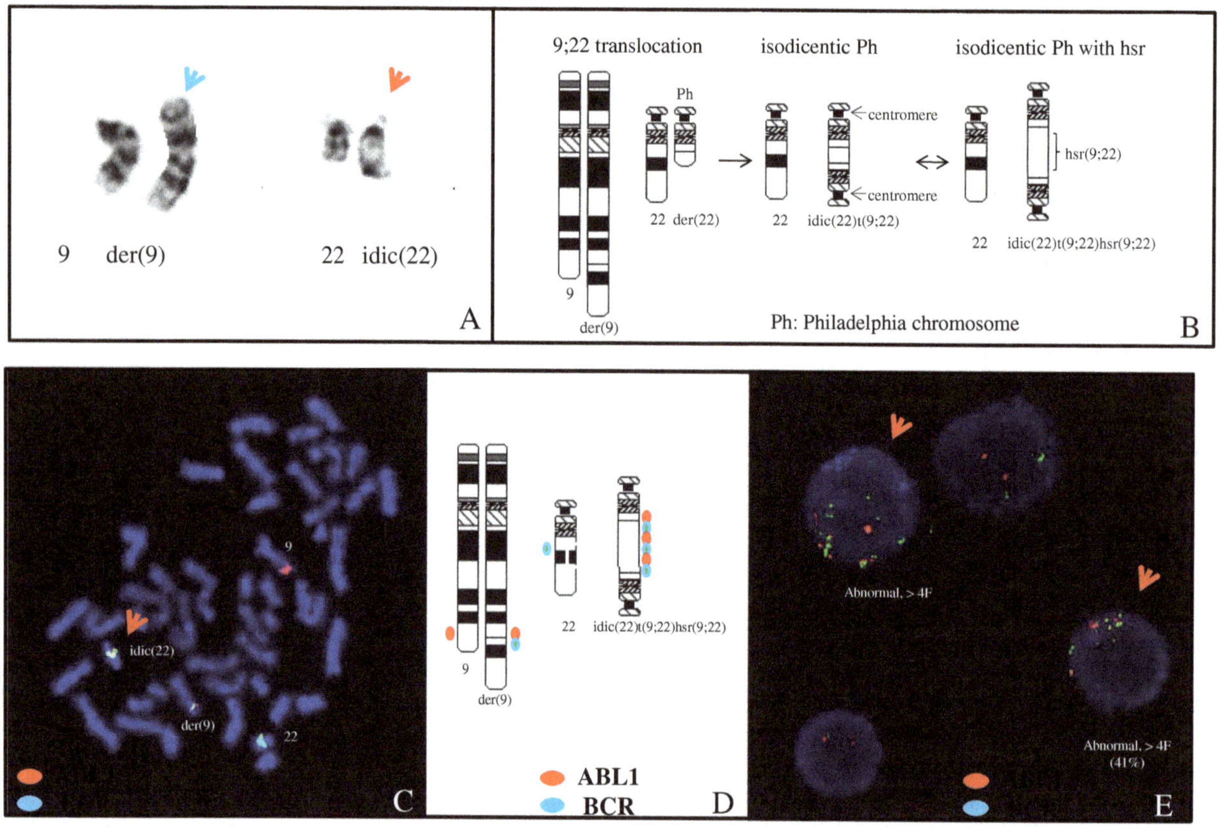


**Fig. 1** Cytogenetic analysis on bone marrow sample of the patient at diagnosis. **a** Partial karyogram showing chromosomes 9 and 22 including a normal chromosome 9, a derivative chromosome 9 (green arrow), a normal chromosome 22, and an isodicentric Philadelphia chromosome 22 (red arrow). **b** Ideograms of G-banding patterns for chromosomes 9 and 22 showing the formation of the isodicentric Philadelphia chromosome 22 with hsr. **c** Metaphase-FISH using dual-color dual-fusion *BCR-ABL1* probes showing multiple copies of *BCR-ABL1* fusions in the isodicentric Philadelphia chromosome 22 (red arrow). **d** Ideograms of FISH signals for *BCR* and *ABL1* genes showing their distributions. **e** Interphase-FISH using dual-color dual-fusion *BCR-ABL1* probes showing multiple copies of *BCR-ABL1* fusion signals in 41% of interphase nucleus analyzed (red arrows)

## Discussion and conclusions

While translocation (9;22) (q34; q11) is most commonly associated with chronic myelogenous leukemia (CML), its presence has been noted in approximately 25% of de novo B-ALL cases, and confers a bad prognosis in the latter, although the use of Imatinib has mitigated this to a degree. In one study, the overall survival of the patients in the Imatinib cohort was 38% whereas the preimatinib group was 22% [9]. The fusion transcripts may yield either a p190 protein (minor breakpoint cluster; e1a2 bcr/abl junction) or a p210 protein (major breakpoint cluster; b2a2 or b3a2 bcr/abl junction). The former is most commonly associated with ALL while the latter is associated with CML. However, p210 transcripts can be seen in low levels in a p190 expressing ALL and vice versa [10, 11]. While this translocation has also previously been reported in T-ALL/LBL, it is exceedingly rare. Among all ALL/LBL cases that demonstrate translocation (9;22), only 2% have a T-cell phenotype [12–14]. Although rearrangement of ABL1 gene is seen commonly in T-ALL/LBL, its fusion partner is most often NUP214 rather than BCR. Interestingly, recent studies have identified that in the majority of NUP214-ABL1 positive cases, there is extrachromosomal amplification of the fusion protein that cannot be detected by conventional cytogenetics. This is due to the presence of extra copies of ABL1 within cytogenetically invisible units known as episomes [6, 12, 14].

Translocation (9;22) occurs very rarely in T-ALL/LBL with an estimated incidence of 2.3% in childhood T-ALL cases and 4.3% in adult T-ALL cases [1]. Although the literature regarding Philadelphia chromosome positive T-ALL is sparse and composed primarily of case reports, like its B-cell counterpart, Philadelphia chromosome positive T-ALL appears to carry a similarly bad prognosis [14–16]. Additionally, previous reports have demonstrated amplifications involving the NUP214-ABL1 fusion gene. The mechanisms of amplification have been heterogeneous. In some cases, there was episomal amplification alone while in others a few of the fusion genes were re-integrated into the chromosome with no subsequent amplification. In the

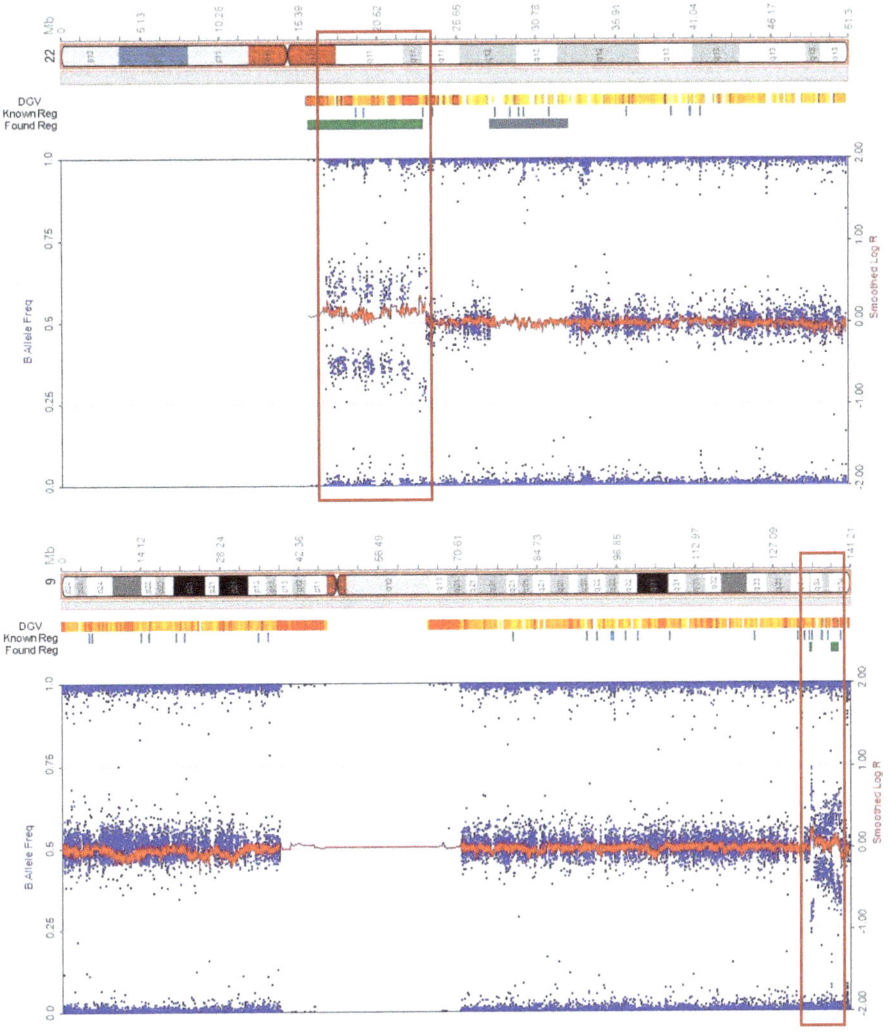


**Fig. 2** SNP microarray analysis of bone marrow sample of patient at diagnosis. SNP array analysis of chromosomes 9 (left) and 22 (right). Gain of 9q34 from genomic position (hg19) 133,624,374–139,394,573 (5.8 Mb) including ABL1, and gain of 22q11 from 16,114,244–23,648,478 (7.5 Mb) including BCR are indicated by the right shift of log R as well as change of B allele frequencies. Loss of heterozygosity at 22q12 (5 Mb) in 100% of the cells is observed, which most likely represents a constitutional change also seen in a few regions on other chromosomes in this patient

cases with purely episomal fusion genes, there was no evidence of the fusion genes on conventional cytogenetic analysis. Therefore, in the absence of specific FISH analysis, these chromosomal fusions may never have come to light. This is of particular interest since there is some suggestion that tyrosine kinase inhibitors may have a role in the treatment of these patients [6]. While clinical experience is limited due to the rarity of these cases, the response of NUP214-ABL1-positive T-ALL patients to tyrosine kinase therapy seems to be highly variable [17–19]. This may be secondary to differences in the catalytic properties of NUP214-ABL1 and BCR-ABL1 as outlined by De Keersmaecker et al. The former was shown to have lower in vitro activity but with increased sensitivity to Imatinib in vitro [20]. Yet another mechanism of amplification was hypothesized to occur whereby the fusion genes within episomes are integrated into chromosomes but then undergo gene amplification [21]. The proposed hypothesis for how this amplification occurs is that the integration occurs downstream of a strong promoter [21].

In the present study, there is intrachromosomal evidence of the BCR-ABL1 fusion gene involving an isodicentric chromosome 22 in approximately 45% of cells. Therefore, we speculate that one of the models previously proposed for the NUP214-ABL1 fusion gene may apply in this case. The demonstration of this translocation in addition to amplification of the fusion gene has, to our knowledge, never been previously reported in T-ALL/LBL. Further detailed analyses of high-resolution sequencing data will provide insights into the mechanism of the BCR-ABL gene amplification in this novel derivative chromosome.

Additionally, due to the presence of this fusion gene, our patient was treated with traditional chemotherapy which was supplemented with a tyrosine kinase inhibitor. She appeared to respond to this therapy. While not relevant to this patient, future annotation of the course of such patients treated with abl-directed therapeutic agents would be of interest to determine if the risk of recurrence in patients with gene amplification is different from those with the fusion gene alone.

### Abbreviations

B-ALL: Precursor B-acute lymphoblastic leukemia; CVVH: Continuous venovenous hemofiltration; FISH: Fluorescence in-situ hybridization; SNP: Single nucleotide polymorphism; T-ALL: Precursor T-acute lymphoblastic leukemia; T-LBL: Precursor T-acute lymphoblastic lymphoma

### Acknowledgments

Not applicable.

### Funding

Not applicable.

### Authors' contributions

RK drafted and finalized the manuscript. NB collected and drafted the clinical history. YZ carried out the cytogenetics and FISH studies in her laboratory. YN performed the SNP microanalysis and interpretation on the diagnostic sample. ES and YZ assisted in critical reading and editing of the manuscript. All authors read and approved the final manuscript.

### Competing interests

The authors declare no competing interests.

### Author details

[1]Department of Pathology, University of Maryland School of Medicine Baltimore, 22 S. Greene St NBW53, Baltimore, MD 21201, USA. [2]Department of Medicine, University of Maryland School of Medicine, 655 W Baltimore S, Baltimore, MD 21201, USA. [3]University of Maryland Marlene and Stewart Greenebaum Cancer Center, Baltimore, MD, USA. [4]Department of Pathology, Johns Hopkins Hospital, Baltimore, MD, USA.

### References

1. Swerdlow S, Campo E, Harris NL, Jaffe ES, Pileri SA, et al. WHO classification of tumours of hematopoietic and lymphoid tissue. 2008.
2. Khalidi HS, Chang KL, Medeiros LJ, Brynes RK, Slovak ML, et al. Acute lymphoblastic leukemia. Survey of immunophenotype, French-American-British classification, frequency of myeloid antigen expression, and karyotypic abnormalities in 210 pediatric and adult cases. Am J Clin Pathol. 1999;111:467–76.
3. Unkun FM, Sather HN, Gaynon PS, Arthur DC, Trigg ME, et al. Clinical features and treatment outcome of children with myeloid antigen positive acute lymphoblastic leukemia: a report from the Children's cancer group. Blood. 1997;90:28–35.
4. Paietta E, Ferrando AA, Neuberg D, Bennett JM, Racevskis J, et al. Activating FLT3 mutations in CD117/KIT (+) T-cell acute lymphoblastic leukemias. Blood. 2004;104(2):558–60.
5. Van Vlierberghe P, Pieters R, Beverloo HB, Meijerink JPP. Molecular-genetic insights in paediatric T-cell acute lymphoblastic leukaemia. Br J Haematol. 2008;143(2):153–68.
6. Graux C, Cools J, Michaux L, Vandenberghe P, Hagemeijer A. Cytogenetics and molecular genetics of T-cell acute lymphoblastic leukemia: from thymocyte to lymphoblast. Leukemia. 2006;20(9):1496–510.
7. Han X, Bueso-Ramos CE. Precursor T-cell acute lymphoblastic leukemia/ lymphoblastic lymphoma and acute biphenotypic leukemias. Am J Clin Pathol. 2007;127:528–44.
8. Cauwelier B, Dastugue N, Poppe B, Herens C, De Paepe A, et al. Molecular cytogenetic study of 126 unselected T-ALL cases reveals high incidence of TCRbeta locus rearrangements and putative new T-cell oncogenes. Leukemia. 2006;20:1238–44.
9. Fielding AK, Rowe JM, Buck G, Foroni L, Gerrard G, et al. UKALLXII/ ECOG2993: addition of imatinib to a standard treatment regimen enhances long-term outcomes in Philadelphia positive acute lymphoblastic leukemia. Blood. 2014;123(6):843–50.
10. Saglio G, Pane F, Gottardi E, Frigeri F, Buonaiuto MR, et al. Consistent amounts of acute leukemia-associated P190BCR/ABL transcripts are expressed by chronic myelogenous leukemia patients at diagnosis. Blood. 1996;87:1075–80.
11. van Rhee F, Hochhaus A, Lin F, Melo JV, Goldman JM, et al. p190 BCR-ABL mRNA is expressed at low levels in p210-positive chronic myeloid and acute lymphoblastic leukemias. Blood. 1996;87:5213–7.
12. Pui CH, Relling MV, Downing JR. Acute lymphoblastic leukemia. N Engl J Med. 2004;350:1535–48.
13. Pui CH, Campana D, Evans WE. Childhood acute lymphoblastic leukaemia – current status and future perspectives. The Lancet Oncology. 2001;2(10):597–607.
14. Arico M, Valsecchi MG, Camitta B, Schrappe M, Chessells J, et al. Outcome of treatment in children with Philadelphia chromosome-positive acute lymphoblastic leukemia. N Engl J Med. 2000;342:998–1006.
15. Brown PA, Shah B, Fathi A, Wieduwilt M, Advani A, et al. NCCN guidelines insights: acute lymphoblastic leukemia, version 1.2017. J Natl Compr Cancer Netw. 2017 Sep;15(9):1091–102.
16. Arican A, Ozbek N, Baltaci V, Haberal M. Philadelphia chromosome (+) T-cell acute lymphoblastic leukaemia after renal transplantation. Nephrol Dial Transplant. 1999;14(8):2054–5. PMID 1046311.
17. Deenik W, Beverloo HB, van der Poel-van de Luytgaarde SC, et al. Rapid complete cytogenetic remission after upfront dasatinib monotherapy in a patient with a NUP214-ABL1-positive T-cell acute lymphoblastic leukemia. Leukemia. 2009;23(3):627–9.
18. Stergianou K, Fox C, Russell NH. Fusion of NUP214 to ABL1 on amplified episomes in T-ALL–implications for treatment. Leukemia. 2005;19(9):1680–1.
19. Clarke S, O'Reilly J, Romeo G, Cooney J. NUP214-ABL1 positive T-cell acute lymphoblastic leukemia patient shows an initial favorable response to imatinib therapy post relapse. Leuk Res. 2011 Jul;35(7):e131–3.
20. De Keersmaecker K, Versele M, Cools J, Superti-Furga G, Hantschel O. Intrinsic differences between the catalytic properties of the oncogenic NUP214-ABL1 and BCR-ABL1 fusion protein kinases. Leukemia. 2008 Dec; 22(12):2208–16.
21. Graux C, Stevens-Kroef M, Lafage M, Dastugue N, Harrison CJ, et al. Heterogeneous patterns of amplification of the NUP214-ABL1 fusion gene in T-cell acute lymphoblastic leukemia. Leukemia. 2009 Jan;23(1):125–33.

# 28

# The decision on the embryo to transfer after Preimplantation Genetic Diagnosis for X-autosome reciprocal translocation in male carrier

Sandrine Chamayou*, Maria Sicali, Debora Lombardo, Carmelita Alecci and Antonino Guglielmino

**Abstract**

**Background:** The aim of Preimplantation Genetic Diagnosis (PGD) on embryos produced *in vitro* is to identify the embryos without genetic or chromosomal defect from those embryos that will develop the genetic disease or are chromosomally abnormal. In case of PGD for structural chromosome indication (PGR-SR), the normal/balanced embryos are transferred in the maternal uterus. This protocol is valid and widely applied for autosomal chromosome translocation. But which embryo should be transferred after preimplantation genetic diagnosis (PGD-SR) for X-3 reciprocal translocation in male patient?

**Case presentation:** The female patient was 26 years old with normal 46,XX karyotype. The male patient had a karyotype with balanced translocation 46,Y,t(X;3)(p11.2;p14)mat, inherited from the mother. The female patient underwent two cycles of ovarian stimulation. In the first cycle, the metaphase II oocytes were vitrified, while in the second cycle they were used as fresh. ICSI was performed on vitrified/warmed and fresh oocytes. Embryos were biopsied at blastocyst stage. Chromosomal analysis was performed by Next Generation Sequencing.
Eleven blastocysts were biopsied from 23 vitrified/warmed and fresh metaphase II oocytes. Two embryos were diagnosed 46,XY; two embryos were diagnosed 46,XX; four embryos were diagnosed with unbalanced translocations and three embryos were diagnosed aneuploid. We knew that the two embryos diagnosed as 46,XX inherited the balanced translocation from the father and the two embryos diagnosed as 46,XY had a normal karyotype. It was explain to the couple that the phenotype of balanced translocated female embryos cannot be predicted because of the random inactivation of X chromosome and that could also occur on the der(X). The couple asked to have a 46,XY embryo transferred. Clinical pregnancy was obtained and non invasive prenatal test confirmed PGD-SR result.

**Conclusions:** Proposing PGD-SR for gonosome-autosome reciprocal translocation implies the risk to exclude balanced translocated female embryos with a normal phenotype for transfer because the early and late normal development at post-natal stage cannot be predicted based on the only chromosomal analysis.

**Keywords:** Genetic counseling, Preimplantation genetic diagnosis, Reciprocal translocation, X-autosome Translocation, X inactivation

* Correspondence: s.chamayou@yahoo.fr
Unità di Medicina della Riproduzione - Centro HERA, via Barriera del Bosco n 51/53 95030 Sant Agata Li Battiati, Catania, Italy

## Background

The primary aim of genetic/chromosomal investigation on embryos produced in vitro is to identify the embryos without genetic/chromosomal defect from those embryos that will develop the genetic disease or are chromosomally unbalanced. The embryos without genetic disease or chromosomally balanced are chosen for embryo-transfer. Preimplantation genetic diagnosis (PGD) is applied in couples with a high risk of inherited defect on offspring such as chromosomal rearrangements including balanced translocations, inversions or deletions [1]. In balanced (Robertsonian or reciprocal) translocations, the carrier parent contains the correct amount of genetic material. If the translocations did not occur within a gene, there is no consequence on carrier phenotype. Nevertheless, the translocated patient has an increased risk for chromosomally unbalanced gametes and conceptions. In case of PGD for structural chromosomal indication (PGD-SR), the embryo diagnosed as diploid for the two entire chromosomes involved in the translocation is chosen for transfer. With the use of the last advanced molecular technologies such as Comparative Genome Hybridization array [2], Single Nucleotide Polymorphism arrays with full molecular karyotyping [3, 4], and Next Generation Sequencing (NGS) [5, 6], a comprehensive chromosomal screening can be performed with a resolution inferior to 1Mb [7, 8]. In routine protocols, these methods do not distinguish an embryo with a normal from an embryo with a balanced translocated karyotype. They remain quantitative on the opposite to banding karyotype.

Among chromosomal translocations, reciprocal translocations that are the product of material exchange between two non-homologous chromosomes are reported with an incidence about 1 in 625 newborns [9]. In particular, balanced gonosome-autosome translocations are very rare, with an incidence estimated in about 1/30,000 live births [10]. Actually, the only available databases that we are aware of on PGD are those from the ESHRE PGD Consortium. On 5247 PGD-SR, only 42 cases due to female or male indications were recorded [11]. In particular, there were listed 16 cases for X-autosome translocation with female indication, 24 cases for Y-autosome translocation with male indication and only 2 cases for X-autosome translocation with male indication [12].

In 1962, Mary Lyon established that one X-chromosome is randomly inactivated in woman to equilibrate the X-linked gene expression between the two sexes [13]. In women with a balanced X-autosome translocation, the normal X chromosome is preferentially inactivated [14] and a normal phenotype is expressed. Nevertheless, the choice of the X chromosome to inactivate is random and can occur on the der(X). In this case, the gene silencing is spread into the autosomal attached segment leading to female patients with genetic disorders with variable gravity.

We presently describe a case of PGD-SR for reciprocal X-3 (p11.2;p14) translocation in male patient. Normal male and balanced translocated female embryos were obtained. We discuss the dilemma of choosing of the embryo to transfer according to sex, in those embryos with unpredictable phenotype. The present work is the first published case of PGD-SR for gonosome-autosome translocation with male indication.

## Case presentation

### Material and methods

#### *Patients*

The female patient was 26 years old at the time of PGD-SR. Karyotype was 46,XX. Basal FSH, LH on day 3 and AMH value were respectively 8.0 IU/l, 6.5 IU/l and 6.3 ng/ml. She had a 30 days ovarian cycle. Uterine cavity and fallopian tubes resulted regular from diagnostic examination. The ovaries had a polycystic ovarian aspect. The patient had no previous pregnancy.

The male patient was 30 years old at the time of PGD-SR. After QFQ-banding karyotype analysis, he was found to have a karyotype with balanced translocation involving X chromosome and autosome 3: 46,Y,t(X;3)(p11.2;p14)mat (Fig. 1).

The X-3 reciprocal translocation was transmitted from the mother that had the karyotype 46,X,t(X;3)(p11.2;p14) in the blood cells. In the family of male patient, the first sibling had a 46,XX normal karyotype (II-1). The third of three siblings (II-5) showed the same karyotype 46,Y,t(X;3)(p11.2;p14)mat of the patient. The parents of the patient were not consanguineous (Fig. 2). His mother and siblings had a normal phenotype.

The male patient had a normal phenotype with normal genital tract.

Semen was characterized by severe oligoasthenoteratozoospermia (Semen concentration: 20.000 sperm /ml; 5% sperm with progressive motility, 2% of normal sperm). From blood cells analysis, the male patient resulted negative for microdeletions of AZFa, AZFb and AZFc regions [15]. The male endocrine was normal for FSH, LH, total Testosterone, Free Testosterone, 17bE2, Prolactin, HCG, aFP. The couple consulted for the first time an infertility center for primary infertility and asked to know 'the state of health' of the embryos as allowed by the Italian law on Medically Assisted Procreation [16].

The following protocols of ovarian stimulation, oocyte and embryo vitrification, ICSI and embryos culture, embryo biopsy and NGS have been described elsewhere and are resumed as follow [17]. Each part of the protocol has been approved by the Institutional Review Board Unità di Medicina della Riproduzione - Centro HERA. The patients signed informed consent forms on all procedures prior application.

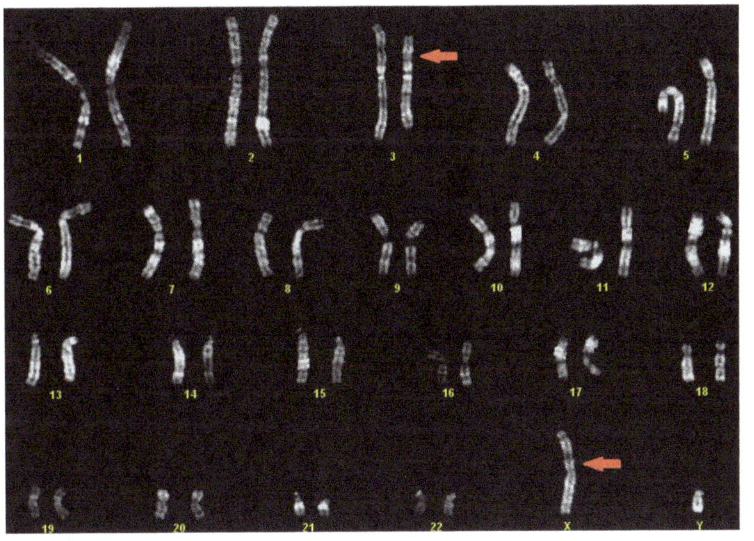

**Fig. 1** Karyotype 46,Y,t(X,3)(p11.2;p14)mat of male patient

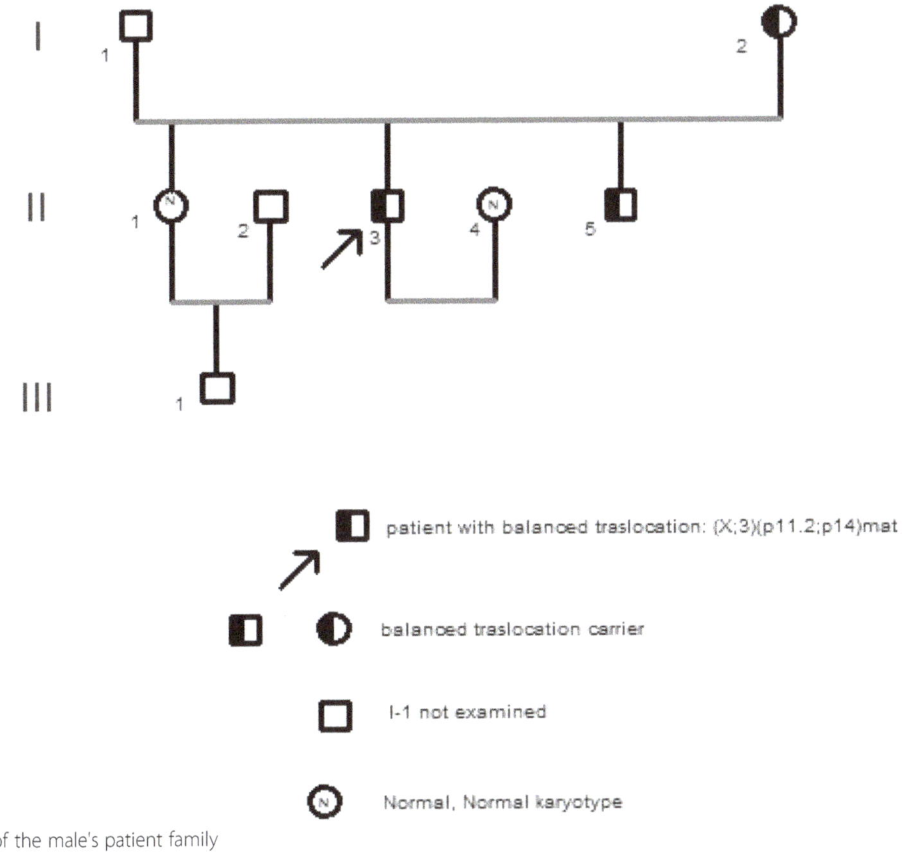


**Fig. 2** Pedigree of the male's patient family

***Ovarian stimulation***

The female patient underwent two cycles of ovarian stimulation. In the first cycle, the metaphase II oocytes were vitrified. In the second cycle the metaphase II oocytes were used as fresh together with the previously vitrified/warmed oocytes.

The first ovarian stimulation was performed by the administration of recombinant FSH and LH (Puregon, MSD, Franklin Lakes, USA and Luveris: Merck-Serono, London, UK) from cycle day 2 in a luteal gonadotrophin-releasing hormone antagonist flexible schema (Orgalutran : MDS). Initial doses were 200 IU/day for FSH and 75 IU/day for LH. Luteal gonadotrophin-releasing hormone antagonist was given when the leader follicle reached 14 mm in diameter with a dosage of 0.25 mg/day. The second ovarian stimulation started on day 2 of the following cycle.

One ICSI session was performed using the accumulated vitrified/warmed oocytes together with the lately produced fresh oocytes and fresh male patient semen.

***ICSI on vitrified/warmed and fresh oocytes and embryo culture***

Vaginal ultrasound-guided aspiration of oocyte–cumulus complex (OPU) was performed 35 hours after human chorionic gonadotrophin administration (HCG 10,000 IU, Gonasi: AMSA, Rome, Italy). ICSI was performed on fresh oocytes 3h after OPU and on cryopreserved oocytes 1 hour after warming and in vitro culture with the same patient's fresh ejaculated spermatozoa sample.

After ICSI, in vitro culture was carried out in Continuous single culture complete medium with human serum albumin (Irvine Scientific, Santa Ana, USA) under mineral oil and in automated incubators with 5% $CO_2$, 5% $O_2$ at 37°C, fitted with time-lapse imaging acquisition (Embryoscope, Unisense, Aarhus, Denmark).

***Embryo biopsy***

Embryo biopsies were performed on day 5 on expanded or hatching blastocysts. Few trophectoderm cells [5 to 10] were removed from a zona pellucida hole using a 1.48 um diode laser (OCTAX, Bruckberg, Germany) and a 20 um inner diameter biopsy pipette. After the biopsy procedure, each embryo was incubated until embryo vitrification and before blastocyst re-expension. The biopsied trophectoderm cells were washed in sterile phosphate buffered saline (PBS) solution and transferred into a 0.2 ml Eppendorf tube containing 4 ul of sterile PBS solution.

***Oocyte/embryo vitrification and warming***

The vitrification and warming protocols for oocyte [18] and embryos [19] were previously described.

***Cell lysis, whole genome amplification and NGS protocol***

The biopsied trophectoderm cells were submitted to alkaline lyses and whole genome amplification according to Repli-g Single Cell protocol (Qiagen, Hilden, Germany). After quantification of amplified DNA, libraries were prepared from 100 ng of each sample and barcoded with IonXpressPlus Fragment and IonXpress Barcode Adapter kits (Life Technologies-Thermo Fisher (Carlsbad, USA). After quantification of the libraries, normalization to 100 pM and mix-up to obtain a final concentration of 8 pM, the eleven enriched libraries were loaded on Chip 16 V2. DNA sequencing was performed on ION PGM HiQ View Sequencing in Ion Personal Genome Machine. The updated Torrent Suite Software was used for base calling and mapping on human genome reference sequence Hg19. For each chromosome read coverage was corrected by guanine-cytosine calculation. Aneuploidy was diagnosed comparing data to baseline values multiple male samples. In all the process, a positive control with normal male DNA and a negative control from biopsy culture media were processed together with the samples to diagnose. Genetic analysis was validated when median absolute pair wise difference (MAPD) was inferior to 0.3. Chromosomal segments as short as 7 Mb could be detected. The protocol was previously validated on single cells from amniocytes with different karyotypes [17].

***Endometrial preparation for embryo transfer***

Warming and single embryo transfer was performed on natural cycle at 7 days after LH surge.

**Results**

***In vitro results***

The results of oocyte vitrification, ICSI, embryo culture and embryo biopsy analysis from vitrified/warmed and fresh oocytes are presented in Table 1.

The patient produced 8 metaphase II oocytes that were vitrified during the first ovarian cycles and 16 metaphase II oocytes in the second ovarian cycle that were used as fresh. Seven of the 8 vitrified oocytes survived to warming and were micro-injected together with the 16 fresh oocytes with the male patient' semen sample and in the same ICSI procedure. The fertilization rates were 71.4% for vitrified/warmed oocytes (5 zygotes/7 micro-injected oocytes) and 75.0% for fresh oocytes (12 zygotes/16 micro-injected oocytes). On day V, 3 expanded or hatching blastocysts from vitrified/warmed oocytes (3 blastocysts/5 zygotes, 60.0%) and 8 expanded or hatching blastocysts from fresh oocytes (8 blastocysts/12 zygotes, 67.0%) were biopsied and vitrified.

***Genetic results***

The genetic analysis were validated and completed respectively in 100% of the biopsied blastocysts from vitrified/warmed and fresh oocytes. Chromosome contents of each blastocyst after PGD-SR are reported in Table 2.

**Table 1** in vitro results of PGD-SR treatment

| | Vitrified/ warmed oocytes (1st ovarian stimulation) | Fresh oocytes (2nd ovarian stimulation) |
|---|---|---|
| Metaphase II oocytes at OPU | 8 | 16 |
| Vitrified oocytes | 8 | - |
| Survived oocytes | 7 | - |
| Micro-injected oocytes | 7 | 16 |
| Zygotes (fertilization rate) | 5 (71.4) | 12 (75.0) |
| Expanded/hatching biopsied Blastocysts (proportion on zygote) | 3 (60.0) | 8 (67.0) |
| Vitrified biopsied blastocysts | 3 | 8 |

According to the karyograms generated by IGV (Integrative Genomics Viewer), it was found that two embryos were diagnosed 46,XY, two embryos were diagnosed 46,XX; four embryos were diagnosed with unbalanced translocations and showed the trisomy 3p14→cen→3qter and monosomy Xp11.2→cen→Xqter, from 2:2 segregation and adjacent-2 disjunction. Three embryos were diagnosed aneuploid (45,X0 ; 45,XY,del [2] ;46,XY,del [8](qter →q22.1). Even if balanced translocation could be detected by NGS analysis, the 2 embryos diagnosed as 46,XX were known to have the balanced translocation inherited by the father and their true karyotype was: 46,X,t(X;3)(Xqter→Xp11.2::3p14→3pter;3qter→3p14::Xp11.2→Xpter)pat. On the same way, the 2 embryos diagnosed as 46,XY had a normal karyotype. Karyograms are shown in Fig. 3.

### *Genetic counseling*

Prior to PGT-SR, a genetic counselling was performed and the couple was informed on the possible karyotypes due to father reciprocal translocation: embryo(s) with normal 46,XY, female(s) with balanced translocation and unpredictable phenotype, embryo(s) with unpredictable complete or partial aneuploidies.

After PGT-SR, the patients were informed on the result of the present PGD-SR. It was explained that among the viable embryos, the 2 male embryos had the true kayotype 46,XY, 2 female embryos had the reciprocal translocation 46,X,t(X;3)(Xqter→Xp11.2::3p14→3pter; 3qter→3p14::Xp11.2→Xpter)pat.

Regarding the 2 female embryos with balanced translocation, it was explained that the phenotype should be normal, due to the preferable silencing of normal X as it seems to have happened in the patient's mother. Consequently, deciding not to transfer balanced translocated female means taking the risk of eliminating from transfer and pregnancy a viable embryo with a normal phenotype.

On the other side, genetic disorders with different degree of gravity (from gonadal digenesis and premature ovarian failure to major genetic disorders and mental retardation) were reported in female patients with balanced reciprocal X-autosome translocations. This risk exists and remains unpredictable. The probability of occurring cannot be calculated.

Finally, one embryo had 45,X0 karyotype. It was explained that Turner Syndrome has a large expressivity [20] and a very high in uterus lethality within the first trimester of pregnancy [21, 22].

It was reminded that de novo balanced translocation could not be detected by the present protocol of NGS.

After counselling, the couple asked to have one 46,XY embryo thawed and transferred.

### *Clinical outcome*

The embryo n. 13 obtained from fresh oocyte, was thawed and transferred. The β-HCG test performed 12 days after embryo transfer was positive. Two weeks later the clinical pregnancy was ascertained by scan of embryonic sac and

**Table 2** Chromosome content of blastocyst after PGD-SR

| Embryo n. | Oocyte origin | Chromosome content | n. Reads | Coverage | MAPD |
|---|---|---|---|---|---|
| 1 | Fresh | Trisomy 3p14→cen→3qter and monosomy Xp11.2→cen→Xqter | 130,326 | 99.90% | 0.170 |
| 3 | Fresh | 46,XY | 106,478 | 99.91% | 0.217 |
| 4 | Fresh | Trisomy 3p14→cen→3qter and monosomy Xp11.2→cen→Xqter | 278,023 | 99.78% | 0.176 |
| 6 | Fresh | Trisomy 3p14→cen→3qter and monosomy Xp11.2→cen→Xqter | 90,688 | 99.92% | 0.226 |
| 12 | Fresh | 46,X,t(X;3)(Xqter→Xp11.2::3p14→3pter;3qter→3p14::Xp11.2→Xpter)pat | 70,759 | 99.95% | 0.226 |
| 13 | Fresh | 46,XY | 124,119 | 99.90% | 0.203 |
| 14 | Fresh | 45,X0 | 125,875 | 99.90% | 0.198 |
| 16 | Fresh | 45,XY,del [2] | 412,006 | 99.66% | 0.153 |
| 17 | Vitrified/warmed | 46,XY,del [8](qter →q22.1) | 157,459 | 99.87% | 0.176 |
| 18 | Vitrified/warmed | Trisomy 3p14→cen→3qter and monosomy Xp11.2→cen→Xqter | 118,589 | 99.90% | 0.200 |
| 22 | Vitrified/warmed | 46,X,t(X;3)(Xqter→Xp11.2::3p14→3pter;3qter→3p14::Xp11.2→Xpter)pat | 133,527 | 99.89% | 0.179 |

*MAPD* median absolute pair wise difference. Coverage:percentage of bases in whole genome covered by at least 20% of the average base coverage depth reads

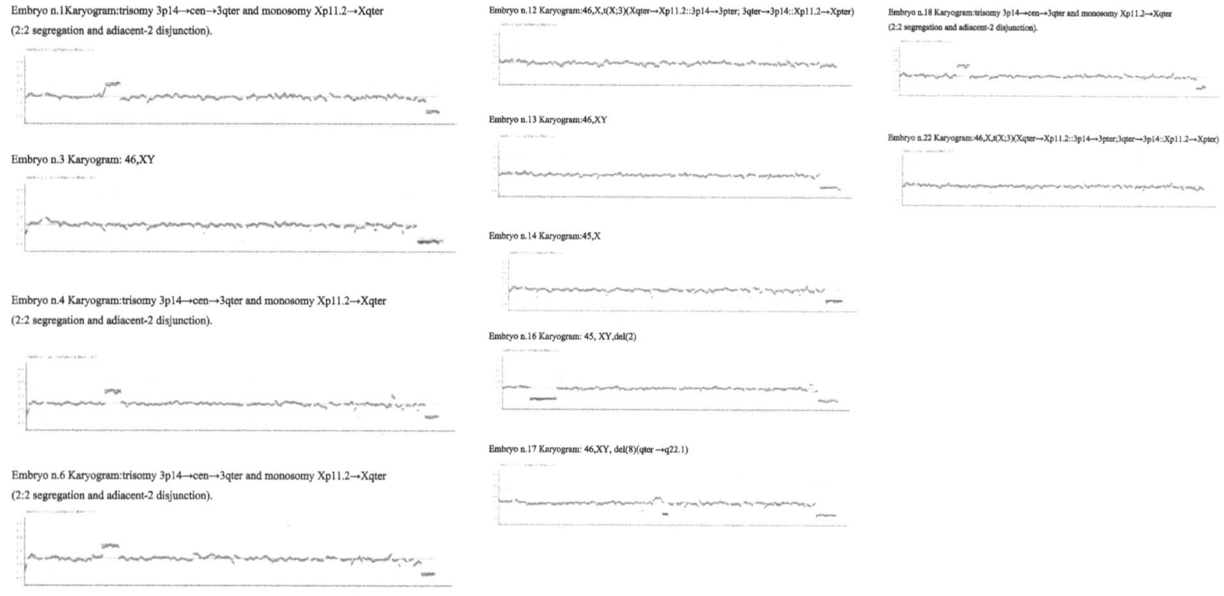


**Fig. 3** Karyograms of diagnosed embryos.

one foetal heart beat was observed. Non invasive prenatal testing (NIPT) for all autosome and gonosome chromosomes was performed on the 15th week of pregnancy and confirmed PGD-SR result.

## Discussion and conclusions

We reported a rare case of PGD-SR for reciprocal X-3 translocation in male patient. The couple came for primary infertility and the male patient discovered to have the karyotype 46,XY,t(X;3)(p11.2;p14)mat in diagnostic phase. The reciprocal translocation was inherited from his mother that had a normal phenotype. The male patient had a severe oligoasthenoteratozoospermia probably due to the structural chromosome abnormality [23]. ICSI was proposed to address the male infertility due to sperm parameters alteration and the couple asked to know 'the state of health of their embryos' as allowed by the Italian law [16]. Consequently, PGD-SR protocol for complete and partial aneuploidie for all chromosomes was applied. On the 11 embryos obtained after two ovarian stimulations and from vitrified/warmed and fresh oocytes, four embryos (36,4%) were diagnosed with a normal karyotype after NGS analysis, two 46,XY and two 46,XX embryos. Even if it was not possible to detect it by NGS, we knew that the two 46,XY embryos had a normal karyotype (excepted if de novo balanced translocations occurred), and the two 46,XX embryos carried the reciprocal translocation inherited from the father and were 46,X,t(X;3)(Xqter→Xp11.2::3p14→3pter;3qter →3p14::Xp11.2→Xpter)pat.

In 2016, Ferfouri et al. presented two cases in which the female patient carried a balanced reciprocal translocation X-autosome [24]. After embryo biopsy on day 3 and FISH analysis, 2/30 (6.7%) embryos resulted normal/balanced. No live birth was obtained after the embryo transfer of two balanced female embryos. In the present case, 4/11 (36.4%) were analysed as chromosomally balanced after embryo biopsy at blastocyst stage.

Among the gonosome-autosome translocations, the X-autosome reciprocal translocations are known to be the most sensitive cases because the phenotype can vary in female carriers. In these cases the normal X chromosome is preferentially inactivated forming the Barr body [25] and the phenotype is normal. Nevertheless, the phenomenon of X inactivation controlled by the X-inactivation centre (XIC) located in Xq13 occurs randomly in one chromosome or the other. In the present case and if lyonisation occurs in the translocated X chromosome, there will be monosomy of autosomic's segment translocated in X chromosome happens on the der(X)t(3pter→3p14::Xp11.2→Xpter) containing Xq13, the der(3)t(Xpter →Xp11.2::3p14→3qter) will not be silenced. Consequently, there will be a double dosage of genes from the portion (Xpter→Xp11.2) and a monosomy of the portion (3pter→3p14).

It has been previously reported that balanced X-autosome translocated females can express an unpredictable phenotype that can vary from gonadal dygenesis and premature ovarian failure to multiple congenital anomalies and mental retardation [26].

In human the X inactivation starts on day 3 due to the silencing process of one X chromosome in female embryos. In the present PGD-SR application, embryo biopsy was performed on day 5 on trophectoderm cells. These cells will generate embryonic annexes and not be part of the embryo. No published data has shown that the study of gene silencing in trophectoderm cells would be representative of gene silencing in the balanced translocated female embryo itself. One of the few alternatives to predict the phenotype of female infants could be the study of X-chromosome inactivation/DNA methylation from foetus blood cells, in prenatal phase [27]. But once again, it remains to demonstrate that X-chromosome inactivation from foetus blood cells would be truly representative of overall gene expression in the infant, the girl and the woman [28].

Regarding the request of the couple to know the state of health of their embryos, we could not answer *in sensus strictus* on the early and late development of the balanced translocated female embryos at post-natal stage as précised during the pre-PGT-SR genetic counselling. At the post-PGT-SR genetic counselling, the couple decided not to consider them as the first choice for embryo transfer. This choice opens an ethical dilemma because, at the same time, embryos with a probably normal phenotype are eliminated from the transfer and possible birth. This would have happened to the male patients' mother at her time! The couple asked to have one 46,XY embryo transferred. They obtained the pregnancy and PGD-SR was confirmed by NIPT.

Among those embryos with abnormal karyotype, there was a 45,X0 embryo with a potential to implant but high probability to miscarriage. The couple rejected its transfer in uterus. There were 6 non-viable embryos left. One embryo with 45,XY,del [2], one embryo with 46,XY,del [8](qter →q22.1) and four embryos with trisomy 3p14→cen→3qter and monosomy Xp11.2→cen→Xqter. The last four embryos were the product of fertilization from a normal haploid 23,X oocyte and an unbalanced 23,der(X)t(X;3)(Xpter→Xp11.2::3p14→3qter) spermatozoon. These spermatozoa were the product of adjacent-2 chromosome segregation of the translocated chromosomes during the first meiotic division. This unbalanced segregation is reported as the most rare in reciprocal translocation [29]. Similar chromosomal abnormalities were observed in embryos from vitrified/warmed (embryos n. 18 and 22) and fresh oocytes (embryos n. 1, 4, 6 and 12). None of the analysed embryos showed mosaicism.

The present case is the first PGD-SR for gonosome-autosome translocation with male indication. Van Echten-Arends et al. previously reported a PGD-SR gonosome-autosome translocation with female indication that resulted in misdiagnosis for technical problem [30]. Comprehensive chromosomal screening by NGS is the method of choice for PGD of structural chromosomal defect.

This present PGD-SR application for reciprocal X-3 translocation in male patient arises the dilemma of balanced embryos excluded for transfer due to their phenotype unpredictability. The present case shows the limits of PGD-SR in helping the couple with a gonosome-autosome translocation to have a healthy child. Other PGD cases are well-known to be unsolvable at preimplantation stage due to the impossibility to predetermine the phenotype and development of the conceptus. Some of them are PGD for rare CFTR mutations and unknown combined phenotype, multifactory disease (heart defects, cancers, diabetes,...), diseases with variable expressivity (Marfan Syndrome, hereditary non-polyposis colorectal cancer,...) and diseases with late onset (ex: Alzheimer's disease). In these cases, proposing PGD implies the elimination of possible normal embryos for transfer.

### Abbreviations

aFP: alpha feto protein; AMH: Anti-Müllerian hormone; AZF: Azoospermic Factor; CFTR: Cystic Fibrosis Transmembrane conductance Regulator; FISH: Fluorescent In Situ hybridization; FSH: Follicle-Stimulating Hormone; HCG: Human chorionic gonadotropin; ICSI: Intra Cytoplasmic Sperm Injection; LH: Luteinizing Hormone; MAPD: Median Absolute Pair wise Difference; NGS: Next Generation Sequencing; NIPT: Non Invasive Prenatal Testing; OPU: Oocyte Pick-UP; PGD: Preimplantation Genetic Diagnosis; PGD-SR: Preimplantation Genetic Diagnosis for Structural chromosomal indication

### Acknowledgements

we thank Dr. Uccellatore for scientific contribution in manuscript revision.

### Funding

The present study was carried out with no fund.

### Authors' contribution

SC: wrote the manuscript, contributed to NGS analysis, is the director of In Vitro Laboratory and NGS laboratories. MS: contributed to manuscript writing, performed NGS analysis. DL: contributed to manuscript writing, performed caryotypes of the couple. CA: contributed to manuscript writing, performed freezing/thawing procedures. AG: contributed to manuscript writing, is the director of Infertility clinic, followed the couple as a clinician. All authors read and approved the final manuscript.

Each part of the protocol has been approved by the Institutional Review Board Unità di Medicina della Riproduzione - Centro HERA. The patients signed informed consent forms on all procedures prior application.

### Competing interests

None of the authors had competing (financial or personal) interest in the application and the publication of the present study. It was just for the pleasure and utility to share science.

### References

1. Scriven PN, Handyside AH, Ogilvie C. Chromosome translocations, segregation modes and strategies for preimplantation genetic diagnosis. Prenat Diagn. 1998;18:1437–49.
2. Handyside AH. 24-chromosome copy number analysis: a comparison of available technologies. Fertil.Steril. 2013;100(3):595–602.
3. Handyside AH, Harton GL, Mariani B, Thornhill AR, Affara N, Shaw MA, Griffin DK. Karyomapping: a universal method for genome wide analysis of genetic disease based on mapping crossovers between parental haplotypes. J Med Genet. 2010;47(10):651–8.

4. Johnson DS, Cinnioglu C, Ross R, Filby A, Gemelos G, Hill M, Ryan A, Smotrich D, Rabinowitz M, Murray MJ. Comprehensive analysis of karyotypic mosaicism between trophectoderm and inner cell mass. Mol Hum Reprod. 2010;16(12):944–9.
5. Wells D, Kaur K, Grifo J, Glassner M, Taylor JC, Fragouli E, Munne S. Clinical utilisation of a rapid low-pass whole genome sequencing technique for the diagnosis of aneuploidy in human embryos prior to implantation. J Med Genet. 2014;51(8):553–62.
6. Fiorentino F, Bono S, Biricik A, Nuccitelli A, Cotroneo E, Cottone G, Kokocinski F, Michel CE, Minasi MG, Greco E. Application of next-generation sequencing technology for comprehensive aneuploidy screening of blastocysts in clinical preimplantation genetic screening cycles. Hum. Reprod. 2014;29(12):2802–13.
7. Fan J, Wang L, Wang H, Ma M, Wang S, Liu Z, Xu G, Zhang J, Cram DS, Yao Y. Theclinical utility of next-generationsequencing for identifying chromosomedisease syndromes in human embryos. ReprodBioMed Online. 2015;31(1):62–70.
8. Ou J, Wang W, Feng T, Liao L, Meng Q, Zou Q, Ding J, Zheng A, Duan C, Li P, Liu Q, Lin C and Li H. Identification of small segmental translocations in patients with repeated implantation failure and recurrent miscarriage using next generationsequencing after in vitro fertilization/intracytoplasmic sperm injection.Mol Cytogenet 2015;8:105, 1-7
9. Van Dyke DL, Weiss L, Roberson JR, Babu VR. The frequency and mutation rate of balanced autosomal rearrangements in man estimated from prenatal genetic studies for advanced maternal age. Am J Hum Genet. 1983;35:301–8.
10. Gupta N, Goel H, Phadke SR. Unbalanced X; Autosome translocation. Indian J Pediatr. 2006;73:840–2.
11. De Rycke M, Goosens V, Kokkali G, Meijer-Hoogeveen M, Coonen E, Moutou C. ESHRE PGD collection XIV-XV: cycles from January 2011 to December 2012 with pregnancy follow-up to October 2013. Hum. Reprod. 2017; 32(10):1974-1994
12. De Rycke M, Belva F, Goossens V, Moutou C, SenGupta SB, Traeger-Synodinos J, Coonen E. ESHRE PGD Consortium data collection XIII: cycles from January to December 2010 with pregnancy follow-up to October 2011. Hum. Reprod. 2015;30(8):1763–89.
13. Lyon MF. Sex chromatin and gene action in the mammalian X-chromosome. Am J Hum Genet. 1962;14:135–48.
14. Schmidt M, De Sart D. Functional disomies of the X chromosome influence the cell selection and hence the X inactivation pattern in females with balanced X-autosome translocations: a review of 122 cases. Am J Med Genet. 1992;42:161–9.
15. Krausz C, Hoefsloot L, Simoni M, Tuttelmann F. EAA/EMQN best practice guidelines for molecular diagnosis of Y-chromosomal microdeletions; state-of-the-art 2013. Andrology. 2014;2:5–19.
16. Parlamento Italiano. Legge n.40: Norme in materia di procreazione medicalmente assistita. Gazzetta ufficiale. 2004; n.45 del 24 febbraio 2004
17. Chamayou S, Sicali M, Alecci C, Ragolia C, Liprino A, Nibali D, Storaci G, Cardea A, Guglielmino A. The accumulation of vitrified oocytes is a strategy to increase the number of euploid available blastocysts for transfer after preimplantation genetic testing. JAssist Reprod Genet. 2017;34(4):479–86.
18. Chamayou S, Bonaventura G, Alecci C, Tibullo D, Di Raimondo F, Guglielmino A, Barcellona ML. Consequences of metaphase II oocyte cryopreservation on mRNA content. Cryobiology. 2011;62:130–4.
19. Kuwayama M. Highly efficient vitrification for cryopreservation of human oocytes and embryos: the Cryotop method. Theriogenology. 2007;67:73–80.
20. Gravholt CH, Andersen NH, Conway GS, Dekkers OM, Geffner ME, Klein KO, Lin AE, Mauras N, Quigley CA, Rubin K, Sandberg DE, Sas TCJ, Silberbach M, Söderström-Anttila V, Stochholm K. van Alfen-van derVelden JA, Woelfe J, Backeljauw. Clinical practice guidelines for the care of girls and women with Turner syndrome: proceedings from the 2016 Cincinnati International Turner Syndrome Meeting. Eur J Endocrinol. 2017;177:G1–G70.
21. Hook EB. Chromosome abnormalities and spontaneous fetal death following amniocentesis: further data and associations with maternal age. Am J Hum Genet. 1983;35:110–6.
22. Hardy K, Hardy P, Jacobs PA, Lewallen K, Hassold TJ. Temporal changes in chromosome abnormalities in human spontaneous abortions: results of 40 years of analysis. AmJ Med Genet. 2016;170A:2671–80.
23. Perrin A, Douet-Guilbert N, Le Bris MJ, Keromnes G, Langlois ML, Barrière P, Amice J, Amice V, De Braekeleer M, Morel F. Segregation of chromosomes in sperm of a t(X;18)(q11;p11.1) carrier inherited from his mother: case report. Hum Reprod. 2008;23(1):117–30.
24. Ferfouri F, Bernicot I, Schneider A, Pharm D, Haquet E, Hédon B, Anahory T. Is the resulting phenotype of an embryo with balanced X-autosome translocation, obtained by means of preimplantation genetic diagnosis, linked to the X inactivation pattern? Fertil Steril. 2016;105(4):1035–46.
25. Barr ML, Bertram EG. A morphologcical distinction between neurons of the male and female, and the behavior of the nucleolar satellite during accelerated nucleoprotein synthesis. Nature. 1949;163:676.
26. McKinlay Gardner RL, Sutherland GR, Shaffer LG. Chromosome abnormalities and genetic counselling. Eds. Oxford monographs on medical genetics. 2012;N.61
27. Ma S, Ho Yuen B, Penaherrera M, Koehn D, Less L, Robinson W. ICSI and the transmission of X-autosomal translocation: a three-generation evaluation of X;20 translocation: Case report. Hum Reprod. 2003;18(7):1377–82.
28. Giorgietti L, Galupa R, Nora EP, Piolot T, Lam F, Dekker J, Tiana G, Heard E. Predictive polymer modeling reveals couples fluctuations in chromosome conformation and transcription. Cell. 2014;157(4):950–63.
29. Jalbert P, Sele B, Jalbert H. Reciprocal translocations: a way to predict the mode of imbalanced segregation by pachytene-diagram drawing. A study of 151 human translocations. Hum Genet. 1980;55:209–22.
30. Van Echten-Arend J, Coonen E, Reuters B, Suijkerbuijk RF, Dul EC, Land JA, van Ravenswaaij-Arts CMA. Preimplantation genetic diagnosis for X; autosome translocations: lessons from a case of misdiagnosis. Hum Reprod. 2013;(11):3141–5.

# Down syndrome associated childhood myeloid leukemia with yet unreported acquired chromosomal abnormalities and a new potential adverse marker: dup(1)(q25q44)

Faten Moassass[1], Abdulsamad Wafa[1], Thomas Liehr[2], Ayman Al-Ablog[1] and Walid AL Achkar[1*]

**Abstract**

**Background:** Children with constitutional trisomy 21, i.e. Down syndrome (DS, OMIM #190685) have a 10 to 20-fold increased risk for a hematopoietic malignancy. They may suffer from acute lymphoblastic leukemia or acute myeloid leukemia (AML). AML referred to as myeloid leukemia of Down syndrome (ML-DS) is observed especially after birth at an early gestational age and characterized by enhanced white blood cell count, failure of spontaneous remission, liver fibrosis or liver dysfunction, and is significantly associated with early death. There are only few studies yet focusing on the clonal cytogenetic changes during evolution of ML-DS.

**Case presentation:** In a 1.4-year-old boy with DS an immunophenotype consistent with AML-M1 according to French-American-British (FAB) classification was diagnoses. Cytogenetic and molecular cytogenetic analyses revealed, besides constitutional free trisomy 21, an unbalanced translocation as der(16)t(1;16)(q25.3;q24), plus a balanced translocation t(3;20)(q25;q13.1). A poor clinical outcome was observed here.

**Conclusions:** To the best of our knowledge, an ML-DS case associated with identical acquired chromosomal abnormalities was not previously reported. Our findings suggest that especially partial trisomy 1q25 to 1q44 may be indicative for a poor prognosis in ML-DS.

**Keywords:** Down syndrome, Trisomy 21, AML, Acquired chromosomal abnormalities (ACAs), Clone evolution, Cytogenetics, Fluorescence in situ hybridization (FISH), Prognostic factors

## Background

Children with trisomy 21 or Down syndrome (DS, OMIM #190685) have a compared to normal population 10- to 20-fold increased risk for developing an acute leukemia; lymphoblastic as well as myeloid leukemia were reported [1, 2]. Acute myeloid leukemia- (AML-) affected children develop a unique type of malignancy, referred to as myeloid leukemia of Down Syndrome (ML-DS), which is recognized as a separate entity in the actual World Health Organization (WHO) classification of leukemia [3]. ML-DS is especially found in children born at early gestational age and is characterized by enhanced white blood cell (WBC) count, failure of spontaneous remission, as well as liver fibrosis or liver dysfunction. Also ML-DS is significantly associated with poor outcome and early death [4–6]. ML-DS cases have, according to French-American-British (FAB) classification, in the majority of the cases M7 morphology, thus they are also called acute megakaryoblastic leukemia (AMKL) cases. As most ML-DS cases are young at diagnosis, the disease occurs almost exclusively in children < 5 years old. A beneficial clinical outcome may occur if treated with reduced intensity chemotherapy protocols without stem cell transplantation [7–9].

* Correspondence: ascientific@aec.org.sy
[1]Molecular Biology and Biotechnology Department, Human Genetics Division, Chromosomes Laboratory, Atomic Energy Commission of Syria, P.O. Box 6091, Damascus, Syria
Full list of author information is available at the end of the article

Even though data on cytogenetics of ML-DS are scarce, it is known that the karyotypic patterns of this entity are different from those observed in AML of children without DS, e.g. translocations t(8;21), t(15;17), t(9;11), inversion inv.(16), as well as AMKL associated translocations t(1;22) and t(1;3) are rather typical for ML-DS [10–12]. The most frequent imbalances in ML-DS are duplications in 1q (16%), or deletions in 7p (10%) and/or 16 (7.4%) [10]. However, the potential clinical impact of these cytogenetic abnormalities is not known, yet. Therefore, the importance of studying and reporting cytogenetic alterations for better classification and risk stratification of ML-DS and non-DS-AML is well recognized [5, 10–14]. There is especially controversial data on the impact of acquired chromosomal abnormalities (ACAs) in ML-DS (see [4, 14] versus [5, 11]).

Here, we describe a typical ML-DS case with two yet unreported ACAs involving chromosomes 1 and 16 as well as 3 and 20, obviously associated with a poor prognosis.

## Case presentation

A 1.4-year-old boy with DS without familial medical history of malignancy presented with 10 days consisting flu and fever, being pallor and unconscious. This patient was the fifth child of healthy, unrelated parents. The mother and the father were at birth of the child, 42 and 54 years old, respectively. Also there was no infection in the pregnant woman during the pregnancy.

At diagnosis the small boy was found to have septicemia, acidosis, dehydration, and lung crackles. Physical examination and ultrasound showed hepatomegaly. His hematological parameters revealed low hemoglobin level (Hgb) (4 g/dl), low platelet count ($47 \times 10^9$/l), and elevated WBC count. Biochemistry determined urea of 118 mg/dl (normal value up to 40 mg/dl) but normal creatinine levels (0.1 mg/dl). Thus, he was diagnosed as ML-DS patient. The patient received blood transfusion repeatedly, stayed in the hospital for 1 week, and then was transferred to hematological malignancy hospital to confirm diagnosis and treatment. Peripheral blood cell analyses revealed a WBC count of $59.08 \times 10^9$/l (18.8% neutrophils, 47.2% lymphocytes, 0.1% eosinophiles, 29.6% monocytes and 4.3% basophiles), red blood cells count of $4.93 \times 10^6/mm^3$, Hgb level of 11.2 g/dl, and platelet count of $24 \times 10^9$/l. Blasts in bone marrow aspiration were present in 32% of analyzed cells. The patient had not received any chemotherapy treatment and died unfortunately died 9 days after diagnosis from the disease due to respiratory arrest, and before cytogenetic and flow-cytometric results were available. His mother agreed with scientific evaluation of the case and the study was approved by the ethical committee of the Atomic Energy Commission, Damascus, Syria.

GTG-banding on peripheral blood sample revealed a karyotype of 47,XY,t(1;16)(?;?),t(3;20)(?;?),+21c[17]/47,XY,+21c[3] (Fig. 1). Further studies were performed by molecular cytogenetics (Fig. 2). Dual-color-FISH (D-FISH) using specific WCP probes for chromosomes #1, #3, #16, and #20 confirmed that no other chromosomes were involved besides #1 and #16 in an imbalanced plus #3 and #20 in a balanced translocation (data not shown). aMCB, using probes for chromosomes #1, #3, #16, and #20 (Fig. 2) revealed the following final karyotype:

47,XY,der(16)t(1;16)(q25.3;q24),t(3;20)(q25;q13.1), +21c[17]/47,XY,+21c[3]

Immunophenotyping of peripheral blood specimen characterized this case as AML-M1 according to FAB classification. The blast cell population (32% of leukocytes) was positive for CD45$^{dim}$, CD7, CD13dim, CD33, HLA-DR, CD38, and CD117 and negative for CD64, CD34, CD10, CD15, CD11b and CD14.

## Discussion and conclusions

The natural history of leukemia in children with DS suggests that trisomy 21 directly contributes to the malignant transformation of hematopoietic cells. Approximately 15% of pediatric AML cases occur in DS children. Thus, ML-DS contribute more than 90% of the most common FAB subtype of DS AML patients and at the same time the majority of cases are diagnosed under the age of 4 years [15–17]. Zipursky et al. [9] have estimated that DS children have a 500-fold increased risk of developing ML-DS compared with non-DS children, highlighting the unique relationship between trisomy 21, leukemogenesis, and a specific leukemia phenotype. Other AML FAB subtypes have also been described in ML-DS including M0, M1/M2, and M6, but less frequently [15–17].

The cytogenetic profiles of ML-DS cases differ significantly from non-DS patients with AML [16, 18, 19]. ML-DS children show more frequently acquired trisomies of chromsomes 8, 11, and 19, dup(1p), del(6q), del(7p), dup(7q), and del(16q) [10]. Typically, the favorable translocations associated with non-DS AML [e.g., t(8;21); t(15;17); inv(16), 11q23 rearrangements] are rarely seen in ML-DS patients [10]. For ML-DS children older than 4 years cytogenetic features, molecular biology findings and response to therapy significantly diverge from younger patients, and are similar to the ones found in non-DS patients with AML [17]. However, recently de Souza et al. [20] reported a new ML-DS case associated with new acquired ACAs and they suggested those were clearly associated with the disease-progress and associated with an adverse risk. The case presented here share some feature with that of de Souza et al. [20]

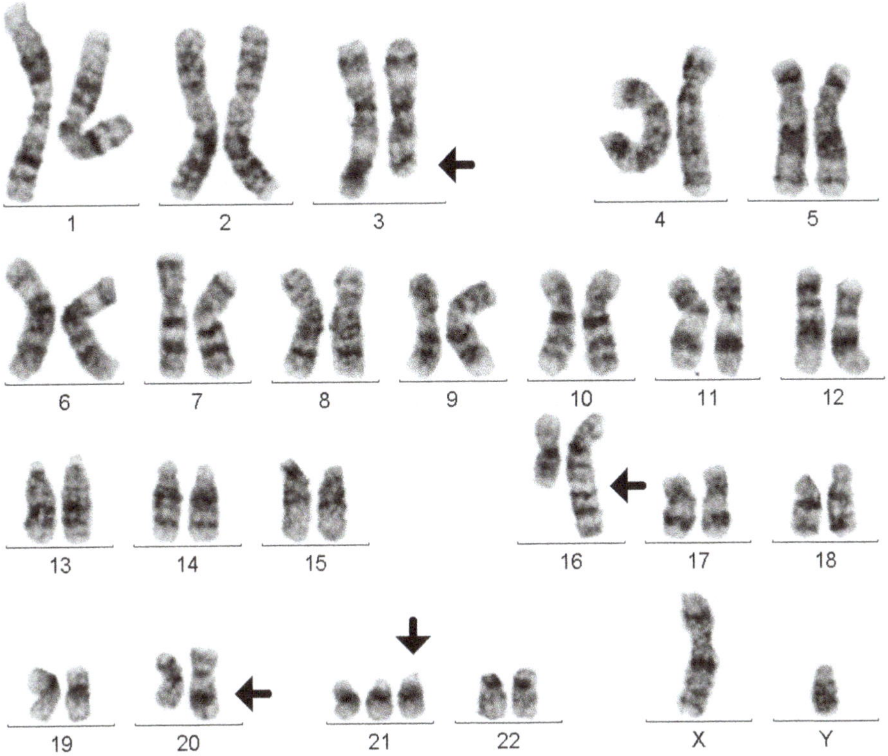


**Fig. 1** GTG-banding revealed an unbalanced translocation t(1;16)(q25.3;q24) and balanced translocation t(3;20)(q25;q13.1) in 17/20 metaphases. All derivative chromosomes are marked and highlighted by arrow heads

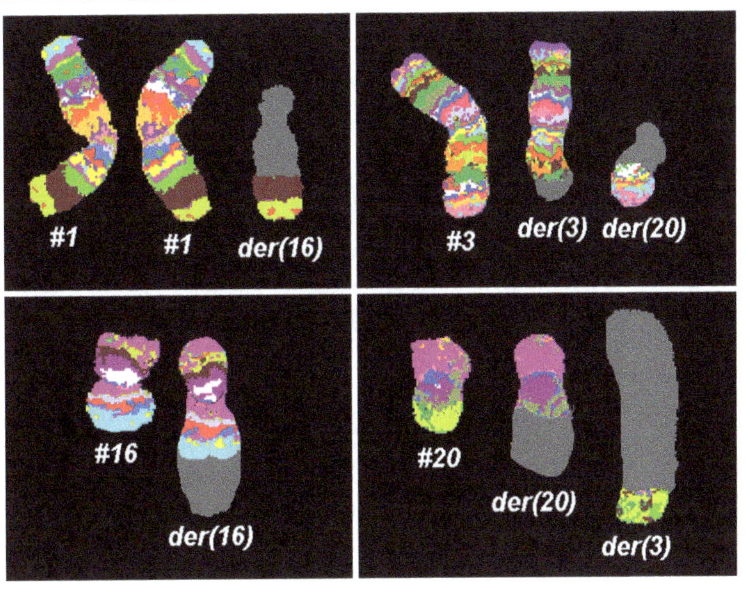


**Fig. 2** Karyotype and chromosomal aberrations were confirmed using molecular cytogenetic approaches. aMCB results are shown. The normal chromosomes (#) are depicted on the left side of each image and the derivative of the other chromosomes on the right side of normal chromosomes. The unstained regions when suing chromosome-specific aMCB-probesets on the derivative chromosomes are shown in gray. Abbreviations: # = chromosome; der = derivative chromosome

such as involvement of chromosomes 1 and 3 was and a poor outcome. Furthermore, chromosomal bands such as 1q25, 3q25, 16q24, and 20q13 are involved in chromosomal rearrangements frequently [21]. Moreover, translocations or inversions involving 3q21 and 3q26 are associated with a high-risk in AML, and these patients usually present with a poor prognosis [17]. However, in our case observed specific translocations der(16)t(1;16)(q25.3;q24) and t(3;20)(q25;q13.1) has never been reported as ACAs in ML-DS or AML cases to date [21].

Several studies have suggested that mutations in the hematopoietic zinc-finger transcription factor gene *GATA-1* (a transcription factor that regulates the differentiation of megakaryocyte and erythrocyte precursors), could be an initiating event in DS leukemogenesis [22, 23]. Besides the involvement of *GATA-1* and trisomy 21 is strongly associated with leukemogenesis [20]. Cytogenetic analyses revealed other acquired recurrent abnormalities associated with gain of chromosome 21. Forestier et al. [10] analyzed 189 ML-DS cases and they confirmed a distinct entity, originating from other genetic pathways than non-DS patients with AML.

Partial trisomy of chromosome 1q is commonly observed in infants with ML-DS and AMKL, which is most often resulting from an unbalanced translocation, like in the present case, or a simple duplication [24]. The long arm of chromosome 1 accommodates genes involved in the control of normal myeloid cell kinetics. Several interesting genes map in this region 1q, including *IL6RA* and *BCL2*-related are located at 1q21, *MNDA* (1q22), *CENPR* (1q32-q41), and *TP53BP2* (1q42.1~q42.2) [25].

For the chromosome 16 related imbalance two genes might specifically be considered: (i) Interferon regulatory factor 8 (IRF8) also known as interferon consensus sequence-binding protein located at 16q24.1, codes for a transcription factor, which plays a critical role in the regulation of lineage commitment and myeloid cell maturation including the checkpoint for a common myeloid progenitor to differentiate into a monocyte precursor cell [26]. (ii) The human *FOXF1* gene located at 16q24.1, previously denominated Forkhead Related ACtivator-1, encodes a homologue of the mouse forkhead box-F1 (*Foxf1*) transcription factor [27]. Gene knockout studies have shown that the function of mouse *Foxf1* is indispensable for organ morphogenesis, including the lung, liver, gallbladder, esophagus, and trachea [28]. Despite the largely unknown role of *FOXF1* in cancer, several lines of evidence have linked human *FOXF1* function to tumorigenesis [29]. Recently, it was suggested that *FOXF1* may play a dual role in tumorigenesis as an oncogene or a tumor suppressor gene depending on tissue cell types and disease stages [30].

As shortly discussed above, age has been recognized as a prognostic factor in ML-DS [31]. In fact, it has been proposed that DS children who present over 4 years of age are suffering from 'normal sporadic AML' occurring in a child with DS, rather than from 'true' ML-DS [32]. In addition, ML-DS patients with a history of transient myeloproliferative disease have a significantly better outcome than children with ML-DS without documented transient myeloproliferative disease [5]. Blink et al. [11] demonstrated that age $\geq 3$ years and high WBC count ($> 20 \times 10^9$) are correlated with poor outcome (event-free survival) in ML-DS. These variables are also known from non-DS pediatric AML studies, in which older age and high WBC predict for poor outcome [33].

According to the literature the here observed partial monosomy 16q24 to 16qter has no clear impact on prognosis, and the meaning of the balanced translocation t(3;20)(q25;q13.1) needs to be delineated by further case studies. However, the present case of ML-DS may have an adverse outcome due to the partial trisomy 1q25.3 to 1qter, as also supported at least by one further similar case [20] and the known adverse effects of distal partial trisomy 1q in other malignancies [32].

## Material and methods

### Cytogenetics and molecular cytogenetics

Chromosomal analysis on peripheral blood sample using GTG-banding according to standard procedures [34] was performed prior blood transfusions. A minimum of 20 metaphase cells was analyzed. The karyotype was described according to the International System for Human Cytogenetic Nomenclature (ISCN 2016) [35].

Fluorescence in situ hybridization (FISH) using whole chromosome painting (WCP) probes for chromosomes 1, 3, 16, and 20 (MetaSystems, Altlussheim, Germany) was done according to manufacturer's instructions [34]. Array-proven multicolor banding (aMCB) probes sets based on microdissection derived region-specific libraries for chromosomes 1, 3, 16, and 20 were hybridized and evaluated as previously reported [36]. A minimum of 10 metaphase spreads were analyzed, each, using a fluorescence microscope (AxioImager.Z1 mot, Carl Zeiss Ltd., Hertfordshire, UK) equipped with appropriate filter sets to discriminate between a maximum of five fluorochromes plus the counterstain DAPI (4′,6-diamino-2-phenylindole). Image capture and processing were performed using an ISIS imaging system (MetaSystems).

### Flow cytometric immunophenotype

Immunophenotyping was performed using a general panel of fluorescent antibodies against the following antigens typical for different cell lineages and cell types: CD1a, CD2, CD3, CD4, CD5, CD8, CD10, CD11b,

CD11c, CD13, CD14, CD15, CD16, CD19, CD20, CD22, CD23, CD32, CD33, CD34, CD38, CD41a, CD45, CD56, CD57, CD64, CD103, CD117, CD123, CD138, CD209, CD235a and CD243; in addition antibodies to Kappa and Lambda light Chains, IgD, sIgM, and HLADr were tested. All antibodies were purchased from BD Biosciences. Samples were analyzed on a BD FACSCalibur™ flow cytometer. Autofluorescence, viability, and isotype controls were included. Flow cytometric data acquisition and analysis were conducted by BD Cellquest™ Pro software.

### Abbreviations

ACAs: Additional cytogenetic abnormalities; aMCB: Array-proven high-resolution multicolor banding; AMKL: Acute megakaryoblastic leukemia; AML: Acute myeloid leukemia; DAPI: 4',6- diamino-2-phenylindole; D-FISH: Dual-color-fluorescence in situ hybridization; DS: Down syndrome; FAB: French–American–British classification; FISH: Fluorescence in situ hybridization; *Foxf1*: Mouse forkhead box-F1 transcription factor; Hgb: Hemoglobin level; *IRF8*: Interferon regulatory factor 8 gene; ISCN 2016: International System for Human Cytogenetic Nomenclature; ML-DS: Myeloid leukemia of Down syndrome; WBC: White blood cell count; WCP: Whole chromosome paint probes; WHO: World Health Organization classification

### Acknowledgements

We thank Prof. I. Othman, the Director General of Atomic Energy Commission of SYRIA (AECS) and Dr. N. Mirali, Head of Molecular Biology and Biotechnology Department for their support.

### Funding

n.a.

### Authors' contributions

FM, AW, AA and WA performed banding cytogenetics and provided the clinical data; FM, AW and TL performed the molecular cytogenetic analyses. AW and TL drafted the paper and all authors worked on the final version of the paper. All authors read and approved the final manuscript.

### Competing interests

The authors declare that they have no competing interests.

### Author details

[1]Molecular Biology and Biotechnology Department, Human Genetics Division, Chromosomes Laboratory, Atomic Energy Commission of Syria, P.O. Box 6091, Damascus, Syria. [2]Jena University Hospital, Institute of Human Genetics, Am Klinikum 1, 07747 Jena, Germany.

### References

1. Rabin KR, Whitlock JA. Malignancy in children with trisomy 21. Oncologist. 2009;14:164–73.
2. Zwaan MC, Reinhardt D, Hitzler J, Vyas P. Acute leukemias in children with Down syndrome. Pediatr Clin N Am. 2008;55:53–70.
3. Hasle H, Niemeyer CM, Chessells JM, Baumann I, Bennett JM, Kerndrup G, Head DR. A pediatric approach to the WHO classification of myelodysplastic and myeloproliferative diseases. Leukemia. 2003;17:277–82.
4. Massey GV, Zipursky A, Chang MN, Doyle JJ, Nasim S, Taub JW, Ravindranath Y, Dahl G, Weinstein HJ, Children's Oncology Group (COG). A prospectivestudy of the natural history of transientleukemia (TL) in neonates with Down syndrome (DS): Children's Oncology Group (COG) study POG-9481. Blood. 2006;107:4606–13.
5. Klusmann JH, Creutzig U, Zimmermann M, Dworzak M, Jorch N, Langebrake C, Pekrun A, Macakova-Reinhardt K, Reinhardt D. Treatment and prognostic impact of transient leukemiain neonates with Down syndrome. Blood. 2008;111:2991–8.
6. Muramatsu H, Kato K, Watanabe N, Matsumoto K, Nakamura T, Horikoshi Y, Mimaya J, Suzuki C, Hayakawa M, Kojima S. Riskfactors for early death in neonates with Down syndrome and transient leukaemia. Br J Haematol. 2008;142:610–5.
7. Creutzig U, Reinhardt D, Diekamp S, Dworzak M, Stary J, Zimmermann M. AML patients with Down syndrome have a high cure rate with AML-BFM therapy with reduced dose intensity. Leukemia. 2005;19:1355–60.
8. Rao A, Hills RK, Stiller C, Gibson BE, de Graaf SS, Hann IM, O'Marcaigh A, Wheatley K, Webb DK. Treatment for myeloid leukaemia of Down syndrome: population-based experience in the UK and results from the Medical Research Council AML 10 and AML 12 trials. Br J Haematol. 2006;132:576–83.
9. Zipursky A, Thorner P, De Harven E, Christensen H, Doyle J. Myelodysplasia and acute megakaryoblastic leukemia in Down's syndrome. Leuk Res. 1994; 18:163–71.
10. Forestier E, Izraeli S, Beverloo B, Haas O, Pession A, Michalova K, Stark B, Harrison CJ, Teigler-Schlegel A, Johansson B. Cytogenetic features of acute lymphoblastic and myeloid leukemias in pediatric patients with Down syndrome: an iBFM-SG study. Blood. 2008;111:1575–83.
11. Blink M, Zimmermann M, von Neuhoff C, Reinhardt D, de Haas V, Hasle H, O'Brien MM, Stark B, Tandonnet J, Pession A, Tousovska K, Cheuk DK, Kudo K, Taga T, Rubnitz JE, Haltrich I, Balwierz W, Pieters R, Johansson B, van den Heuvel-Eibrink MM, Zwaan CM. Normal karyotype is a poor prognostic factor in myeloid leukemia of Down syndrome: a retrospective, international study. Haematologica. 2014;99:299–307.
12. Bhatnagar N, Nizery L, Tunstall O, Vyas P, Roberts I. Transient abnormal myelopoiesis and AML in Down syndrome: an update. Curr Hematol Malig Rep. 2016;11:333–41.
13. Arber DA, Orazi A, Hasserjian R, Thiele J, Borowitz MJ, Le Beau MM, Bloomfield CD, Cazzola M, Vardiman JW. The 2016 revision to the World Health Organization classification of myeloid neoplasms and acute leukemia. Blood. 2016;127:2391–405.
14. Picos Cárdenas VJ, Meza Espinoza JP, Garibaldi Covarrubias RF, Barajas Torres RL, González García JR. Transient myeloproliferative disorder progression and acquired chromosomal abnormalites in children with Down syndrome. Pediatr Blood Cancer. 2012;59:962–3.
15. Ravindranath Y, Yeager AM, Chang MN, Steuber CP, Krischer J, Graham-Pole J, Carroll A, Inoue S, Camitta B, Weinstein HJ. Autologous bone marrow transplantation versus intensive consolidation chemotherapy for acute myeloid leukemia in childhood. Pediatric Oncology Group. N Engl J Med. 1996;334:1428–34.
16. Lange BJ, Kobrinsky N, Barnard DR, Arthur DC, Buckley JD, Howells WB, Gold S, Sanders J, Neudorf S, Smith FO, Woods WG. Distinctive demography, biology, and outcome of acute myeloid leukemia and myelodysplastic syndrome in children with Down syndrome: children's Cancer Group Studies 2861 and 2891. Blood. 1998;91:608–15.
17. Gamis AS, Woods WG, Alonzo TA, Buxton A, Lange B, Barnard DR, Gold S, Smith FO. Increased age at diagnosis has a significantly negative effect on outcome in children with Down syndrome and acute myeloid leukemia: a report from the Children's Cancer Group Study 2891. J Clin Oncol. 2003;21:3415–22.
18. Zeller B, Gustafsson G, Forestier E, Abrahamsson J, Clausen N, Heldrup J, Hovi L, Jonmundsson G, Lie SO, Glomstein A, Hasle H, Nordic Society of Paediatric Haematology and Oncology (NOPHO). Acute leukaemia in children with Down syndrome: a population-based Nordic study. Br J Haematol. 2005;128:797–804.
19. Creutzig U, Ritter J, Vormoor J, Ludwig WD, Niemeyer C, Reinisch I, Stollmann-Gibbels B, Zimmermann M, Harbott J. Myelodysplasia and acute myelogenous leukemia in Down's syndrome. A report of 40 children of the AML-BFM Study Group. Leukemia. 1996;10:1677–86.
20. de Souza DC, de Figueiredo AF, Ney Garcia DR, da Costa ES, Othman MAK, Liehr T, Abdelhay E, Silva MLM, de Souza Fernandez T. A unique set of complex chromosomal abnormalities in an infant with myeloid leukemia associated with Down syndrome. Mol Cytogenet. 2017;10:35.
21. Mitelman F, Johansson B, Mertens F, editors: Mitelman database of chromosome aberrations and gene fusions in cancer (2017). http://cgap.nci.nih.gov/Chromosomes/Mitelman. Accessed 18 Sept 2017.
22. Gurbuxani S, Vyas P, Crispino JD. Recent insights into the mechanisms of myeloid leukemogenesis in Down syndrome. Blood. 2004;103:399–406.
23. Hitzler JK, Zipursky A. Origins of leukaemia in children with Down syndrome. Nat Rev Cancer. 2005;5:11–20.

24. Silva ML, Pombo-de-Oliveira MS, Raimondi SC, Mkrtchyan H, Abdelhay E, de Figueiredo AF, de Souza MT, Garcia DR, de Ventura EM, de Sousa AM, Liehr T. Unbalanced chromosome 1 abnormalities leadingto partial trisomy 1q in four infants with Downsyndrome and acute megakaryocytic leukemia. Mol Cytogenet. 2009;2:7.
25. Cho HS, Kim M, Hyun MS. Triplication of 1q in a patient with myelodysplastic syndrome. Korean J Hematol. 2006;41:56–60.
26. Weisz A, Marx P, Sharf R, Appella E, Driggers PH, Ozato K, Levi BZ. Human interferon consensus sequence binding protein is a negative regulator of enhancer elements common to interferon-inducible genes. J Biol Chem. 1992;267:25589–96.
27. Hellqvist M, Mahlapuu M, Samuelsson L, Enerback S, Carlsson P. Differential activation of lung-specific genes by two forkhead proteins, FREAC-1 and FREAC-2. J Biol Chem. 1996;271:4482–90.
28. Kalinichenko W, Zhou Y, Bhattacharyya D, Kim W, Shin B, Bambal K, Costa RH. Haploinsufficiency of the mouse Forkhead Box f1 gene causes defects in gall bladder development. J Biol Chem. 2002;277:12369–74.
29. Lo PK, Lee JS, Liang X, Han L, Mori T, Fackler MJ, Sadik H, Argani P, Pandita TK, Sukumar S. Epigenetic inactivation of the potential tumor suppressor gene FOXF1 in breast cancer. Cancer Res. 2010;70:6047–58.
30. Lo PK, Lee JS, Chen H, Reisman D, Berger FG, Sukumar S. Cytoplasmic mislocalization of overexpressed FOXF1 is associated with the malignancy and metastasis of colorectal adenocarcinomas. Exp Mol Pathol. 2013;94:262–9.
31. Sorrell AD, Alonzo TA, Hilden JM, Gerbing RB, Loew TW, Hathaway L, Barnard D, Taub JW, Ravindranath Y, Smith FO, Arceci RJ, Woods WG, Gamis AS. Favorable survival maintained in children who have myeloid leukemia associated with Down syndrome using reduced-dose chemotherapy on Children's Oncology Group trial A2971: a report from the Children's Oncology Group. Cancer. 2012;118:4806–14.
32. Hasle H, Abrahamsson J, Arola M, Karow A, O'Marcaigh A, Reinhardt D, Webb DK, van Wering E, Zeller B, Zwaan CM, Vyas P. Myeloid leukemia in children 4 years or older with Down syndrome often lacks GATA1 mutation and cytogenetics and risk of relapse are more akin to sporadic AML. Leukemia. 2008;22:1428–30.
33. Wechsler J, Greene M, McDevitt MA, Anastasi J, Karp JE, Le Beau MM, Crispino JD. Acquired mutations in GATA1 in the megakaryoblastic leukemia of Down syndrome. Nat Genet. 2002;32:148–52.
34. AL-achkar W, Wafa A, Nweder MS. A complex translocation t(5;9;22) in Philadelphia cells involving the short arm of chromosome 5 in a case of chronic myelogenous leukemia. J Exp Clin Cancer Res. 2007;26:411–5.
35. McGowan-Joran J, Simons A, Schmid MS. ISCN 2016: an international system of human cytogenomic nomenclature. Unionville: S. Karger Publications, Inc; 2016.
36. Liehr T, Heller A, Starke H, Rubtsov N, Trifonov V, Mrasek K, Weise A, Kuechler A, Claussen U. Microdissection based high resolution multicolor banding for all 24 human chromosomes. Int J Mol Med. 2002;9:335–9.

# X-derived marker chromosome in patient with mosaic Turner syndrome and Dandy-Walker syndrome

Alena S. Telepova[1,2], Svetlana A. Romanenko[1,2], Natalya A. Lemskaya[1], Yulia V. Maksimova[3,4], Asia R. Shorina[4] and Dmitry V. Yudkin[1,2*]

**Abstract**

**Background:** Small supernumerary marker chromosomes can be derived from autosomes and sex chromosomes and can accompany chromosome pathologies, such as Turner syndrome.

**Case presentation:** Here, we present a case report of a patient with mosaic Turner syndrome and Dandy-Walker syndrome carrying a marker chromosome. We showed the presence of the marker chromosome in 33.8% of blood cells. FISH of the probe derived from the marker chromosome by microdissection revealed that it originated from the centromeric region of chromosome X. Additionally, we showed no telomeric sequences and no XIST sequence in the marker chromosome. This is the first report of these two syndromes accompanied by the presence of a marker chromosome.

**Conclusion:** Marker chromosome was X-derived and originated from centromeric region. Patient has mild symptoms but there is no XIST gene in marker chromosome.

**Keywords:** Marker chromosome, Turner syndrome, Dandy-Walker syndrome, X-chromosome

## Background

Small supernumerary marker chromosomes (sSMC) are structurally abnormal chromosomes. The size of sSMC is smaller than chromosome 20 on metaphase spread [1]. sSMC can be derived from autosomes and sex chromosomes. Occasionally, sSMC can accompany chromosome pathologies, such as Turner syndrome [2]. Turner syndrome is a genetic disorder caused by karyotype 45,X with or without mosaicism [3]. Described by Henry Turner in 1938, it consists of a constellation of phenotypic findings: short stature, sexual infantilism, webbed neck, and cubitus valgus. Usually, sSMC in Turner syndrome ($sSMC^T$) are derived from sex chromosomes [4]. Most $sSMC^T$(X) form ring-chromosomes, but rare $sSMC^T$(Y) are inverted duplicated/isodicentric ones. The frequency of $sSMC^T$ is 1:100,000 in a population [3]. The phenotypic variability of these mosaics is largely dependent on the size of the marker chromosome and the presence of a functioning XIST gene in the X-inactivation center (Xq13). If the marker chromosome undergoes inactivation, patients with $sSMC^T$ have a mild Turner variant phenotype [5].

In this case report we described an exceptional patient with both Turner and Dandy-Walker syndromes carrying a $sSMC^T$ derived from the centromere region of the X chromosome. The combination of a Dandy-Walker syndrome and $sSMC^T$ was described for the first time.

## Materials and methods

### Clinical study

The clinical study of the patient included consultations with medical specialists such as clinical psychologists, neurologists, speech therapists and MRI research.

* Correspondence: dim@mcb.nsc.ru
[1]Institute of Molecular and Cellular Biology SB RAS, Lavrentieva ave. 8/2, Novosibirsk 630090, Russia
[2]Novosibirsk State University, Novosibirsk 630090, Russia
Full list of author information is available at the end of the article

### Metaphase preparation and GTG banding

Metaphase chromosome preparations were obtained from lymphocyte cultures according to standard procedures [6]. GTG banding was carried out as described previously [7]. Metaphase spreads were analyzed using an Olympus BX 53 microscope and the "VideoTest Karyo 3.1" (Zenit, Russia) software.

### Microdissection and FISH

Marker chromosomes were dissected as described earlier [8] using an Olympus IX 51 microscope and the micromanipulator of Eppendorf Transferman NK2. DNA of microdissected chromosomes was amplified by GenomePlex Complete Whole Genome Amplification (WGA) Kit (Sigma-Aldrich, USA). Probes were labeled with digoxigenin. Every library was obtained from one copy of marker chromosome.

FISH of microdissected probes, sorted human chromosome probes and telomeric probes was carried out as described [8]. Slides were analyzed using an Olympus BX 53 fluorescence microscope and the "VideoTest FISH 2.0" (Zenit, Russia) software.

### PCR screening

PCR screening of painting probes was carried out with primers: XISTF 5'AGTGTACCTACCGCTTTGGC3' and XISTR 5'TCCTCTGCCTGACCTGCTAT3' (ref. seq. NG_016172.1) for XIST, CHXF 5'TTCTCTGTCCTGCG ACCTTG3' and CHXR 5'GCTCAAAAGACTGGGCA CCT3' (ref. seq. NC_000023.11) for centromeric region of chromosome X and CH3F 5'GTGACTTCCCAACCTGGA TTCT3' and CH3R 5'GATCATCCCAAAGGACATCA ACT3' (ref. seq. NG_047144.1) for CNTN6 gene on chromosome 3. Painting probes of microdissection-derived marker chromosomes and sorted chromosomes X and 3 were used as a template.

## Case presentation

### Clinical study

The patient is a 13-year-old female with growth retardation (nanism, 137 cm), a short neck, low hair growth on the neck, widely spaced nipples, a shield chest, secondary sexual characteristics deficiency, and the presence of episodic hyperglycemia. Her body mass index is 25. The parents of the patient have normal growth (mother – 175 cm, father – 180 cm). MRI study revealed Dandy-Walker syndrome and hydrocephaly. Hypoplasia of segment A1 of the anterior cerebral artery and segment P1 of the posterior cerebral artery were revealed.

### Karyotypic study

The patient has karyotype 45,X/46,X,+mar. The marker chromosome was found in 33.8% of the metaphase spreads ($N$ = 80). It was small and comparable in size with chromosome 20. Although DAPI staining showed that this chromosome looks such as a small acrocentric chromosome, localization of the telomeric probe revealed no signals on it (Fig. 1). However, as shown previously, the absence of telomeres cannot indicate unambiguously that the chromosome is a ring [9]. FISH of the set of human whole chromosomes-specific probes showed the localization of chromosome X painting probe on the whole length of the marker chromosome (Fig. 2a). To visualize the boundaries of the derivate formation, the marker chromosome was microdissected, and the derived probe was localized on chromosomes of the patient and a healthy control. In total, we obtained 4 libraries. In the patient cells each probe painted the marker chromosome and the centromeric region of chromosome X (Fig. 2b). In the healthy control, probes painted the centromeric region of chromosome X only (Fig. 2c, d). This localization showed the marker chromosome was derived from region Xp11.23-q13.2. (Fig. 2c – box).

### PCR screening for XIST gene

To test whether XIST gene presents in marker chromosome or not we made PCR screening of two separate copies of microdissection-derived probes of the marker chromosome (mar1 and mar2) and painting probes of chromosomes X and 3 as controls (see Materials and Methods). Both analyzed marker chromosomes do not contain XIST sequences whereas X centromeric sequences are presented in marker chromosomes painting probes (Fig. 3).

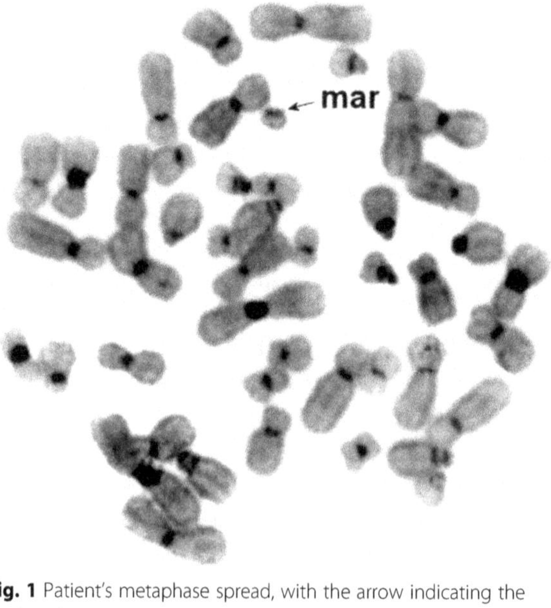


**Fig. 1** Patient's metaphase spread, with the arrow indicating the marker chromosome

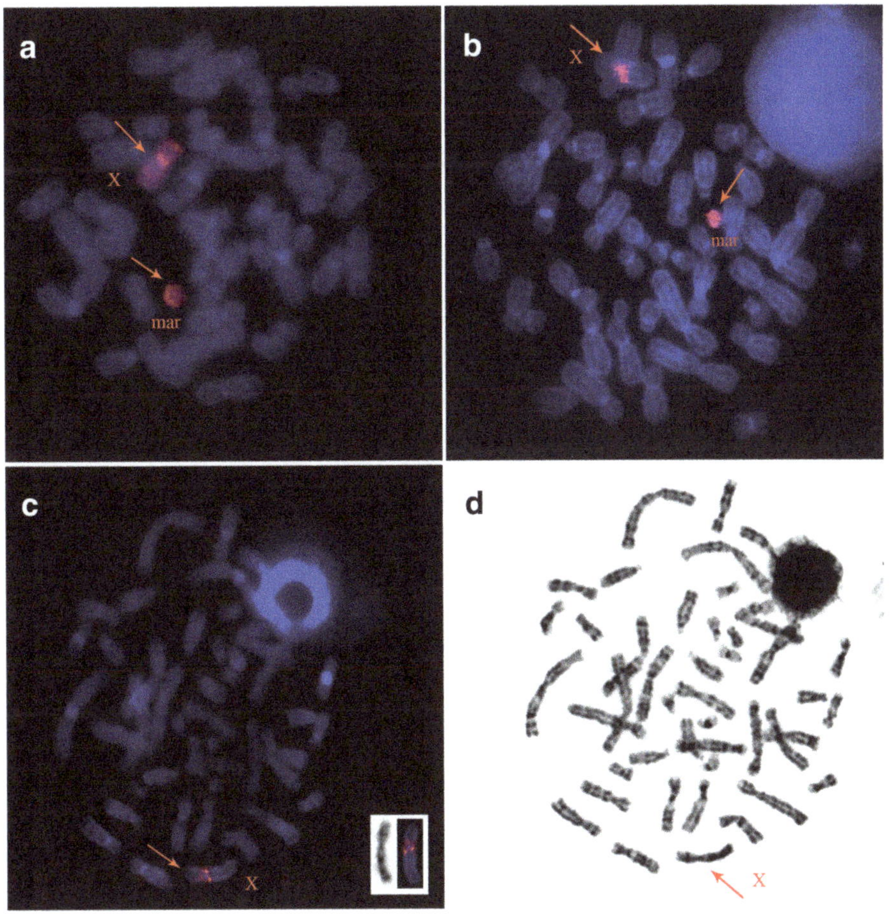


**Fig. 2** Examples of fluorescent in situ hybridization: **a** Localization of human chromosome X painting probe (red) on chromosomes of the patient. **b** Localization of microdissected probe of marker chromosome on chromosomes of the patient. **c** Localization of microdissected probe of marker chromosome on chromosomes of the healthy control after G-banding (**d**). Box on (**c**) is localization of signal on G-banded chromosome X. Arrows indicate signal localization

## Discussion

In 2014, Mazzaschi R. et al. described a female patient with sSMC[T] derived from the centromere region of the chromosome X. In that case, the proband had poor growth, global developmental delay, type I diabetes, clonic seizures, cardiomyopathy, hepatic adenomas, and skeletal dysplasia. Moreover, she had delayed secondary sexual characteristic development and ovarian failure and growth hormone deficiency [5]. The clinical symptoms of the patient in our research differed from those described above. The manifestations of Turner's syndrome in our case were milder; the patient had not expressed cognitive failure, clonic seizures or damage to other organs. However, she had Dandy-Walker syndrome. Dandy-Walker syndrome is defined by hypoplasia of the cerebellar vermis and dilation of the fourth ventricle [10]. Patients with this syndrome often have motor deficits such as delayed motor development, hypotonia and ataxia; further, approximately half have mental retardation and some have hydrocephalus [11]. Based on the results of an MRI study of the brain, hydrocephalus was diagnosed in this case as well.

A female patient with symptoms similar to the case was described earlier. The ten-year-old girl had typical manifestations of Turner's syndrome – short stature, webbing of neck, cubitus valgus, shield chest, congenital dislocation of hip, renal anomalies, clinodactyly, unilateral simian crease on right palm, acyanotic congenital heart disease and small patent ductus arteriosus. However, intellectual insufficiency did not occur in that patient, and further analysis revealed that the marker chromosome in her karyotype was derived from chromosome 14 [2].

Combining the conventional karyotyping and FISH data allowed us to characterize the genetic content of the marker chromosome. The derivate corresponds to Xp11.23-q13.2 region, which contains the gene XIST. This gene is responsible for the X chromosome

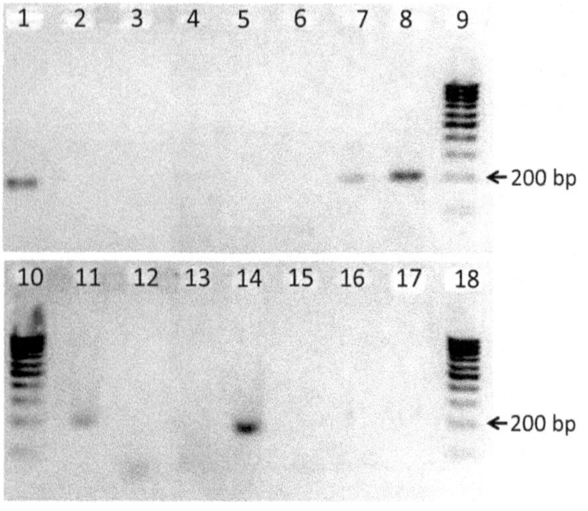


**Fig. 3** Results of PCR screening of marker chromosomes for XIST gene presence. Primers: CH3R/F on lines 1-5; CHXR/F on lines 6-8, 11, 12; XISTF/R on lines 13-17. DNA templates: chromosome 3 painting probe on lines 1, 6, 13; chromosome X painting probe on lines 2, 7, 14; microdissection-derived marker chromosome (mar1) on lines 3, 8, 15; microdissection-derived marker chromosome (mar2) on lines 4, 11, 16; negative controls on lines 5, 12, 17; 100 bp ladder on lines 9, 10, 18

inactivation, which is necessary to realize the epigenetic mechanism of dosage compensation. The structurally abnormal chromosome X without XIST could not be inactivated, which led to an increase in the dose of genes and, consequently, to the appearance of features of Turner's syndrome. This, in turn, led to a more severe phenotype of Turner's syndrome [5]. In the case report we found no XIST gene in X derived marker chromosome that means other reason of mild symptoms.

## Conclusion

In this clinical case we described the patient with a mild phenotype of Turner's syndrome. The proband does not have intellectual disability or severe diseases of internal organs in absence of XIST gene in X-derived marker chromosome.

**Acknowledgements**

We thank Professor Malcolm A. Ferguson-Smith at the University of Cambridge for provided human chromosomes painting probes.

**Funding**

The study is supported by Russian Science Foundation Grant 15-15-10001.

**Authors' contributions**

AST, DVY – study concept. AST, NAL – cell growing, metaphase preparation, GTG banding, FISH experiments. SAR – microdissection. YVM, ARS – all clinical procedures and study. DVY – manuscript preparation. All authors read and approved the final manuscript.

**Competing interests**

The authors declare that they have no competing interests.

**Author details**

[1]Institute of Molecular and Cellular Biology SB RAS, Lavrentieva ave. 8/2, Novosibirsk 630090, Russia. [2]Novosibirsk State University, Novosibirsk 630090, Russia. [3]Novosibirsk State Medical University, Novosibirsk 630091, Russia. [4]Novosibirsk City Clinical Hospital No.1, Novosibirsk 630047, Russia.

**References**

1. Liehr T, Mrasek K, Hinreiner S, Reich D, Ewers E, Bartels I, et al. Small supernumerary marker chromosomes (sSMC) in patients with a 45,X/46,X,+mar karyotype-17 new cases and a review of the literature. Sex Dev. 2007;1:353–62.
2. Sheth F, Ewers E, Kosyakova N, Weise A, Sheth J, Desai M, et al. A small supernumerary marker chromosome present in a turner syndrome patient not derived from X- or Y-chromosome: a case report. Mol Cytogenet. 2009;2:22.
3. Wang H, Wang T, Yang N, He Y, Chen L, Hong L, et al. The clinical analysis of small supernumerary marker chromosomes in 17 children with mos 45,X/46,X,+mar karyotype. Oncol Lett. 2017;13:4385–9.
4. Zhong Q, Layman LC. Genetic considerations in the patient with turner syndrome—45,X with or without mosaicism. Fertil Steril. 2012;98:775–9.
5. Mazzaschi RLP, Taylor J, Robertson SP, Love DR, George AMA. Turner syndrome patient carrying a mosaic distal X chromosome marker. Case Reports in Genetics. 2014;2014:597314.
6. Yudkin D, Hayward BE, Aladjem MI, Kumari D, Usdin K. Chromosome fragility and the abnormal replication of the FMR1 locus in fragile X syndrome. Hum Mol Genet. 2014;23:2940–52.
7. Seabright MA. Rapid banding technique for human chromosomes. Lancet. 1971;2:971–2.
8. Liehr T. Fluorescence in situ hybridization (FISH) – application guide. 2nd ed. Berlin, Heidelberg: Springer-Verlag; 2017.
9. Guilherme RS, Klein E, Venner C, Hamid AB, Bhatt S, Melaragno MI, et al. Human ring chromosomes and small supernumerary marker chromosomes – do they have telomeres? Chromosom Res. 2012;20:825–35.
10. Love K, Huddleston L, Olney P, Wrubel D, Visootsak J. Developmental outcomes of down syndrome and Dandy-Walker malformation. J Pediatr Neurol. 2011;9:405–8.
11. Ecker J, Shipp T, Bromley B, Benacerraf B. The sonographic diagnosis of Dandy-Walker and Dandy-Walker variant: associated findings and outcomes. Prenat Diagn. 2000;20:328–32.

# Monosomy chromosome 21 compensated by 21q22.11q22.3 duplication in a case with small size and minor anomalies

Meng Su[1], Paul J. Benke[2], Guney Bademci[3], Filiz Basak Cengiz[3], Xiaomei Ouyang[1], Jinghong Peng[1], Carmen E. Casas[1], Mustafa Tekin[3] and Yao-Shan Fan[1*]

**Abstract**

**Background:** Partial monosomy 21 is a rare finding with variable sizes and deletion breakpoints, presenting with a broad spectrum of phenotypes.

**Case presentation:** We report a 10-month-old boy with short stature, minor anomalies and mild motor delay. The patient had a monosomy 21 and duplication of the 21q22.11q22.3 region on the remaining derivative chromosome 21 which represents a partial 21q uniparental disomy of paternal origin, upd(21q22.11q22.3)pat. The abnormalities were characterized by karyotyping, FISH, chromosomal microarray, and genotyping.

**Conclusions:** This is the first case showing a monosomy 21 compensated by upd(21q22.11q22.3) as a mechanism of genomic rescue. Because there is no strong evidence showing imprinting on chromosome 21, the uniparental disomy itself is not associated with abnormal phenotype but has reduced phenotype severity of monosomy 21. We reviewed the previously published cases with isolated 21q deletions and identified a common deletion of 5.7 Mb associated with low birth weight, length and head circumference in the 21q21.2 region.

**Keywords:** Chromosome 21, Partial monosomy, Deletion, Duplication, Partial uniparental disomy

## Background

Full monosomy 21 has been rarely reported and is likely to be lethal in utero [1]. Even in a case of a live born with molecularly confirmed monosomy 21 [2], mosaicism could not be ruled out. It was suggested that full monosomy 21 may not exist in live born and those reported cases of monosomy 21 are likely to be either mosaicism or partial monosomy 21 resulting from a cryptic unbalanced translocation [1, 3]. Some cases previously reported were identified prior to the era of high resolution G-banding and molecular cytogenetics. Several cases described as full monosomy 21 initially by conventional karyotyping were later re-classified as partial monosomy by molecular cytogenetics or other molecular techniques [4–6]. Among the more than 30 cases previously reported with a partial monosomy 21, about half were isolated chromosome 21 segmental monosomy without other abnormalities identified [7, 8]. The remaining half had rearrangements involving other chromosomes in addition to chromosome 21 [7, 9–14]. Each partial monosomy 21 case represents a rare and unique finding with variable deletion breakpoints, and therefore the cases with partial monosomy 21 have a broad spectrum of phenotypes.

Here, we present a patient with monosomy 21 and a duplication in the 21q22.11q22.3 region on the remaining derivative chromosome 21 which represent a partial uniparental disomy (UPD), with discussions on the possible mechanisms with which the abnormality arose in this case and the genotype-phenotype correlation of 21q deletions.

* Correspondence: YFan@med.miami.edu
[1]Department of Pathology and Laboratory Medicine, University of Miami Miller School of Medicine, 1601 NW 12th Avenue, Miami, FL 33136, USA
Full list of author information is available at the end of the article

## Methods

### DNA extraction and chromosomal microarray analysis (CMA)

CMA was performed using a combined comparative genomic hybridization (CGH) and single nucleotide polymorphism (SNP) microarray platform SurePrint G3 4x180K CGH + SNP microarray chip (Agilent). The CMA platform is composed of approximately 120,000 oligonucleotide probes for CGH analysis and 60,000 oligonucleotide probes for SNP analysis with an average resolution of 5~ 10 Mb for absence of heterozygosity (AOH)/UPD detection. Probes were annotated against NCBI Build 37 (UCSC hg19, February 2009). The data was analyzed using Agilent C microarray scanner and CytoGenomics Edition 4.0.2.21 software.

### Chromosome analysis

Peripheral blood samples of the patient and his parents were cultured and slides were prepared according to standard laboratory protocol. Chromosome analysis was performed on 20 G-banded metaphase cells at the resolution level of 500–550 bands per haploid set, using standard technology. Chromosome abnormalities were described using An International System for Human Cytogenomic Nomenclature [15].

### Fluorescence in-situ hybridization (FISH)

FISH was performed on metaphase chromosome slides according to a protocol recommended by the manufacturer of the FISH probes used in this study. A mixture of AneuVysion Vysis locus-specific indicator (LSI) 13 and 21 probes (Abbott, Abbott Park, IL) was used and these two probes were designed to hybridize to the 13q14 and the 21q22.13q22.2 regions respectively. 10 metaphases and 200 interphase cells were analyzed.

### Genotyping

Genotyping was done by Sanger sequencing on DNA samples of the patient and his parents. Briefly, genomic DNA was extracted and purified from peripheral blood samples using QIAamp DNA Blood Midi Kit (Qiagen). Primers specific for four highly polymorphic single nucleotide polymorphisms (SNPs) (rs2776109, rs68172960, rs6517210, and rs9968008) across the chromosome 21 were designed using Primer3 (http://primer3.ut.ee/, version 4.0.0) and UCSC In-Silico PCR (University of California Santa Cruz, Santa Cruz, CA). The targeted regions were amplified with a touchdown thermal cycling program, which was 3 min at 94 °C followed by 5 s at 94 °C; 30 s at 65 °C (minus 2 °C every two cycles); 60 s at 72 °C, then 7 min at 72 °C. The PCR products were purified using SOPE resin (Edge Biosystems, Gaithersburg, MD) combined with Sephadex Plate. Afterward, the purified amplicons were bidirectionally sequenced using BIG DYE Terminator Ready Reaction Mix v3.1 on an ABI 3130 system (Applied Biosystems, Foster City, CA). The results were analyzed using Sequencher (version 5.4.5, Ann Arbor, MI).

## Case presentation

An Hispanic male infant was referred to genetics clinic at three months of age by his neurologist for short stature and minor facial findings. A prenatal ultrasound scan at 20 weeks of gestation showed intrauterine growth restriction (IUGR). Labor was medically induced at 38 weeks because of the small size and an emergency Caesarean section was performed due to heart deceleration during induction. His weight was 2.183 kg (< 1%ile), length was 40.5 cm (< 1%ile), and head circumference was 32.5 cm (1%ile) at birth. He was otherwise healthy and discharged from the hospital after 3 days. By twelve months of age, his length was 68.6 cm (< 1%ile) and weight was 7.7 kg (2%ile), but head circumference had increased dramatically and reached 45.7 cm (36%ile).

The patient's bone age was delayed. At 11 months of age, his bone age was between three and six months. His motor skills were mildly delayed about two to three months. At four months of age, he was mildly hypertonic and was late lifting up. His left eye had difficulty with upward gaze, and he had problems tracking objects. At eight months of age, he was able to sit with support and grab at objects. He could roll front to back, but not yet back to front. He had shoulder stiffness and difficulty reaching his arms over his head. He had minor facial dysmorphic features including a broad, prominent forehead, mildly depressed nasal bridge, thin upper lip, small chin, and boarder-line low set ears (Fig. 1a). He was happy, smiling, engaged, and had good eye contact. His mental development was normal for age. Both his 35 years old mother and 47 years old father were healthy and did not show similar findings.

The CGH array detected a 15.98 Mb deletion in the 21q11.2q21.3 chromosome region, arr[GRCh37] 21q11.2q21.3(15143552_31118908)× 1 (Fig. 1b). The SNP array confirmed the deletion and also showed absence of heterozygosity (AOH) at 21q22.11q22.3 with a size of approximately 14.32 Mb (chr21:33,080,313_47,399,375, GRCh37/hg19) (Fig. 1b). Chromosome analysis revealed an abnormal karyotype, 45,XY,-21,der(21)dup(21)(q22.11q22.3) (Fig. 1c), that is a loss of an entire chromosome 21 and duplication of the 21q22.11q22.3 region on the derivative 21. This duplication was subsequently confirmed by FISH showing the two signals on the der(21) (Fig. 1d). Chromosome analysis by G-banding demonstrated a normal karyotype in both parents. Genotyping clearly demonstrated paternal origin of the der(21) (Fig. 1e).

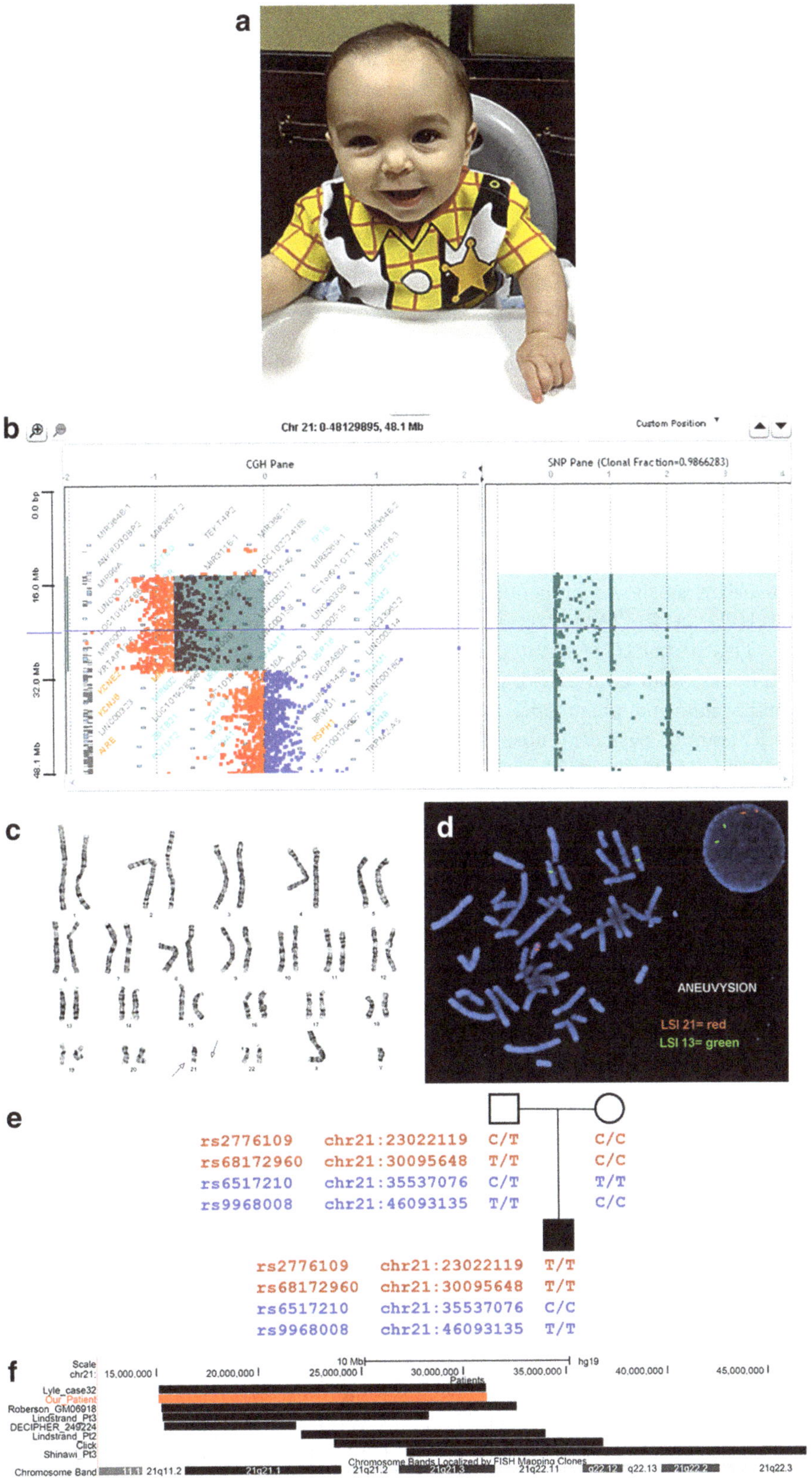


Fig. 1 (See legend on next page.)

(See figure on previous page.)

**Fig. 1** Clinical presentation and molecular cytogenetics analysis of the present patient. **a** Clinical presentation of the patient at 8 months of age. He had minor facial dysmorphic features including a broad, prominent forehead, mildly depressed nasal bridge, thin upper lip, small chin, and boarder-line low set ears. **b-d** Cytogenetic analysis identified a deletion and an AOH resulted by duplication in chromosome 21. **b** CGH and SNP array profile of chromosome 21. The numbers in the CGH pane are indicating log2 ratio of the intensity of fluorescence of the patient versus control genome. In the SNP pane, the numbers indicate the number of B allele. **c** Karyotype of the patient. **d** FISH analysis in both metaphase and interphase cells using probes designed for testing presence or absence of the 21q22.11q22.3 region (red). **e** Genotyping by Sanger sequencing indicating the paternal origin of the derivative chromosome 21. SNPs rs2776109 and rs68172960 (shown in red) are located in the 21q11.2q21.3 region, and rs6517210 and rs9968008 (shown in blue) covered the 21q22.11q22.3 UPD region. **f** Genomic location of the 21q deletions in the present patient and previously published cases. The red bar indicates the 15.98 Mb deletion at 21q11.2q21.3 (chr21:15,143,552_31,118,908, GRCh37/hg19) in our patient. The black bars represent the deletion regions of previously reported cases with isolated deletion at 21q overlapping with our patient, without any other chromosomal structural abnormality. Genomic locations are showed by UCSC genome browser

## Discussion and conclusions

Combining the results of chromosome analysis, FISH, CGH/SNP microarray and genotyping, this patient has a single copy of the 21q11.2q21.3 region with a size of approximately 16 Mb, and two copies of the remaining chromosome 21q22.11q22.3 region, resulting from loss of one entire chromosome 21 and duplication of the 21q22.11q22.3 in the derivative 21 chromosome. The derived 21 is paternal in origin as shown by genotyping, representing a partial UPD in 21q22.11q22.3 region, upd(21q22.11q22.3)pat. This partial UPD in the der(21) has compensated for the loss of an entire chromosome 21, thus leading to a mildly abnormal phenotype.

Among the over 30 patients of partial monosomy 21 published previously, none of them share common breakpoints of their deletion regions, and their phenotype shows a broad spectrum [7, 12, 14]. Therefore, each partial monosomy 21 case is a unique finding and more patients are warranted to further elucidate the genotype-phenotype correlation and unveil the possible consequences of the deletions. To date, this is the first patient reported with a monosomy 21 associated with a partial upd(21)pat in the most gene-rich region [16]. Because there is no strong evidence showing imprinting on chromosome 21 and upd(21) is not associated with an abnormal phenotype [17, 18], the partial upd(21), upd(21q22.11q22.3)pat in our case has reduced phenotype severity of monosomy 21.

A well accepted model proposed by Lyle et al. [12] divided chromosome 21 into three regions: Region 1 (~ 31.2 Mb, 21q11.2-q22.11) harboring more than 50 genes, Region 2 (31.2–36 Mb, 21q22.11-q22.12) containing more than 80 genes, and Region 3 (~ 36–37.5 Mb to 21qter, 21q22.12-q22.3) encompassing more than 130 genes. Phenotypic severity associated with these three regions are severe, lethal, and mild, respectively. In the present patient, the missing of an entire chromosome 21 and the duplication on the derivative chromosome 21 have resulted in a deletion of about 16 Mb in the 21q11.2q21.3 region, which is within Region 1. Lyle et al. [12] proposed that deletions of Region 2 lead to a much more severe phenotype and are not compatible with survival. Nonetheless, Roberson et al. [14] suggested to expand Region 1 to merge with Region 2, because four patients they reported along with one patient reported by Lindstrand et al. [19] and three DECIPHER cases (DECIPHER patient 2609, 4976, 249,393) all had deletions overlapping part of Region 2. The severity of clinical presentation for deletions in this region was variable and seems comparable with that of Region 1. However, even though the above-mentioned cases had deletions overlapping part of Region 2, there were no non-mosaic cases reported that spanned the entire Region 2. There was one case in the literature with a deletion spanning Region 2 which was 15% mosaic [20]. Deletion of Region 3 is associated with a mild phenotype. In the present patient, there is no deletion in Region 2 and Region 3. Instead, there is a UPD in the derivative chromosome 21 that spans the whole Region 2 and Region 3.

We suggest that monosomy rescue is the most likely mechanism of the chromosome abnormalities observed in our patient. One possibility is that a normal sperm fertilized an ovum with nullisomy 21, and then the paternal chromosome 21 duplicated its q22.1q23.3 region in the zygote. The q22.1q23.3 region contains the most biologically important genes to compensate the loss of an entire maternal chromosome 21. The second possibility is a somatic event: A loss of the maternal chromosome 21 occurred in the first mitotic cell division after a normal fertilization, followed by duplication of the q22.1q23.3 region in the paternal chromosome 21. The phenomenon of monosomy rescue supports the hypothesis that a deletion spanning the gene dense region in chromosome 21 cannot be tolerated [12] and a pure monosomy 21 cannot exist in live born [1, 3]. Our findings re-emphasize the importance of Region 2 in chromosome 21.

Genotype-phenotype correlation in patients with partial monosomy 21 has always been challenging because of the variable sizes of the deletions [7]. Such correlation can be more complicated due to presence of complex abnormalities such as unbalanced rearrangements involving other chromosomes which are usually associated with more severe phenotypes and are more complex to interpret [12, 14, 19].

Among previously published cases with isolated chromosome 21 segmental monosomy without other abnormalities, we compared their breakpoints with our patient and discovered seven of them had deletions overlapped with the deletion region observed in our patient (Fig. 1f). The phenotypes of these seven patients and our patient are summarized in Table 1. Our patient shares some of the most common abnormal phenotypes observed in this group (Table 1). The patient reported by Lyle et al. (case 32) [12] had a deletion similar to that of the present case. The common features of these two patients include developmental delay and microcephaly. The 21q21.2 region with a size of 5.7 Mb (chr21: 22,560,763 to 28,265,000) encompassing 22 genes was commonly deleted in 4 of these 7 patients (Patient 2 and 3 in Lindstrand's report, the case reported by Click et al., and the present case). All these 4 patients had low birth weight, length and head circumference. It was noted that the weight and length of the Patient 3 in the Lindstrand's report reached to the normal range at 5 years and 10 months of age. In our patient at 12 months of age, no obvious improvement was observed in the measurements besides that of head circumference. These observations may suggest association of 21q21.2 deletion with a low birth weight, length and head circumference.

Intellectual disability and congenital heart malformations are the most common features in partial monosomy 21 but were not found in our patient. Previous studies have suggested association of intellectual disability with the *ITSN1* gene, and proposed *KCNE1, RCAN1, CLIC6* and *RUNX1* as candidate genes for congenital heart malformations [19]. All of these genes are located in Region 2 and none was lost in our case.

In summary, the deletion in the present case encompasses 63 genes, and none of them are known dosage sensitive genes. The 15.98 Mb deletion in the 21q11.2q21.3 region is caused by loss of the entire maternal chromosome 21 which was compensated by a 14.32 Mb paternal duplication of the 21q22.11q22.3

**Table 1** Summary of phenotypes of isolated chromosome 21 deletion patients with overlapping regions with our patient

| | Present patient | Lyle case 32 | Lindstrand Pt 2 | Lindstrand Pt 3 | Roberson GM06918 | Click | Shinawi Pt 3 | DECIPHER 249224 | # of abnormal phenotypes |
|---|---|---|---|---|---|---|---|---|---|
| intellectual disability | | yes | yes | yes | yes | | yes | | 5 |
| low birth weight | yes | | yes | yes | | yes | | | 4 |
| broad or depressed nasal bridge | | yes | | | yes | yes | yes | | 4 |
| short stature | yes | yes | | | yes | | | | 3 |
| low anterior or posterior hairline | | yes | | | yes | yes | | | 3 |
| low set ears | yes | | yes | | | yes | | | 3 |
| downward slanting palpebral fissures | | | yes | | yes | yes | | | 3 |
| hypertelorism | yes | | yes | | | | yes | | 3 |
| congenital heart defect | | | yes | yes | | yes | | | 3 |
| delayed speech and language development | | | | yes | | | | yes | 2 |
| hypotonia | yes | yes | | | | | | | 2 |
| microcephaly | yes | yes | | | | | | | 2 |
| large ears | | yes | | | | yes | | | 2 |
| high or cleft palate | | yes | | | yes | | | | 2 |
| strabismus | | | | | | yes | yes | | 2 |
| feeding difficulties | | | yes | | | | | | 1 |
| hypertonia | | yes | | | | | | | 1 |
| distal limbs abnormalities | | | | yes | | | | | 1 |

Abnormal phenotypes are listed from the most common to least common ones

region in the derivative chromosome 21. Although the deletion is within the 21q Region 1 (q11.2q22.1), the smaller deletion is associated with relatively mild developmental disabilities. Deletion of the 21q21.2 region is associated with a low birth weight and short stature as shown by several reported cases.

### Abbreviations

AOH: Absence of heterozygosity; CGH: Comparative genomic hybridization; CMA: Chromosomal microarray analysis; FISH: Fluorescence in-situ hybridization; IUGR: Intrauterine growth restriction; SNP: Single nucleotide polymorphism; UPD: Uniparental disomy

### Acknowledgements

We would like to thank the child and his family for their support and consent to publication of this paper.

### Funding

This work was supported by University of Miami Miller School of Medicine.

### Authors' contributions

PJB provided the clinical information of this case; XO, JP, and CEC performed the cytogenetic analysis including G-banding, FISH, and microarray analysis; GB, FBC, and MT performed genotyping; MS and YSF analyzed and interpreted the results; MS, PJB, MT, and YSF wrote and revised the manuscript; YSF supervised the study and did most of the editing for the manuscript. All authors read and approved the final manuscript.

### Competing interests

The authors declare that they have no competing interests.

### Author details

[1]Department of Pathology and Laboratory Medicine, University of Miami Miller School of Medicine, 1601 NW 12th Avenue, Miami, FL 33136, USA. [2]Department of Genetics, Joe DiMaggio Children's Hospital and the Charles E Schmidt College of Medicine, 1150 N 35th Avenue, Hollywood, FL 33021, USA. [3]John P. Hussman Institute for Human Genomics, University of Miami Miller School of Medicine, 1501 NW 10th Avenue, Miami, FL 33136, USA.

### References

1. Schinzel A. Letter: Does full monosomy 21 exist? A comment to the paper: A male infant with monosomy 21 by Y. Kaneko, T. Ikeuchi, M. Sasaki, Y. Satake and S. Kuwajima Humangenetik 29, 1–7 (1975). Hum Genet. 1976; 32(1):105–7.
2. Shah MG, Franco A, Wills KM, Kulharya AS, Buckler BS, Bhatia JJS. A rare case of complete monosomy 21 with multiple osseous, cardiac, and vascular anomalies. Eur J Radiol Extra. 2010;76:e65–8.
3. Burgess T, Downie L, Pertile MD, Francis D, Glass M, Nouri S. Monosomy 21 seen in live born is unlikely to represent true monosomy 21: a case report and review of the literature. Case Rep Genet. 2014;2014:965401.
4. Iqbal MA, Ahmed MZ, Wu D, Sakati N. A case of presumptive monosomy 21 re-diagnosed as unbalanced t(5p;21q) by FISH and review of literature. Am J Med Genet. 1997;70(2):174–8.
5. Gill P, Uhrich S, Disteche C, Cheng E. Fetal t(5p;21q) misdiagnosed as monosomy 21: a plea for in situ hybridization studies. Am J Med Genet. 1994;52(4):416–8.
6. Hertz B, Brandt CA, Petersen MB, Pedersen S, Konig U, Stromkjaer H, Jensen PK. Application of molecular and cytogenetic techniques to the detection of a de novo unbalanced t(11q;21q) in a patient previously diagnosed as having monosomy 21. Clin Genet. 1993;44(2):89–94.
7. Jespersgaard C, Damgaard IN, Cornelius N, Bache I, Knabe N, Miranda MJ, Tümer Z. Proximal 21q deletion as a result of a de novo unbalanced t(12;21) translocation in a patient with dysmorphic features, hepatomegaly, thick myocardium and delayed psychomotor development. Mol Cytogenet. 2016;9(1):11.
8. Vorsanova SG, Iourov IY, Voinova-Ulas VY, Weise A, Monakhov VV, Kolotii AD, Soloviev IV, Novikov PV, Yurov YB, Liehr T. Partial monosomy 7q34-qter and 21pter-q22.13 due to cryptic unbalanced translocation t(7;21) but not monosomy of the whole chromosome 21: a case report plus review of the literature. Mol Cytogenet. 2008;1:13.
9. Zheng Z, Yao RE, Geng J, Jin X, Shen Y, Ying D. A unique combination of 17pter trisomy and 21qter monosomy in a boy with developmental delay, severe intellectual disability, growth retardation and dysmorphisms. Gene. 2013;516:301–6.
10. dos Santos AP, Vieira TP, Simioni M, Monteiro FP, Gil-da-Silva-Lopes VL: Partial monosomy 21 (q11.2-->q21.3) combined with 3p25.3-->pter monosomy due to an unbalanced translocation in a patient presenting dysmorphic features and developmental delay. Gene 2013, 513(2):301–304.
11. Szabo GP, Knegt AC, Ujfalusi A, Balogh E, Szabo T, Olah E. Subtelomeric 6.7 Mb trisomy 10p and 5.6 Mb monosomy 21q detected by FISH and array-CGH in three related patients. Am J Med Genet A. 2012;158A:869–76.
12. Lyle R, Bena F, Gagos S, Gehrig C, Lopez G, Schinzel A. Genotype-phenotype correlations in Down syndrome identified by array CGH in 30 cases of partial trisomy and partial monosomy chromosome 21. Eur J Hum Genet. 2009;17:454–66.
13. Katzenstein JM, Oghalai JS, Tonini R, Baker D, Haymond J, Caudle SE. Neurocognitive functioning of a child with partial trisomy 6 and monosomy 21. Neurocase. 2009;15:97–100.
14. Roberson ED, Wohler ES, Hoover-Fong JE, Lisi E, Stevens EL, Thomas GH. Genomic analysis of partial 21q monosomies with variable phenotypes. Eur J Hum Genet. 2011;19:235–8.
15. International Standing Committee on Human Cytogenomic Nomenclature, McGowan-Jordan J, Simons A, Schmid M: ISCN: an international system for human cytogenomic nomenclature (2016).
16. Hattori M, Fujiyama A, Taylor TD, Watanabe H, Yada T, Park HS, Toyoda A, Ishii K, Totoki Y, Choi DK, et al. The DNA sequence of human chromosome 21. Nature. 2000;405(6784):311–9.
17. Blouin JL, Avramopoulos D, Pangalos C, Antonarakis SE. Normal phenotype with paternal uniparental isodisomy for chromosome 21. Am J Hum Genet. 1993;53(5):1074–8.
18. Rogan PK, Sabol DW, Punnett HH. Maternal uniparental disomy of chromosome 21 in a normal child. Am J Med Genet. 1999;83(1):69–71.
19. Lindstrand A, Malmgren H, Sahlen S, Schoumans J, Nordgren A, Ergander U. Detailed molecular and clinical characterization of three patients with 21q deletions. Clin Genet. 2010;77:145–54.
20. Shinawi M, Erez A, Shardy DL, Lee B, Naeem R, Weissenberger G. Syndromic thrombocytopenia and predisposition to acute myelogenous leukemia caused by constitutional microdeletions on chromosome 21q. Blood. 2008;112:1042–7.

# 7p15 deletion as the cause of hand-foot-genital syndrome: a case report, literature review and proposal of a minimum region for this phenotype

Emiy Yokoyama[1], Dennise Lesley Smith-Pellegrin[1], Silvia Sánchez[2], Bertha Molina[2], Alfredo Rodríguez[2], Rocío Juárez[3], Esther Lieberman[1], Silvia Avila[4], José Luis Castrillo[4], Victoria del Castillo[1*] and Sara Frías[2,5*]

**Abstract**

**Background:** Hand-foot-genital syndrome (HFGS) is a rare condition characterized by congenital malformations in the limbs and genitourinary tract. Generally, this syndrome occurs due to point mutations that cause loss of function of the *HOXA13* gene, which is located on 7p15; however, there are some patients with HFGS caused by interstitial deletions in this region.

**Case presentation:** We describe a pediatric Mexican patient who came to the Medical Genetics Department at the National Institute of Pediatrics because he presented with genital, hand and feet anomalies, facial dysmorphisms, and learning difficulties. Array CGH reported a 12.7 Mb deletion that includes *HOXA13*.

**Conclusions:** We compared our patient with cases of HFGS reported in the literature caused by a microdeletion; we found a minimum shared region in 7p15.2. By analyzing the phenotype in these patients, we suggest that microdeletions in this region should be investigated in all patients with clinical characteristics of HFGS who also present with dysplastic ears, mainly low-set implantation with a prominent antihelix, as well as a low nasal bridge and long philtrum.

**Keywords:** Hand-foot-genital syndrome, *HOXA13*, 7p15 deletion

## Background

Hand-foot-genital syndrome (HFGS; OMIM #140000) is an autosomal dominant condition that has been reported in 23 families [1–8] and 5 sporadic cases [9–12]. It is characterized by congenital limb malformations, mainly affecting the hands, such as short thumbs, and feet, as well as the genitourinary tract, such as hypospadias and cryptorchidism in males or urogenital septum and bicorne uterus in females [13]. HFGS is produced by mutations that cause loss of function of the *HOXA13* gene, which is located on 7p15 and is important for the development of fetal limbs and the urinary tract. The mutations responsible for HFGS include missense mutations, nonsense mutations, polyalanine expansions, and in very few cases, interstitial deletions at 7p15. We describe a Mexican patient with HFGS caused by a 12.7 Mb deletion on chromosome 7, ranging from p15.3 to p14.3, including the *HOXA13* gene. We compared previously reported patients with the purpose of determining a minimum shared region, as well as clinical characteristics that could guide the diagnosis of HFGS caused by a microdeletion.

* Correspondence: vdelcastilloruiz@yahoo.com.mx; sarafrias@biomedicas.unam.mx
[1]Departamento de Genética Humana, Instituto Nacional de Pediatría, Insurgentes Sur 3700-C, Colonia Insurgentes Cuicuilco, Coyoacán, Ciudad de México, CDMX, Mexico
[2]Laboratorio de Citogenética, Departamento de Investigación en Genética Humana. Instituto Nacional de Pediatría, Avenida IMAN no. 1, Torre de Investigación, Colonia Insurgentes Cuicuilco, Coyoacán, Ciudad de México, CDMX, Mexico
Full list of author information is available at the end of the article

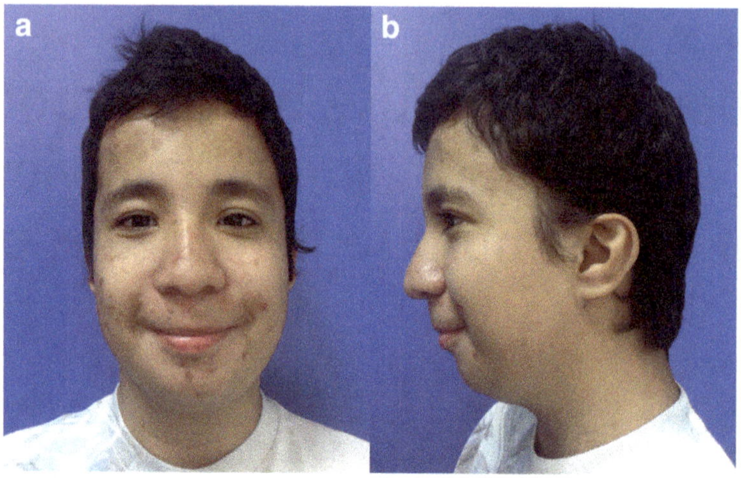


**Fig. 1** **a**. Facial phenotype of patient with midface hypoplasia, broad and prominent front, mild hypertelorism, strabism, broad nasal bridge, long and smooth philtrum, thin upper lip. **b**. Posteriorly rotated ears and prominent antihelix

## Case presentation

The patient is a 14-year-old male, the third child of a 21-year-old mother and a 30-year-old father, both of whom are healthy and non-consanguineous. He has two healthy brothers aged 20 and 18 years old. He was born after an uneventful pregnancy; his birth weight was 2300 g (<3th percentile), and his height was 49 cm (>15th percentile).

At 7 years old, the patient was referred to our hospital due to genital anomalies. Upon admission, a global developmental delay was detected, which was most profound in the area of language. He also presented with short stature, microcephaly, facial dysmorphisms, such as facial asymmetry, midface hypoplasia, a broad and prominent forehead, mild hypertelorism, strabismus, a broad nasal bridge, a long and smooth philtrum, a thin upper lip, a high palate (Fig. 1a), and low-set ears with a prominent antihelix (Fig. 1b). Additionally, we observed subglandular hypospadias and cryptorchidism, hands with fifth finger clinodactyly, abnormal palmar creases, and severe bilateral hallux valgus (Fig. 2a, b and 3a).

The patient's brain MRI was normal, while auditory evoked potentials revealed normal left hearing and right conductive superficial hearing loss (secondary to serous otitis media). An X-ray of the hands showed a three-year delayed bone age, feet with an absence of mid-foot bone structures, such as cuneiform bones, only cuboid and navicular bones were observed, as well as bilateral hallux valgus, which was surgically repaired at 13 years old (Figs. 2c and 3b). Karyotype and Array CGH *Agilent 60 K* reported a 12.7 Mb deletion at 7p14.2p15.3 (Fig. 4a and b; ISCN 2016), which was confirmed by FISH with a specific 54.95Kb probe targeted to 7p15.2 inside the deleted region (Fig. 4c). The specific nomenclature is as follows: 46,XY.ish del(7)(p15.2)(D7Z1+,HOXA6 –,HOXA13–).arr[GRCh37/hg19] 7p15.3p14.3(22574164_35288260)x1dn (Fig. 5; ISCN 2016). Both parents were normal. Analysis of the

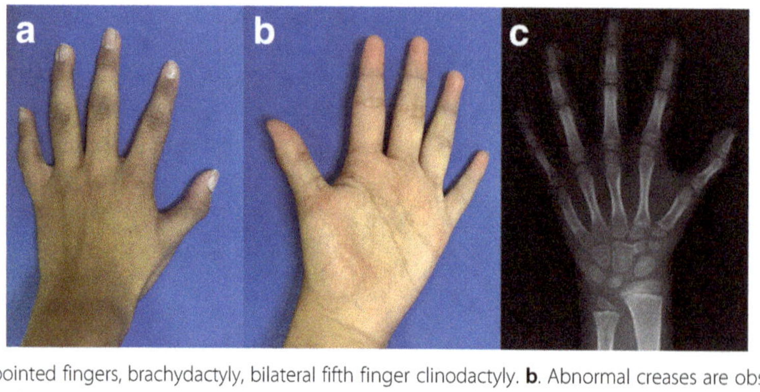


**Fig. 2** **a**. Small hands with pointed fingers, brachydactyly, bilateral fifth finger clinodactyly. **b**. Abnormal creases are observed. **c**. Small distal phalanges, metacarpal shortening

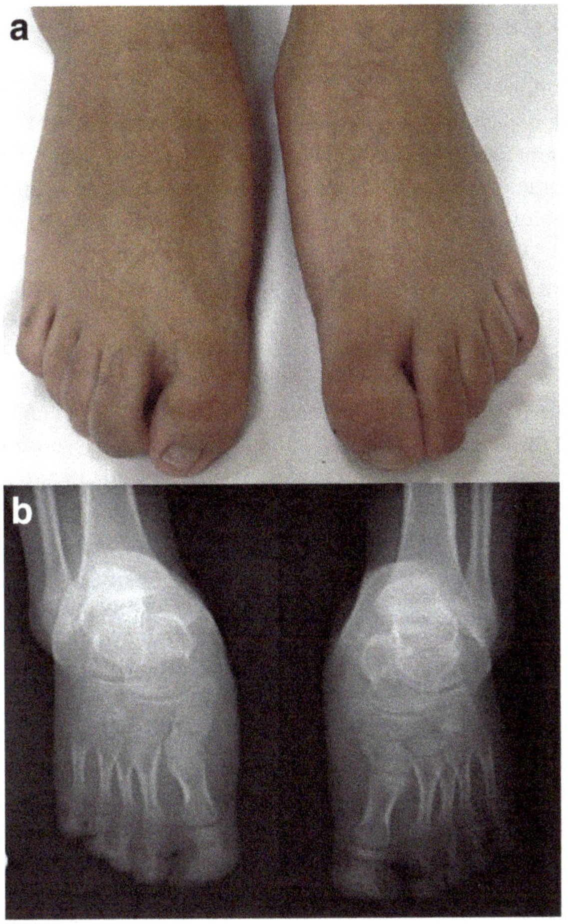


**Fig. 3** **a**. Feet with brachydactyly and severe bilateral hallux valgus. **b**. Metatarsal shortening and hypoplastic phalanges of all toes. Most notable is the thumb, which presents with valgus deviation of the last phalange

genomic alterations and the genotype-phenotype correlation enabled a diagnosis of hand-foot-genital syndrome.

## Discussion and conclusions

### Clinical aspects of hand-foot-genital syndrome

Some of the most frequent limb anomalies in HFGS are short thumbs, medial phalanges, small feet and clinodactyly of the fifth finger [13]. Hallux valgus is an important diagnostic sign, when present [11]. These anomalies have complete penetrance, but they can be so mild that imaging studies may be necessary to observe them. Short phalanges and pointed thumbs, hypoplasia of the first metacarpus and metatarsus, a small calcaneus, trapezium-scaphoid fusion, and cuneiform-navicular fusion can be observed radiologically [10]. Occasional findings include fusion of the medial and distal phalanges to the second to fifth toes [14], as well as delayed ossification [8].

It is estimated that half of the affected patients show urogenital malformations with variable expressivity. Male patients show hypospadias and cryptorchidism, while women present with a double uterus and partial or complete longitudinal urogenital septum. In the presence of any of these findings, HFGS must be investigated due to a 0.5–4% prevalence of the fusion of müllerian structures in the general population [8]. Fertility is conserved in HFGS, though there is an increased risk of spontaneous abortion, preterm birth, and stillbirth [2, 10, 11, 13].

In both genders, common findings include chronic urinary tract infections, ectopic ureteric orifices, vesicoureteral reflux, and pelviureteric junction. Additionally, the disease is associated with complications, such as

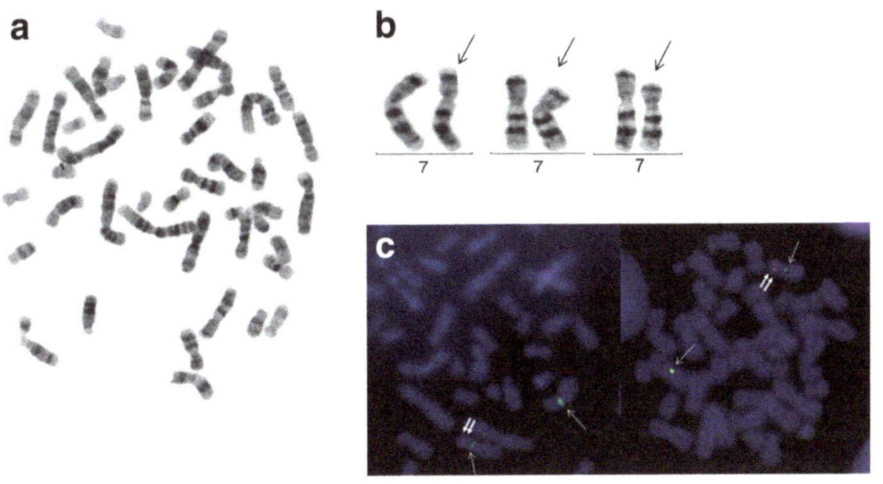


**Fig. 4** **a**. Karyotype with G-banding. **b**. Normal and deleted chromosome 7 (arrows) from different metaphases; **c**. FISH for the 7p15 region on metaphase chromosomes; alpha satellite probe for chromosome 7 centromere (D7Z1) marked with green fluorochrome Q-BIOgene (one thin arrow), and locus specific probe for 7p15.2 (where the *HOXA6-HOXA13* genes are normally located) marked with red fluorochrome-SureFiSH, Agilent (two thick arrows). Note that deleted chromosomes only have the green fluorescent probe and are missing the red fluorescent probe

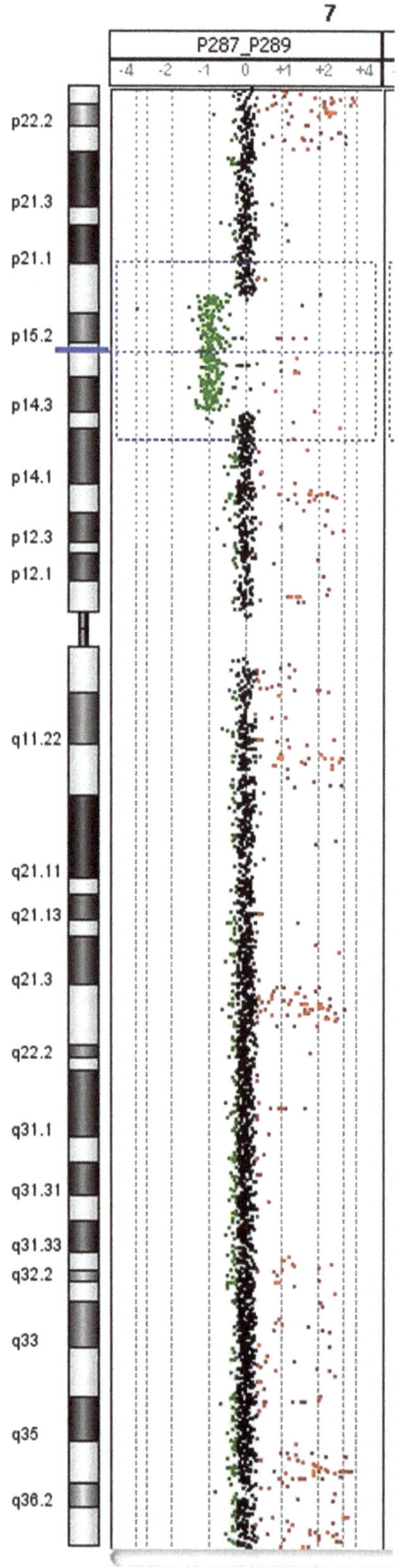


**Fig. 5** Array CGH of the patient. Array Agilent SurePrint G3 Human CGH microarray kit, 8x60K 46,XY.array [GRCh37/hg19] 7p15.3p14.3(22574164_35288260)x1dn (12,714,097 bp)

chronic pyelonephritis and renal failure, which may require transplant. Psychomotor development and cognitive abilities are within normal range [11].

Differential diagnosis to be considered are Fanconi anemia syndrome, Rothmund Thomson syndrome, Holt-Oram syndrome, SALL4-related disorders, Nager syndrome, Townes-Brocks syndrome, and Lacrimo-auriculo-dento-digital (LADD) syndrome, due to the thumb hypoplasia. Incomplete Müllerian fusion and/or longitudinal vaginal septum should be cause for consideration of acro-renal-mandibular, Bardet-Biedl, Beckwith-Wiedemann, Fraser, Fryns, Halal, and Meckel syndromes. Heterozygous mutations in the *HOXA13* gene cause HFGS, however the specific c.1112A > T (p.Gln371Leu) mutation causes Guttmacher syndrome which shares some, but not all, features of HFGS and includes postaxial polydactyly of the hands, preaxial hand and foot deficiencies, short second toes, and glandular hypospadias [14]. Moreover, when patients present with short or absent nails and absent or hypoplastic distal phalanges without genital anomalies, brachydactyly type B1 and Cooks syndrome, must be considered [14].

### Genetics of HFGS

HOX genes are evolutionarily conserved; they participate in developmental processes and maintain their expression until adulthood [14]. They are organized into four clusters, *HOXA*, *HOXB*, *HOXC*, and *HOXD*, localized in 7p15.2, 17q21.32, 12q13.2, and 2q31.1, respectively. They contain between 9 and 11 genes each and codify transcription factors essential for morphogenesis [2]. In particular, *HOXA13* has 2 exons: exon 1 contains five polyalanine regions, and exon 2 has a homeobox domain that is involved in the development of distal limbs and the fetal urogenital tract [12]. *HOXA13* was proposed as candidate gene for HFGS and its involvement in limb development was corroborated in murine models [15].

The first identified pathogenic variant that causes HFGS in humans was the nonsense mutation c.1107G > A (p.Trp369Ter) [15]. Since then, there have been reports of pathogenic variants in both familial and de novo cases, including missense mutations (p.Arg326Gly, p.Asn372His, p.Gln371 Leu), nonsense mutations (p.Ser1360Ter, p.Gln1960Ter, p.Gln3650Ter and p.Trp3690Ter), and triplet expansions that code for a polyalanine region (6, 8–12, and 14 additional polyalanines) [7, 12]. Approximately 35% of these variants are localized within the coding region and, of these, 50 to 60% are found in the polyalanine regions [13, 15]. The missense pathogenic variants produce a gain of function mechanism associated with a more severe phenotype, while the nonsense mutations and polyalanine expansion variants are responsible for loss of protein function, presenting a milder phenotype [15].

**Table 1** Clinical features of patients with deletion including 7p15 region and point mutations in *HOXA13*

| | Patients with microdeletion in 7p15 region | | | | | | | | | Patients with point mutations in *HOXA13* | | | |
|---|---|---|---|---|---|---|---|---|---|---|---|---|---|
| | Patient 1 Present case | Patient 2 [9] (Devriendt et al., 1999)[c] | Patient 3 [18] (Dunø et al., 2004)[b] | Patient 4 [18] (Dunø et al., 2004)[b] | Patient 5 [19] (Kosaki et al., 2005) [c] | Patient 6 [20] (Jun et al., 2011) | Patient 7 [21] (Fryssira et al., 2011) | Patient 8 [17] (Hosoki et al., 2012) | Patient 9 [16] (Pezzani et al., 2016) | Patient A [2] (Mortlock & Innis, 1997) | Patient B [3] (Goodman et al., 2000) | Patient C [10] (Parker et al., 2011) | Patient D [12] (Imagawa et al., 2014) |
| Chromosomal region (size) or mutation in *HOXA13* gene | 7p14.3p15.3 (12.7 Mb) | 7p14.2p15.3 (?) | 7p14.3p15.3 (9.8 Mb) case 1 | 7p14.2p15.2 (9.0 Mb) case 2 | 7p15.2p21 (?) | 7p15.1p15.3 (5.6 Mb) | 7p14.3p21.1 (13 Mb) | 7p15.1p15.3 (6.9 Mb) | 7p14.3p15.2 (2.5 Mb) | p.Trp369Ter | p.Asn372His | p.Arg326Gly | p.Ile368Phe |
| Neurodevelopmental delay | + | Borderline | + | + | + | + | + | + | + | – | – | – | – |
| Height | Short stature | Normal | Normal at birth | Normal at birth | NR | Low weight at birth, short stature with relative macrocephaly | Low weight, short stature, and low cephalic perimeter | Postnatal short stature | Short stature with relative macrocephaly | NR | NR | Normal | Normal |
| Frontal bossing | + | NA | NA | NA | NA | + | – | – | + | – | – | – | – |
| Depressed nasal bridge | + | NA | + | – | +[a] | +[a] | + | + | + | – | – | – | – |
| Mild hypertelorism | + | NA | +[a] | -[a] | +[a] | NA | + | – | + | – | – | – | – |
| Long philtrum | + | NA | +[a] | +[a] | +[a] | NA | + | – | + | – | – | – | – |
| Ear anomalies | Posteriorly rotated and dysplastic | Low-set and malformed | ND | Small and dysplastic | Prominent crus hélix | Posteriorly rotated, low-set, external audi tory canal stenosis | Low-set, hypoplastic helix, prominent antihelix and antitragus | Posteriorly rotated, dysplastic, and low-set | Prominent antihelix, upslanted lobule | – | – | – | – |
| Hand anomalies | Small, bilateral fifth finger clinodactyly | Small, bilateral fifth finger clinodactyly, short distal phalange of second finger | Small, right fourth finger clinodactyly | Small, bilateral fifth finger clinodactyly | Bilateral fifth finger hypoplasia, with single crease on left side | Small, hypoplastic thumb, extension limitation of thumbs, second and third fingers, nail dysplasia, abnormal creases | Small, mesomelic shortening and fifth finger hypoplasia with bilateral clinodactyly, abnormal creases | Small, bilateral fifth finger clinodactyly, small distal phalanges | Small[a], Thumb and second finger distal phalanges hypoplasia, conic fingers | Small, thenar hypoplasia, abnormal left thumb, right fifth finger clinodactyly, left palmar transverse crease | Small[a], hypoplastic thumbs, bilateral fifth finger clinodactyly | Hypoplastic thumbs with proximal insertion, fifth finger clinodactyly | Small[a] hypoplastic thumbs, importantly affected distal phalanges |
| Feet anomalies | Severe hallux valgus | Hypoplastic thumb, laterally deviated | Small and broad thumb | Small thumb, pes planus | NA | Small feet, thumb hypoplasia, nail dysplasia, abnormal creases | Brachydactyly of toes II–IV with a long and broad hallux, medially deviated | Hallux valgus, short and broad thumb | Small feet and short toes | Small feet, right foot smaller than left foot, bilateral abnormal and small thumbs | Absent thumb | Hallux valgus | Absent thumbs, distal phalanges affected |
| | | | NA | – | | Hypospadias | | – | – | – | Hypospadias | | |

**Table 1** Clinical features of patients with deletion including 7p15 region and point mutations in *HOXA13 (Continued)*

| | Patients with microdeletion in 7p15 region | | | | | | | | | Patients with point mutations in *HOXA13* | | | |
|---|---|---|---|---|---|---|---|---|---|---|---|---|---|
| | Patient 1 Present case | Patient 2 [9] (Devriendt et al., 1999)[c] | Patient 3 [18] (Dunø et al., 2004)[b] | Patient 4 [18] (Dunø et al., 2004)[b] | Patient 5 [19] (Kosaki et al., 2005) [c] | Patient 6 [20] (Jun et al., 2011) | Patient 7 [21] (Fryssira et al., 2011) | Patient 8 [17] (Hosoki et al., 2012) | Patient 9 [16] (Pezzani et al., 2016) | Patient A [2] (Mortlock & Innis, 1997) | Patient B [3] (Goodman et al., 2000) | Patient C [10] (Parker et al., 2011) | Patient D [12] (Imagawa et al., 2014) |
| Genital anomalies | Cryptorchidism, hypospadias | Cryptorchidism, ventral-bowed penis | | | Rectoperineal fistula | | Hypospadias left cryptorchidism and scrotum hypoplasia | | | | | Double uterus and cérvix | Bicornis hypoplastic uterus |
| Other dismorphias | Facial asymmetry strabism, thin upper lip | Anteverted nares, retrognathia, wide mouth, short uvula, short soft palate | Anteverted nares, broad lips, upslanted palpebral fissures, broad nose | Broad neck, upslanted short palpebral fissures | Depressed supraorbital ridge on the left, maxillary hypoplasia, craniosynostosis, anal atresia | Accessory nipples | Craniosynostosis, short palpebral fissures, epicanthus, ptosis, anteverted nostrils, micrognathia[a], high palate and soft-palate cleft, short neck, widely spaced nipples | Bifrontal narrowing | Thin lips, micrognathia, short neck | – | – | – | – |

**Superscript numbers indicate the references**
***NR*** **Not reported**
***NA*** **Not available**
**[a] Observed in clinical picture but not referred in the corresponding article; [b]CGH; [c]Karyotype**

**Microdeletions in HFGS**

Interstitial deletions including the 7p15 region are a rare cause of hand-foot-genital syndrome. To date, there are few reported patients with de novo deletions, which mostly occur between 7p15 and 7p21, with a variable size ranging from 2.5 to 12.7 Mb [9, 16–21]. We compared previously reported patients in the literature according to the genetic cause of the syndrome, polyalanine expansions, point mutations, and microdeletions; our patient was included in the latter group (Table 1). We found clinical features in patients with microdeletions that are not shared with patients carrying point mutations or those with polyalanine expansions (data not shown). Likewise, we found a minimum deleted region of 584,758 bp located at 7p15.2 that is shared by patients with HFGS. This region contains the *HOXA* cluster, the *SKAP2* and *EVX1* genes, and miRNA196b (Fig. 6).

From this analysis, we derived important phenotypic data that might suggest the presence of a microdeletion in the 7p15 region, which include the following: a) Neurodevelopmental delay or intellectual disability present in all patients with the microdeletion. *HOXA1* gene is localized in the minimum shared region and is associated with central nervous system development [22]. Also, in this region is miRNA196b (Fig. 6; green circle) [22], in which the gene target *NRC2* is implicated in neuronal development [23]. b) Short stature is shared by more than half of the patients (5 of 9) with the microdeletion. Both *HOXA5* and *HOXA11* are located within the *HOXA* cluster (Fig. 6; orange circle), dysregulation of which might affect growth and consequently generate short stature [22, 24]. c) Facial dysmorphias that are not present in patients with point mutations are found in 9 out of 9 patients with the microdeletion; the most common finding is dysplastic ears, particularly low-set ears with a prominent antihelix, observed in 8 out of 9 reported patients (in the ninth patient, the ears were not phenotypically described). Other facial features shared by most patients with microdeletion are a depressed nasal bridge and a long philtrum. The *HOXA* cluster is located within the minimum shared region and includes the *HOXA1* and *HOXA2* genes (Fig. 6; blue circle), both of which are related to external ear development. This has been verified in mouse models, where high *Hoxa1* and *Hoxa2* messenger expression levels and low mmu-miR-10a (a modulator of *Hoxa1* expression during ear development) levels have been reported [25].

These genes, as members of the *HOX* gene family, play an important role in embryonic patterning and organogenesis, specifically in the developing region of the rhombencephalus and branchial arch [26–28]. Mouse *Hoxa2* knockout models, as well as pig models with nonsense mutations in *Hoxa1*, have been associated with congenital microtia [29, 30].

Deleted region sizes are variable, so we looked for a minimum shared region in patients with HFGS caused by a 7p15 microdeletion to compare phenotypes and to determine if larger genomic losses cause more dysmorphisms or more severe phenotypes. We found that the patient that had the smallest deletion (2.5 Mb; including the 584,758 bp minimum shared region; Fig. 6)

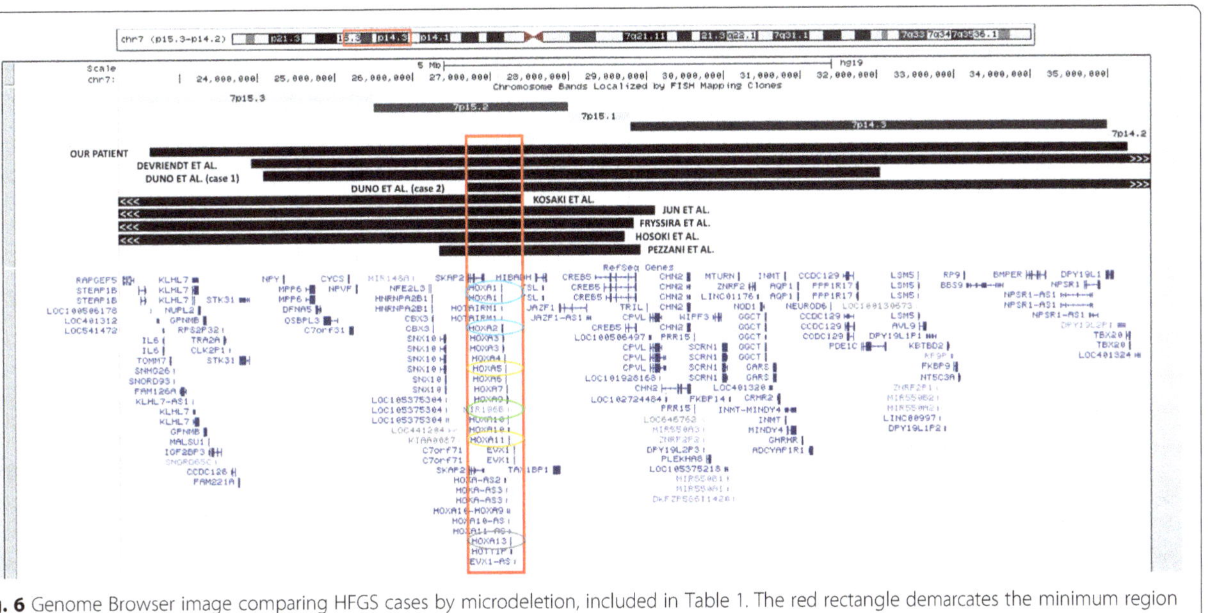


**Fig. 6** Genome Browser image comparing HFGS cases by microdeletion, included in Table 1. The red rectangle demarcates the minimum region (including the HOXA cluster) proposed as responsible for the phenotype of these patients. The most important genes that correlate with the proposed phenotype are: the *HOXA13* gene (gray circle), the *HOXA1* and *HOXA2* genes (blue circle), the *HOXA5* and *HOXA11* genes (orange circle), and miRNA196b (green circle)

[17], as well as our patient, who has the largest deletion reported so far (12.7 Mb), the classical clinical characteristics of HFGS were sufficient evidence to suggest haploinsufficiency of *HOXA13*, despite the absence of several other genes, responsible of a more severe phenotype, making diagnosis more difficult.

According to the information reviewed in every previously reported patient and the characteristics of our patient, we can suggest that a microdeletion in the 7p15 region must be investigated in every HFGS patient that presents with dysplastic ears, mainly low-set ears with a prominent antihelix, as well as a depressed nasal bridge and a long philtrum. Finally, the patient's follow-up and management was based on the literature reports [16], and independent of the etiology, the recurrence risk for each pregnancy is 50% for carrier parents and less than 1% for healthy parents.

**Acknowledgements**
The aCGH was carried out at Genetadi Laboratory (Bilbao, Spain).

**Funding**
This study was partially supported by CONACYT FOSSIS-S0008-2008-C01-87792 and Fondos Federales 2013, Instituto Nacional de Pediatría (México). The funding body did not participate in the design of the study, in the collection, analysis, or interpretation of the data, or in the writing of the manuscript.

**Authors' contributions**
EY and SF contributed to the design and development of the protocol, analyzed the results and wrote the manuscript. DLSP wrote the early manuscript and interpreted results. SS and AR performed FISH and designed the figs. BM and RJ performed the G-banded karyotype. EL contributed to the clinical description and revised the English language usage in the manuscript. SA and JLC performed the array-CGH. VC contributed to the design of the protocol, clinical description and analysis of results. All authors read and approved the final version and are responsible for all aspects of the manuscript. SF and VC share the responsibility of corresponding authors for this paper.

**Competing interests**
The authors declare that they have no competing interests.

**Author details**
[1]Departamento de Genética Humana, Instituto Nacional de Pediatría, Insurgentes Sur 3700-C, Colonia Insurgentes Cuicuilco, Coyoacán, Ciudad de México, CDMX, Mexico. [2]Laboratorio de Citogenética, Departamento de Investigación en Genética Humana. Instituto Nacional de Pediatría, Avenida IMAN no. 1, Torre de Investigación, Colonia Insurgentes Cuicuilco, Coyoacán, Ciudad de México, CDMX, Mexico. [3]Laboratorio de Genética y Cáncer. Departamento de Genética Humana, Instituto Nacional de Pediatría, Avenida IMAN no. 1, Torre de Investigación, Colonia Insurgentes Cuicuilco, Coyoacán, México D.F, Mexico. [4]Laboratorio GENETADI, Bilbao, Spain. [5]Departamento de Medicina Genómica y Toxicología Ambiental. Instituto de Investigaciones Biomédicas, UNAM, Avenida IMAN no. 1, Torre de Investigación, Colonia Insurgentes Cuicuilco, Coyoacán. Ciudad de México, CDMX., México D.F, Mexico.

**References**

1. Stern AM, Gall JC Jr, Perry BL, Stimson CW, Weitkamp LR, Poznanski AK. The hand-foot-uterus syndrome: a new hereditary disorder characterized by hand and foot dysplasia, dermatoglyphic abnormalities, and partial duplication of the female genital tract. J Pediatr. 1970;77:109–16.
2. Mortlock DP, Innis JW. Mutation of HOXA13 in hand-foot-genital syndrome. Nat Genet. 1997;15:179–80. 10.1038/ng0297-179.
3. Goodman FR, Bacchelli C, Brady AF, Brueton LA, Fryns JP, Mortlock DP, et al. Novel HOXA13 mutations and the phenotypic spectrum of hand-foot-genital syndrome. Am J Hum Genet. 2000;67:197–202.
4. Debeer P, Bacchelli C, Scambler PJ, De Smet L, Fryns JP, Goodman FR. Severe digital abnormalities in a patient heterozygous for both a novel missense mutation in HOXD13 and a polyalanine tract expansion in HOXA13. J Med Genet. 2002;39:852–6.
5. Utsch B, Becker K, Brock D, Lentze MJ, Bidlingmaier F, Ludwig M. A novel stable polyalanine [poly(a)] expansion in the HOXA13 gene associated with hand-foot-genital syndrome: proper function of poly(a)-harbouring transcription factors depends on a critical repeat length? Hum Genet. 2002;110:488–94.
6. Frisén L, Lagerstedt K, Tapper-Persson M, Kockum I, Nordenskjöld A. A novel duplication in the HOXA13 gene in a family with atypical hand-foot-genital syndrome. J Med Genet. 2003;40:e49. 10.1136/jmg.40.4.e49.
7. Innis JW, Mortlock D, Chen Z, Ludwig M, Williams ME, Williams TM, et al. Polyalanine expansion in HOXA13: three new affected families and the molecular consequences in a mouse model. Hum Mol Genet. 2004;13:2841–51.
8. Jorgensen EM, Ruman JI, Doherty L, Taylor HS. A novel mutation of HOXA13 in a family with hand-foot-genital syndrome and the role of polyalanine expansions in the spectrum of Müllerian fusion anomalies. Fertil Steril. 2010;94:1235–8. 10.1016/j.fertnstert.2009.05.057.
9. Devriendt K, Jaeken J, Matthijs G, Van Esch H, Debeer P, Gewillig M, Fryns JP. Haploinsufficiency of the HOXA gene cluster, in a patient with hand-foot-genital syndrome, velopharyngeal insufficiency, and persistent patent Ductus botalli. Am J Hum Genet. 1999;65:249–51.
10. Parker L, Mangwani J, Wakeling E, Singh D. Hallux valgus interphalangeus and a novel mutation in HOXA13. Part of the broadening spectrum of hand-foot-genital syndrome. Foot Ankle Surg. 2011;17:e28–30. 10.1016/j.fas.2010.12.003.
11. Wallis M, Tsurusaki Y, Burgess T, Borzi P, Matsumoto N, Miyake N2, True D, Patel C. Dual genetic diagnoses: atypical hand-foot-genital syndrome and developmental delay due to de novo mutations in HOXA13 and NRXN1. Am J Med Genet A. 2016;170:717–24. 10.1002/ajmg.a.37478.
12. Imagawa E, Kayserili H, Nishimura G, Nakashima M, Tsurusaki Y, Saitsu H, Ikegawa S, Matsumoto N, Miyake N. Severe manifestations of hand-foot-genital syndrome associated with a novel HOXA13 mutation. Am J Med Genet A. 2014;164A:2398–402. 10.1002/ajmg.a.36648.
13. Tas E, Sebastian J, Madan-Khetarpal S, Sweet P, Yatsenko AN, Pollock N, et al. Familial deletion of the HOXA gene cluster associated with hand-foot-genital syndrome and phenotypic variability. Am J Med Genet A. 2017;173:221–4. 10.1002/ajmg.a.37981.
14. Quinonez SC, Innis JW. Human HOX gene disorders. Mol Genet Metab. 2014;111:4–15. 10.1016/j.ymgme.2013.10.012.
15. Watson CM, Crinnion LA, Harrison SM, Lascelles C, Antanaviciute A, Carr IM, Bonthron DT, Sheridan E. Chromosome 7 Pericentric inversion defined at single-nucleotide resolution using diagnostic whole genome sequencing in a patient with hand-foot- genital syndrome. PLoS One. 2016;11:e0157075. 10.1371/journal.pone.0157075.
16. Pezzani L, Milani D, Manzoni F, Baccarin M, Silipigni R, Guerneri S, Esposito S. HOXA genes cluster: clinical implications of the smallest deletion. Ital J Pediatr. 2015;41:31. 10.1186/s13052-015-0137-3.
17. Hosoki K, Ohta T, Fujita K, Nishigaki S, Shiomi M, Niikawa N, Saitoh S. Hand-foot-genital syndrome with a 7p15 deletion: clinically recognizable syndrome. Pediatr Int. 2012;54:e22–5. 10.1111/j.1442-200X.2011.03550.x.
18. Dunø M, Hove H, Kirchhoff M, Devriendt K, Schwartz M. Mapping genomic deletions down to the base: a quantitative copy number scanning approach used to characterise and clone the breakpoints of a recurrent 7p14.2p15.3 deletion. Hum Genet. 2004;115:459–67.
19. Kosaki R, Higuchi M, Mitsui N, Matsushima K, Ohashi H, Kosaki K. Deletion involving the *TWIST* locus and the *HOXA* cluster: a contiguous gene syndrome on 7p? Congenit Anom. 2005;45:35–8.
20. Jun KR, Seo EJ, Lee JO, Yoo HW, Park IS, Yoon HK. Molecular cytogenetic and clinical characterization of a patient with a 5.6-Mb deletion in 7p15 including HOXA cluster. Am J Med Genet A. 2011;155:642–7.
21. Fryssira H, Makrythanasis P, Kattamis A, Stokidis K, Menten B, Kosaki K, Willems P, Kanavakis E. Severe developmental delay in a patient with 7p21.

1-p14.3 microdeletion spanning the *TWIST* gene and the *HOXA* gene cluster. Mol Syndromol. 2011;2:45–9.
22. UCSC Genome Browser Database. https://genome.ucsc.edu/cgi-bin/hgTracks?db=hg19&lastVirtModeType=default&lastVirtModeExtraState=&virtModeType=default&virtMode=0&nonVirtPosition=&position=chr7%3A26706135-27290892&hgsid=598513081_4nTQV0mYW5UIO52GaWMNBnraE8RI. Accessed 5 jun 2017.
23. NCBI Gene Database. https://www.ncbi.nlm.nih.gov/gene?cmd=Retrieve&dopt=full_report&list_uids=7182. Accessed 5 jun 2017.
24. Foucher I, Volovitch M, Frain M, Kim JJ, Souberbielle JC, Gan L, Unterman TG, Prochiantz A, Trembleau A. Hoxa5 overexpression correlates with IGFBP1 upregulation and postnatal dwarfism: evidence for an interaction between Hoxa5 and Forkhead box transcription factors. Development. 2002;129:4065–74.
25. Torres L, Juárez U, García L, Miranda-Ríos J, Frias S. External ear microRNA expression profiles during mouse development. Int J Dev Biol. 2015;59:497–503. https://doi.org/10.1387/ijdb.150124sf.
26. Trainor PA, Krumlauf R. Hox genes, neural crest cells and branchial arch patterning. Curr Opin Cell Biol. 2001;13:698–705.
27. Barrow JR, Stadler HS, Capecchi MR. Roles of Hoxa1 and Hoxa2 in patterning the early hindbrain of the mouse. Development. 2000;127:933–44.
28. O'Gorman S. Second branchial arch lineages of the middle ear of wild-type and Hoxa2 mutant mice. Dev Dyn. 2005;234:124–31.
29. Qiao R, He Y, Pan B, Xiao S, Zhang X, Li J, et al. Understanding the molecular mechanisms of human microtia via a pig model of HOXA1 syndrome. Dis Model Mech. 2015;8:611–22. 10.1242/dmm.018291.
30. Minoux M, Kratochwil CF, Ducret S, Amin S, Kitazawa T, Kurihara H, et al. Mouse Hoxa2 mutations provide a model for microtia and auricle duplication. Development. 2013;140:4386–97. 10.1242/dev.098046.

# 33

# Down syndrome phenotype in a boy with a mosaic microduplication of chromosome 21q22

Franziska Schnabel[1*], Mateja Smogavec[1], Rudolf Funke[2], Silke Pauli[1], Peter Burfeind[1] and Iris Bartels[1]

**Abstract**

**Background:** Down syndrome, typically caused by trisomy 21, may also be associated by duplications of the Down syndrome critical region (DSCR) on chromosome 21q22. However, patients with small duplications of DSCR without accompanying deletions have rarely been reported.

**Case presentation:** Here we report a 5½-year-old boy with clinical features of Down syndrome including distinct craniofacial dysmorphism and sandal gaps as well as developmental delay. Conventional karyotype was normal, whereas interphase FISH analysis revealed three signals for DSCR in approximately 40% of lymphocytes and 80% of buccal mucosa cells. Array-CGH analysis confirmed a 2.56 Mb duplication of chromosome 21q22.13q22.2 encompassing *DYRK1A*.

**Conclusion:** This presents one of the smallest duplications within DSCR leading to a Down syndrome phenotype. Since the dosage sensitive gene *DYRK1A* is the only duplicated candidate DSCR gene in our patient, this finding supports the hypothesis that *DYRK1A* contributes to dysmorphic and intellectual features of Down syndrome even in a mosaic state.

**Keywords:** Down syndrome, Down syndrome critical region, Microduplication, Mosaicism, *DYRK1A*

## Background

Down syndrome (DS), typically caused by complete trisomy 21, is associated with a wide range of clinical phenotypes including cognitive deficits, craniofacial dysmorphism, neurological, cardiovascular, immunological defects as well as ophthalmologic and hearing problems. DS is acknowledged as a gene dosage disease where overexpression of genes located on chromosome 21 distorts the balance of gene products. It has been known for decades that not the complete duplicated chromosomal region in trisomy 21 patients contributes equally to the DS phenotype. Particularly genotype-phenotype studies on partial trisomies performed by Sinet et al. [1] revealed that the genes which are essential in producing the main DS features cluster within a relatively small region in chromosomal bands 21q22.2q22.3. The minimum extent of this Down Syndrome Critical Region (DSCR), however, has been a matter of discussion. Until the year 2000, the technical options to establish a genotype-phenotype correlation were limited to targeted analyses and methods of restricted resolution, e.g. fluorescence in situ hybridization (FISH). Today, whole-genome array technologies allow to perform high-resolution breakpoint mapping and to rule out complex imbalances. DS patients with microduplications without concomitant imbalances are extremely rare. Here, we describe a 5½-year-old boy with a 21q22.13q22.2 microduplication in a mosaic state and distinctive clinical features of DS.

* Correspondence: franziska.schnabel@med.uni-goettingen.de
[1]Institute of Human Genetics, University Medical Center, Heinrich-Düker-Weg 12, 37073 Göttingen, Germany
Full list of author information is available at the end of the article

### Case presentation

A 5½-year-old boy was referred to clinical genetic service for evaluation concerning DS. The patient is the first child of healthy non-consanguineous parents. His mother was 28 years old and his father was 31 years old when he was born. His younger sister showed no clinical abnormalities. The patient was born by vaginal delivery after a 9-week period of premature labor at 37 weeks of gestation with a birth weight of 3290 g (70th centile), length of 50 cm (50th centile) and occipitofrontal circumference of 32.5 cm (10th centile). Postnatally, the patient presented with muscular hypotonia, hyperopia and astigmatism. Throughout the first years a significant developmental delay was observed.

Kiphard developmental test [2] was performed at the age of 36 months and 58 months in order to evaluate the stage of development at different levels. Optical perception was estimated as age-appropriate at both time points (39/36 and 58/58 months), whereas a delayed developmental age was observed in speech (34/36 and 45/58 months), auditory perception (35/36 and 42/58 months) and social contact (37/36 and 47/58 months). The most recent testing performed in the department of neuropediatrics at 6 years of age by Wechsler Preschool and Primary Scale of Intelligence (wppsi-III) showed a low-average overall IQ of 80. However, there were significant differences regarding specific abilities as expressive speech (VT-IQ = 88) reached just average score, whereas the ability to reason (HT-IQ = 81) and the processing speed (VG-IQ = 60) were in the low-average range. Motor development was quite normal, as he walked with support at 16 months and freely at 20 months. Echocardiography showed no abnormalities with a fractional shortening of 42%. At the age of 5½ years, his height was 113 cm (30th centile), his weight was 20.2 kg (50th centile) and his head circumference was 51 cm (25th centile). The patient presented with craniofacial dysmorphism including posterior plagiocephaly, flat face, epicanthus, upslanted palpebral fissures and anteverted nares (Fig. 1a). Furthermore he has a fused left upper lateral incisor and maxillary canine as well as sandal gaps.

## Methods

The karyotype of the patient was ascertained by standard cytogenetic analysis. Metaphase and interphase FISH analyses were performed using a DNA probe LSI 21 that binds to the DSCR region (21q22.13q22.2) and LSI13 RB1(13q14) as a control (Vysis, Abbott Molecular). The distribution of mosaicism was investigated on nuclei preparations from lymphocytes and non-cultured buccal cells by cohybridization of the two probes.

Genomic DNA was extracted from EDTA peripheral blood samples from the patient and his parents. The trio was investigated by microarray typing. Array comparative genomic hybridization (array-CGH) was performed on genomic DNA using the Human Genome 180 K CGH Microarray (Agilent Technologies, Waldbronn, Germany) according to the manufacturer's recommendations. The results were scanned with the SureScan Dx Microarray scanner G5761A (Agilent Technologies, USA). Image analysis was carried out using the Feature Extraction Software V10.7 (Agilent Technologies, USA) and data analysis was performed using Cytogenomics V2.9.2.4 (Agilent Technologies, USA). Interpretation was based on Human Genome Assembly 37 (GRCh37/hg19).

## Results

Conventional chromosome analysis showed no numerical or structural aberration. Due to the persistent indication of DS, FISH was performed using a commercial DSCR-specific DNA probe. In approximately half of the metaphases a duplication was detected in the same cytogenetic band (karyotype: 46,XY.ish dup(21)(q22.13q22.2)(DSCR++)). Interphase FISH revealed a mosaic pattern with three signals for DSCR in approximately 40% of lymphocytes and in approximately 80% of buccal mucosa cells (Fig. 1c).

Array-CGH analysis detected a duplication at 21q22.13q22.2, spanning about 2.56 Mb (arr[GRCh37] 21q22.13q22.2(38668355_41187454)× 3 dn) (Fig. 1b), which was confirmed by qPCR. The duplication encompassed 15 OMIM genes (*DYRK1A*, *KCNJ6*, *DSCR4*, *DSCR8*, *KCNJ15*, *ERG*, *LINC00114*, *ETS2*, *PSMG1*, *BRWD1*, *HMGN1*, *WRB*, *SH3BGR*, *B3GALT5* and *IGSF5*). The duplication was not found in the parents of the patient.

## Discussion

In trisomy 21, not all loci are necessarily duplicated for the manifestation of DS. The concept of a DSCR on chromosome 21 is almost 30 years old [3]. Many studies were performed to define the minimum DSCR and identify those genes or contiguous genes whose overexpression provokes particular features of DS. It seems that duplications on chromosome 21 proximal from approximately 31 Mb [4] and distal from approximately 43 Mb [5] are not related to an abnormal phenotype.

Delabar et al. [6] narrowed down the critical region on chromosome 21q to a region between markers D21S17 and MX1, corresponding to approximately 35.89–41.72 Mb, whereas Lyle et al. [7] identified a minimum region of 37.94–38.64 Mb encompassing the genes *KCNJ6*, *DSCR4* and *KCNJ15* and a second one from the centromere to 26.96 Mb related to intellectual disability.

Most of the phenotype-genotype data for partial trisomy 21 were collected at pre-array days when additional imbalances due to unbalanced reciprocal translocations could not be ruled out [7, 8]. In this discussion, we focus on patients with pure microduplication of less than 5 Mb in size, which were investigated by array-CGH. All chromosomal coordinates were transformed to GRCh37(hg19). Microduplications with their respective sizes are summarized in Table 1. In addition to our patient, two other corresponding microduplications of chromosome 21q with a DS phenotype could be found in the literature [9, 10]. Furthermore, two microduplications of chromosome 21q without a DS phenotype have also been reported [11, 12]. Within the range of microduplication in 21q22 the physical size of the duplicated region itself does not seem to play a major role. While mother and daughter reported by Ronan et al. [9] show DS appearance and learning disabilities, mother and daughter reported by Su et al. [12] do not show this disease phenotype. Both families present with a 4.4 to 4.5 Mb duplication. Instead, the implementation of specific genes in the duplicated region is relevant for the phenotype.

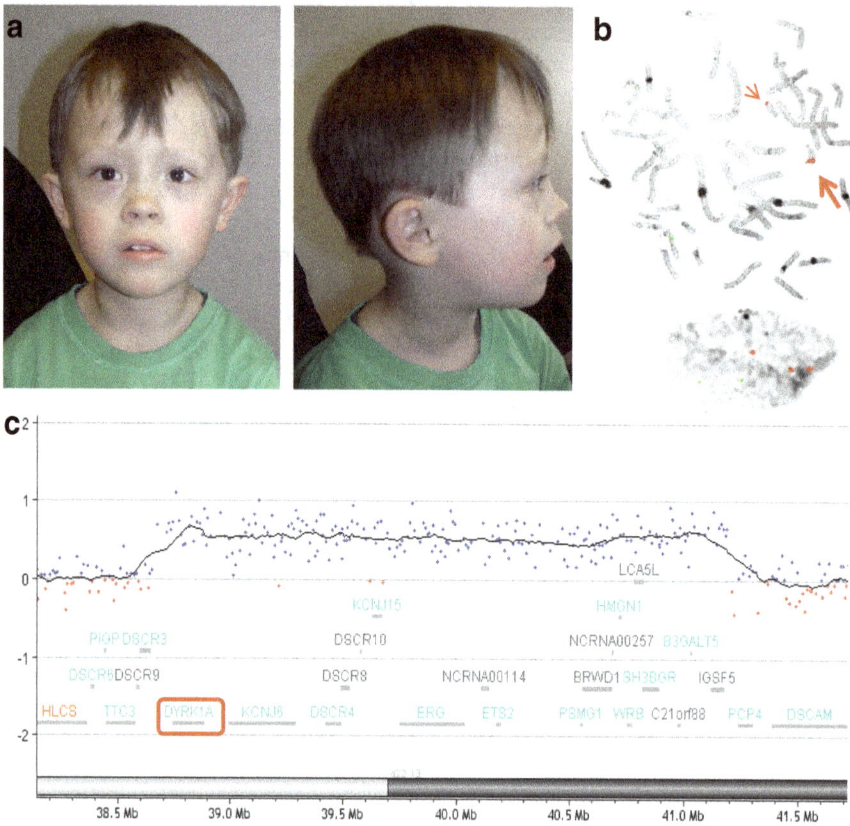


**Fig. 1** The facial appearance, FISH results and array CGH profile for the patient. **a** Frontal and lateral view of the patient at the age of 5½ years displays some distinctive clinical features of DS including posterior plagiocephaly, flat face, epicanthus, upslanted palpebral fissures and anteverted nares. **b** FISH result on metaphase spreads and interphase preparation using a probe for DSCR on chromosome 21 (orange signals) and RB-1 as a control probe on chromosome 13 (green). The fluorescence signal on one chromosome 21 is stronger as compared to the signal on the other chromosome 21 (arrows). Three orange signals for chromosome 21 are visible on interphase nuclei. **c** Array CGH result (Agilent, 180 K array). Zoom view of the 2.56 Mb mosaic microduplication and gene content at 21q22.13q22.2 encompassing *DYRK1A* (red box) as duplicated candidate DSCR gene

Candidate genes for the key clinical features of DS (classical DSCR) are *APP, DSCR1 (RCAN1), DYRK1A* and *DSCAM* [1, 6]. Our patient presented with a 2.56 Mb microduplication in the 21q22.13q22.2 region in a mosaic state which overlaps in part with the distal region of the 4.3 Mb microduplication in the three members of a family described by Ronan et al. [9]. Both microduplications encompass *DYRK1A* but none of the other classical DSCR genes (Fig. 1b and Table 1). The four patients share similar DS dysmorphic features and mild intellectual disability but no cardiac or other malformations.

*DYRK1A* (Dual Specificity Tyrosine Phosphorylation Regulated Kinase 1A) is a highly conserved proline-directed protein kinase with multiple domains, a high substrate diversity and known to be involved in neuronal processes [13, 14]. From mice data it was proposed that *DYRK1A* contributes together with *DSCR1* to the typical DS phenotype only in a synergistic way [15]. In both, the family

**Table 1** Summary of reported patients with pure microduplications 21q22.13q22.2 (< 5 Mb)

| Publication | Size (Mb) | Segregation | DS phenotype | *APP* | *DSCR1* | *DYRK1A* | *DSCAM* |
|---|---|---|---|---|---|---|---|
| This Case | 2.56 | De novo | + | – | – | + | – |
| Ronan et al., 2007 | 4.3 | Inherited from affected mother | + | – | – | + | – |
| Weisfeld-Adams et al., 2016 | 2.78 | De novo | + | – | – | – | – |
| Eggermann et al., 2010 | 0.46 | Inherited from healthy father | – | – | + | – | – |
| Su et al., 2006 (Case 1) | 4.4 | Inherited from healthy mother | – | – | – | – | – |

Duplicated (+) and non-duplicated (–) classical DSCR genes (Delabar et al., [6]; Sinet et al., [1])

studied by Ronan et al. [9] and our patient with DS phenotype, only *DYRK1A* is duplicated, but not *DSCR1*. Thus, the duplication of *DYRK1A* alone seems to be sufficient to impair normal intellectual development in those two families. *DYRK1A* belongs to the haploinsufficient genes on chromosome 21, meaning that loss-of-function mutations in *DYRK1A* can lead to a dominant form of intellectual disability [16]. On the assumption that haploinsufficient genes are sensitive to overexpression in partial trisomy, *DYRK1A* is a candidate gene for the intellectual phenotype in DS [17]. Overexpression of *DYRK1A* in transgenic mice induces dramatic deficits of serotonin levels in the brain [18] and has been shown to contribute to DS craniofacial dysmorphology [19].

All these findings on *DYRK1A* suggest that certain kinase inhibitors, such as polyphenol epigallocatechin-3-gallate, feature potential pharmacotherapy for cognitive impairment in DS. There are already therapeutic attempts and even clinical trials for the evaluation of *DYRK1A* kinase inhibitors [19–21]. Children with a microduplication involving *DYRK1A* such as described in our patient and the patients reported by Ronan et al. [9] could benefit from the development of new therapeutic options.

However, the pathogenesis of DS cannot be simply reduced to *DYRK1A*. Weisfeld-Adams et al. [10] reported a child with intellectual disability and distinct dysmorphic features of DS without heart defect. Array-CGH revealed a de novo 2.78 Mb microduplication on chromosome 21q22.11 involving none of the DSCR candidate genes. This duplication does not overlap with the duplicated region in our patient. This supports the hypothesis that more than the duplication of a single gene is causative for the DS phenotype. It seems that also other genes or other mechanisms contribute to the pathogenesis of DS. As further candidate genes, Weisfeld-Adams et al. [10] suggested *SOD1*, *SYNJ1* and/or *ITSN1*, which were included in the duplicated region in their patient.

In our patient the microduplication on chromosome 21q was present in a mosaic state. Mosaicism for trisomy 21 has been known since decades [22]. It has been even proposed that a low-grade mosaicism of trisomy 21 is present in the general population without any phenotypical resemblance of DS. Furthermore, the incidence of both, trisomy and microdeletions/-duplications in different tissues are underestimated and may contribute to different medical problems [23]. To our knowledge a mosaic microduplication with a DS phenotype has not been reported to date. The mosaic pattern of trisomic cells in our patient had a ratio of approximately 40% in lymphocytes and approximately 80% in buccal mucosa cells. A phenotype-genotype study showed that the trisomy level in mucosa cells is strongly correlated with phenotypic findings of ectodermal origin, whereas the trisomy level in lymphocytes is associated with heart malformations [24]. This might explain the intellectual impairment without heart phenotype in our patient.

## Conclusion

In summary, to the best of our knowledge this is the first report on a patient with a DS phenotype resulting from mosaicism for a microduplication of chromosome 21q. Since *DYRK1A* is the only duplicated candidate DSCR gene in our patient, this result reinforces the hypothesis that *DYRK1A* duplication contributes essentially to the intellectual phenotype even in a mosaic state. Current progress in the development of drugs such as *DYRK1A* kinase inhibitors may provide promising therapeutic options for such patients.

### Abbreviations

CGH: Comparative genome hybridization; DS: Down syndrome; DSCR: Down syndrome critical region; DYRK1A: Dual Specificity Tyrosine Phosphorylation Regulated Kinase 1A; FISH: Fluorescence in situ hybridization

### Acknowledgements

We thank the patient and his family for their interest and support.

### Funding

We acknowledge support by the German Research Foundation and the Open Access Publication Funds of the Goettingen University. No further funding was received.

### Authors' contributions

RF and FS contributed to clinical evaluation. MS, FS and SP counselled the parents. IB, BP and MS performed genetic testing and interpretation. FS, MS and IB structured and drafted the manuscript. All authors read and approved the final manuscript.

### Competing interests

The authors declare that they have no competing interests.

### Author details

[1]Institute of Human Genetics, University Medical Center, Heinrich-Düker-Weg 12, 37073 Göttingen, Germany. [2]Department of Neuropediatrics, Sozialpädiatrisches Zentrum, Mönchebergstr. 41-43, 34125 Kassel, Germany.

### References

1. Sinet PM, Théophile D, Rahmani Z, Chettouh Z, Blouin JL, Prieur M, et al. Mapping of the Down syndrome phenotype on chromosome 21 at the molecular level. Biomed Pharmacother. 1994;48(5–6):247–52.
2. Kiphard EJ. Wie weit ist ein Kind entwickelt. 12th ed. Verlag modernes lernen: Dortmund; 2006.
3. Rahmani Z, Blouin JL, Créau-Goldberg N, Watkins PC, Mattei JF, Poissonnier M, et al. Down syndrome critical region around D21S55 on proximal 21q22. 3. Am J Med Gen. 1990;7:98–103.
4. Capkova P, Misovicova N, Vrbicka D. Partial trisomy and tetrasomy of chromosome 21 without Down syndrome phenotype and short overview of genotype-phenotype correlation. A case report. Biomed Pap Med Fac Univ Palacky Olomouc Czech Repub. 2014;158(2):321–5.
5. Gijsbers ACJ, van Haeringen A, Bosch CAJ, Hansson K, Verschuren M, Bakker E, et al. A subtle familial translocation t(3;21)(p26.3;q22.3): an apparently healthy boy with a 3p deletion and 21q duplication. Cytogenetic Genome Res. 2010;128(4):245–9.

6. Delabar JM, Theophile D, Rahmani Z, Chettouh Z, Blouin JL, Prieur M, et al. Molecular mapping of twenty-four features of Down syndrome on chromosome 21. Eur J Hum Gen. 1993;1(2):114–24.
7. Lyle R, Béna F, Gagos S, Gehrig C, Lopez G, Schinzel A, et al. Genotype-phenotype correlations in Down syndrome identified by array CGH in 30 cases of partial trisomy and partial monosomy chromosome 21. Eur J Hum Gen. 2009;17(4):454–66.
8. Pelleri MC, Cicchini E, Locatelli C, Vitale L, Caracausi M, Piovesan A, et al. Systematic reanalysis of partial trisomy 21 cases with or without Down syndrome suggests a small region on 21q22.13 as critical to the phenotype. Hum Mol Genet. 2016;25(12):2525–38.
9. Ronan A, Fagan K, Christie L, Conroy J, Nowak NJ, Turner G. Familial 4.3 Mb duplication of 21q22 sheds new light on the Down syndrome critical region. J Med Genet. 2007;44(7):448–51.
10. Weisfeld-Adams JD, Edelmann L, Gadi IK, Mehta L. Phenotypic heterogeneity in a family with a small atypical microduplication of chromosome 22q11.2 involving TBX1. Eur J Hum Gen. 2012;55(12):732–6.
11. Eggermann T, Schönherr N, Spengler S, Jäger S, Denecke B, Binder G, et al. Identification of a 21q22 duplication in a silver-Russell syndrome patient further narrows Down the Down syndrome critical region. Am J Med Gen A. 2010;152A(2):356–9.
12. Su M-T, Kuan L-C, Chou Y-Y, Tan S-Y, Kuo T-C, Kuo P-L. Partial trisomy of chromosome 21 without the Down syndrome phenotype. Prenat Diagn. 2016;36(5):492–5.
13. Dowjat WK, Adayev T, Kuchna I, Nowicki K, Palminiello S, Hwang YW, Wegiel J. Trisomy-driven overexpression of DYRK1A kinase in the brain of subjects with Down syndrome. Neurosci Lett. 2007;413(1):77–81.
14. Park J, Song W-J, Chung KC. Function and regulation of Dyrk1A: towards understanding Down syndrome. Cell Mol Life Sci. 2009;66(20):3235–40.
15. Arron JR, Winslow MM, Polleri A, Chang CP, Wu H, Gao X, et al. NFAT dysregulation by increased dosage of DSCR1 and DYRK1A on chromosome 21. Nature. 2006;441(7093):595–600.
16. Ji J, Lee H, Argiropoulos B, Dorrani N, Mann J, Martinez-Agosto JA, et al. DYRK1A haploinsufficiency causes a new recognizable syndrome with microcephaly, intellectual disability, speech impairment, and distinct facies. Eur J Hum Gen. 2015;23(11):1473–81.
17. Antonarakis SE. Down syndrome and the complexity of genome dosage imbalance. Nat Rev Genet. 2017;18(3):147–63.
18. London J, Rouch C, Bui LC, Assayag E, Souchet B, Daubigney F, et al. Overexpression of the DYRK1A gene (dual-specificity tyrosine phosphorylation-regulated kinase 1A) induces alterations of the serotoninergic and dopaminergic processing in murine brain tissues. Mol Neurobiol. 2018;55(5):3822–31.
19. McElyea SD, Starbuck JM, Tumbleson-Brink DM, Harrington E, Blazek JD, Ghoneima A, et al. Influence of prenatal EGCG treatment and Dyrk1a dosage reduction on craniofacial features associated with Down syndrome. Hum Mol Genet. 2016;25(22):4856–69.
20. de la Torre R, de Sola S, Hernandez G, Farré M, Pujol J, Rodriguez J, et al. Safety and efficacy of cognitive training plus epigallocatechin-3-gallate in young adults with Down's syndrome (TESDAD): a double-blind, randomised, placebo-controlled, phase 2 trial. Lancet Neurol. 2016;15(8):801–10.
21. Stringer M, Goodlett CR, Roper RJ. Targeting trisomic treatments: optimizing Dyrk1a inhibition to improve Down syndrome deficits. Mol Genet Genomic Med. 2017;5(5):451–65.
22. Clarke CM, Edwards JH, Smallpeice V. 21-trisomy/normal mosaicism in an intelligent child with some mongoloid characters. Lancet. 1961;1(7185): 1028–30.
23. Hulten MA, Jonasson J, Iwarsson E, Uppal P, Vorsanova SG, Yurov YB, et al. Trisomy 21 mosaicism: we may all have a touch of Down syndrome. Cytogenet Genome Res. 2013;139:189–92.
24. Papavassiliou P, York TP, Gursoy N, Hill G, Nicely LV, Sundaram U, et al. The phenotype of persons having mosaicism for trisomy 21/Down syndrome reflects the percentage of trisomic cells present in different tissues. Am J Med Gen A. 2009;149A(4):573–83.

# Permissions

All chapters in this book were first published in MC, by BioMed Central; hereby published with permission under the Creative Commons Attribution License or equivalent. Every chapter published in this book has been scrutinized by our experts. Their significance has been extensively debated. The topics covered herein carry significant findings which will fuel the growth of the discipline. They may even be implemented as practical applications or may be referred to as a beginning point for another development.

The contributors of this book come from diverse backgrounds, making this book a truly international effort. This book will bring forth new frontiers with its revolutionizing research information and detailed analysis of the nascent developments around the world.

We would like to thank all the contributing authors for lending their expertise to make the book truly unique. They have played a crucial role in the development of this book. Without their invaluable contributions this book wouldn't have been possible. They have made vital efforts to compile up to date information on the varied aspects of this subject to make this book a valuable addition to the collection of many professionals and students.

This book was conceptualized with the vision of imparting up-to-date information and advanced data in this field. To ensure the same, a matchless editorial board was set up. Every individual on the board went through rigorous rounds of assessment to prove their worth. After which they invested a large part of their time researching and compiling the most relevant data for our readers.

The editorial board has been involved in producing this book since its inception. They have spent rigorous hours researching and exploring the diverse topics which have resulted in the successful publishing of this book. They have passed on their knowledge of decades through this book. To expedite this challenging task, the publisher supported the team at every step. A small team of assistant editors was also appointed to further simplify the editing procedure and attain best results for the readers.

Apart from the editorial board, the designing team has also invested a significant amount of their time in understanding the subject and creating the most relevant covers. They scrutinized every image to scout for the most suitable representation of the subject and create an appropriate cover for the book.

The publishing team has been an ardent support to the editorial, designing and production team. Their endless efforts to recruit the best for this project, has resulted in the accomplishment of this book. They are a veteran in the field of academics and their pool of knowledge is as vast as their experience in printing. Their expertise and guidance has proved useful at every step. Their uncompromising quality standards have made this book an exceptional effort. Their encouragement from time to time has been an inspiration for everyone.

The publisher and the editorial board hope that this book will prove to be a valuable piece of knowledge for researchers, students, practitioners and scholars across the globe.

# List of Contributors

**Ilse P. J. van Heel, Malgorzata I. Srebniak, Laura J. C. M. van Zutven, Diane Van Opstal and Karin E. M. Diderich**
Department of Clinical Genetics, Erasmus MC, Ee2475, Wytemaweg 80, 3015 CN Rotterdam, The Netherlands

**Florence Petit**
Department of Clinical Genetics, University Hospital, Lille, France

**Sonia Bouquillon**
Department of Cytogenetics, University Hospital, Lille, France

**Jerome M. J. Cornette**
Department of Obstetrics and Gynecology, subdivision Obstetrics and Prenatal Medicine, Erasmus MC, Rotterdam, The Netherlands

**Maarten F. C. M. Knapen**
Department of Obstetrics and Gynecology, subdivision Obstetrics and Prenatal Medicine, Erasmus MC, Rotterdam, The Netherlands
Stichting Prenatale Screening Zuidwest Nederland, Wytemaweg 80, Na-1509, 3015GE Na-1503 Rotterdam, The Netherlands

**Andreas Kremer**
Department of Bioinformatics Erasmus MC, Rotterdam, The Netherlands

**Siying Liang, Nan Jiang, Shuo Li and Dongyi Yu**
Genetic Testing Center, Qingdao Women and Children's Hospital, Qingdao University, #217, Liaoyangxi Road, Qingdao 266034, China

**Xiaohu Jiang**
Qingdao Women and Children's Hospital, Qingdao University, Qingdao, China

**Malgorzata I. Srebniak, Karin E. M. Diderich, Lutgarde C. P. Govaerts, Marieke Joosten, Marnix J. Bos, Gerda A. G. Looye-Bruinsma, Mieke Koningen, Robert Jan H. Galjaard and Diane Van Opstal**
Department of Clinical Genetics, Erasmus Medical Center, Wytemaweg 80, 3015, CN, Rotterdam, The Netherlands

**Attie T. J. I. Go and Merel C. de Wit**
Department of Obstetrics and Gynecology, Erasmus Medical Center, Wytemaweg 80, 3015, CN, Rotterdam, The Netherlands

**Maarten F. C. M. Knapen**
Department of Obstetrics and Gynecology, Erasmus Medical Center, Wytemaweg 80, 3015, CN, Rotterdam, The Netherlands
Foundation Prenatal Screening Southwest region of The Netherlands, Wytemaweg 80, Na-1509, 3015, CN, Rotterdam, The Netherlands

**Arianna Tucci, Claudia Ciaccio, Giulietta Scuvera, Susanna Esposito and Donatella Milani**
Pediatric Highly Intensive Care Unit, Department of Pathophysiology and Transplantation, Università degli Studi di Milano, Fondazione IRCCS Ca' Granda Ospedale Maggiore Policlinico, Via Commenda 9, 20122 Milano, Italy

**Donia Mili, Kaouthar Abid, Imed Rjiba and Abderraouf Kenani**
UR 12ES08 "Signalisation Cellulaire et Pathologies" Faculté de Médecine Monastir, Université de Monastir, Monastir, Tunisie

**Jing Liu, Hao Hu, Na Ma, Zhengjun Jia, Yuchun Zhou, Jiancheng Hu and Hua Wang**
Prenatal Diagnosis Center of Province Hunan, The Maternal and Child Health Care Hospital of Hunan province, Changsha, Hunan 410008, People's Republic of China

**Zhishuo Ou, Sally J. Kochmar and Shafagh Parsazad**
Center for Clinical Genetics and Genomics, Pittsburgh Cytogenetics Laboratory, Magee-Womens Hospital of UPMC, Pittsburgh, PA 15213, USA

**Jie Hu**
Center for Clinical Genetics and Genomics, Pittsburgh Cytogenetics Laboratory, Magee-Womens Hospital of UPMC, Pittsburgh, PA 15213, USA
Department of Obstetrics, Gynecology & Reproductive Sciences, University of Pittsburgh School of Medicine, Pittsburgh, PA 15213, USA

**Elena Infante and Suneeta Madan-Khetarpal**
Department of Genetics, Children's Hospital of Pittsburgh of UPMC, Pittsburgh, PA 15224, USA

**Lori Hoffner**
Department of Pathology, University of Pittsburgh School of Medicine, Pittsburgh, PA 15213, USA

**Urvashi Surti**
Center for Clinical Genetics and Genomics, Pittsburgh Cytogenetics Laboratory, Magee-Womens Hospital of UPMC, Pittsburgh, PA 15213, USA
Department of Obstetrics, Gynecology & Reproductive Sciences, University of Pittsburgh School of Medicine, Pittsburgh, PA 15213, USA
Department of Pathology, University of Pittsburgh School of Medicine, Pittsburgh, PA 15213, USA

**Bárbara Marques, Cristina Ferreira, Filomena Brito, Sónia Pedro, Cristina Alves and Hildeberto Correia**
Unidade de Citogenética, Departamento de Genética Humana, Instituto Nacional de Saúde Doutor Ricardo Jorge, I.P, Avenida Padre Cruz, 1649-016 Lisboa, Portugal

**Teresa Lourenço and Marta Amorim**
Serviço de Genética Médica, Hospital de Dona Estefânia, Centro Hospitalar de Lisboa Central, Rua Jacinta Marto, 1169-045 Lisboa, Portugal

**Anna Poluha and Ilona Jaszczuk**
Department of Pediatric Hematology, Oncology and Transplantation Children's University Hospital, Lublin, Poland

**Joanna Bernaciak, Marta Kędzior and Beata Anna Nowakowska**
Department of Medical Genetics, Cytogenetics, Institute of Mother and Child, Kasprzaka 17, A 01-211 Warsaw, Poland

**Kyungsoo Ha**
Department of Molecular Physiology and Biophysics, Baylor College of Medicine, Houston, TX 77030, USA
Section of Reproductive Endocrinology, Infertility & Genetics, Department of Obstetrics & Gynecology, Augusta University, Augusta, GA 30912, USA

**Tyler Graves**
Section of Reproductive Endocrinology, Infertility & Genetics, Department of Obstetrics & Gynecology, Augusta University, Augusta, GA 30912, USA

**Yiping Shen**
Department of Neurology, Massachusetts General Hospital, Harvard Medical School, Boston, MA 02114, USA

**Hyung-Goo Kim**
Section of Reproductive Endocrinology, Infertility & Genetics, Department of Obstetrics & Gynecology, Augusta University, Augusta, GA 30912, USA
Department of Neuroscience and Regenerative Medicine, Augusta University, 1120 15th Street, Augusta, GA 30912, USA

**Bingshan Liu**
School of Basic Medical Sciences, Zhengzhou University, Zhengzhou, Henan 450000, China

**Xiaodong Lyu**
School of Basic Medical Sciences, Zhengzhou University, Zhengzhou, Henan 450000, China
Central Laboratory, the Affiliated Cancer Hospital of Zhengzhou University; Henan Cancer Hospital, Zhengzhou, Henan 450000, China

**Xianwei Wang, Jieying Hu, Bing Liu, Yu Zhao, Ruihua Fan and Zhen Guo**
Central Laboratory, the Affiliated Cancer Hospital of Zhengzhou University; Henan Cancer Hospital, Zhengzhou, Henan 450000, China

**Yongping Song and Jingke Yang**
Department of Hematology, the Affiliated Cancer Hospital of Zhengzhou University; Henan Cancer Hospital, Zhengzhou, Henan 450000, China

**Jiasun Su, Jin Wang, Xin Fan, Chunyun Fu, ShuJie Zhang, Yue Zhang, Zailong Qin, Hongdou Li, Jingsi Luo, Chuan Li and Tingting Jiang**
Department of Genetic and Metabolic Central Laboratory, Guangxi Maternal and Child Health Hospital, Guangxi Birth Defects Prevention and Control Institute, No 59, Xiangzhu Road, Nanning, China

**Yiping Shen**
Department of Genetic and Metabolic Central Laboratory, Guangxi Maternal and Child Health Hospital, Guangxi Birth Defects Prevention and Control Institute, No 59, Xiangzhu Road, Nanning, China
Department of Laboratory Medicine, Boston Children's Hospital, Harvard Medical School, 300 Longwood Avenue, Boston, MA 02115, USA

**Ioannis Papoulidis**
Access To Genome - ATG P.C, Clinical Laboratory Genetics, 33A Ethn. Antistaseos str, 55134 Thessaloniki, Greece

**Elena Papageorgiou, Elisavet Siomou and Vassilis Paspaliaris**
Access To Genome - ATG P.C, Clinical Laboratory Genetics, 33A Ethn. Antistaseos str, 55134 Thessaloniki, Greece
Access To Genome - ATG P.C, Clinical Laboratory Genetics, 8 Sisini str, 11528 Athens, Greece

**Themistoklis Dagklis**
3rd Department of Obstetrics and Gynecology, Aristotle University of Thessaloniki, Hippokration Hospital, Thessaloniki, Greece
Embryomitriki, Prenatal Diagnostic Center, Thessaloniki, Greece

**Christina Zerva**
Embryomitriki, Prenatal Diagnostic Center, Thessaloniki, Greece

**Panagiotis Chatzis**
2nd Department of Obstetrics and Gynecology, Aristotle University of Thessaloniki, Hippokration Hospital, Thessaloniki, Greece

**Loretta Thomaidis**
Developmental assessment unit, 2nd department of pediatrics, P. & A. Kyriakou children's hospital, School of medicine, National and Kapodistrian University of Athens, Athens, Greece

**Emmanouil Manolakos**
Access To Genome - ATG P.C, Clinical Laboratory Genetics, 33A Ethn. Antistaseos str, 55134 Thessaloniki, Greece
Access To Genome - ATG P.C, Clinical Laboratory Genetics, 8 Sisini str, 11528 Athens, Greece
Developmental assessment unit, 2nd department of pediatrics, P. & A. Kyriakou children's hospital, School of medicine, National and Kapodistrian University of Athens, Athens, Greece
Department of Medical Genetics, University of Cagliari, Binaghi Hospital, Cagliari, Italy

**H. Fryssira, E. Tsoutsou and S. Psoni**
Medical genetics, School of Medicine, National and Kapodistrian University of Athens, "Aghia Sophia" Children's Hospital, Athens, Greece

**S. Amenta**
"Mitera" Maternity Hospital, Athens, Greece

**A. Ntouflia and I. Papoulidis**
"Access to Genome" Clinical Laboratory Genetics, Athens Thessaloniki, Greece

**N. Chaliasos**
Child Health Department, University Hospital of Ioannina (UHI), Ioannina, Greece

**Ch Skentou**
"Mitera kai emvrio" Medical centre, Larisa, Greece

**T. Liehr**
Institute of Human Genetics, Jena University Hospital, Friedrich Schiller University, Jena, Germany

**E. Anastasakis**
Hellenic Navy Hospital, Deinokratous 70, Athens 11521, Greece

**E. Manolakos**
"Access to Genome" Clinical Laboratory Genetics, Athens Thessaloniki, Greece
Department of Medical Genetics, Binaghi Hospital, University of Cagliari, Cagliari, Italy

**Abdulsamad Wafa, Faten Moassass and Walid Al Achkar**
Human Genetics Division, Department of Molecular Biology and Biotechnology, Atomic Energy Commission of Syria, Damascus, Syria

**Thomas Liehr and Samarth Bhatt**
Jena University Hospital, Institute of Human Genetics, Kollegiengasse 10, D-07743 Jena, Germany

**Abdulmunim Aljapawe**
Molecular Biology and Biotechnology Department, Mammalians Biology Division, Flow-cytometry Laboratory, Atomic Energy Commission of Syria, Damascus, Syria

**Stuti Tewari, Naznin Lubna, Krati Shah, Jayesh Sheth and Frenny Sheth**
FRIGE's Institute of Human Genetics, FRIGE House, Jodhpur Gam Road, Satellite, Ahmedabad 380009, India

**Raju Shah**
Ankur Institute of Child Health, Ashram Road, Ahmedabad 380009, India

**Ahmed B. H. Al-Rikabi**
Institute of Human Genetics, Am Klinikum 1, 07747 Jena, Germany

**Yuan Tian, Linlin Zhang, Weifang Tian, Jinshuang Gao and Liting Jia**
Department of Clinical Laboratory, The Third Affiliated Hospital of Zhengzhou University, No. 7 Front Kangfu Street, Er'qi District, Zhengzhou 450052, China

**Shihong Cui**
Department of gynaecology and obstetrics, The Third Affiliated Hospital of Zhengzhou University, No. 7 Front Kangfu Street, Er'qi District, Zhengzhou 450052, China

**Roberta La Starza, Tiziana Pierini, Elisa Albi, Caterina Matteucci, Barbara Crescenzi, Franca Falzetti, Paolo Sportoletti and Cristina Mecucci**
Molecular Medicine Laboratory, Hematology and Bone Marrow Transplantation Unit, University of Perugia, Hospital S. Maria della Misericordia, Piazzale Menghini n.9, 06132 Perugia, Italy

**Lorenza Pastorino**
Department of Internal Medicine and Medical Specialties (DiMI), University of Genova and IRCCS AOU San Martino-IST, Viale Benedetto XV n.6, 16132 Genova, Italy

**Piero Covarelli**
Department of Surgery, University of Perugia, Piazzale Menghini n.1, 06132 Perugia, Italy

**Giovanni Roti**
C.S. Ematology and Center of bone marrow transplants, University and Hospital of Parma, Via Gramsci n.14, Parma 43126, Italy

**Stefano Ascani**
Institute of Pathology, University of Perugia and Hospital S. Maria di Terni, Viale Tristano di Joannuccio n.1, 05100 Perugia, Italy

**Emiy Yokoyama, Victoria Del Castillo and María José Navarro**
Departamento de Genética Humana, Instituto Nacional de Pediatría, Ciudad de México, México

**Silvia Sánchez, Sandra Ramos, Bertha Molina, Leda Torres and Benilde García-De Teresa**
Laboratorio de Citogenética, Departamento de Genética Humana, Instituto Nacional de Pediatría, Ciudad de México, México

**Sara Frías**
Laboratorio de Citogenética, Departamento de Genética Humana, Instituto Nacional de Pediatría, Ciudad de México, México
Departamento de Medicina Genómica y Toxicología Ambiental, Instituto de Investigaciones Biomédicas, Universidad Nacional Autónoma de México, Avenida IMAN no. 1, Torre de Investigación, Colonia Insurgentes Cuicuilco, Coyoacán, Ciudad de México, Mexico

**Silvia Avila and José Luis Castrillo**
Laboratorio GENETADI, Bilbao, Spain

**Bárbara Asch**
Laboratorio Diagen, Hospital ABC Santa Fe, Cuidad de México, México

**Luca Lovrecic and Borut Peterlin**
Clinical Institute of Medical Genetics, University Medical Center Ljubljana, Ljubljana, Slovenia

**Chiara Gnan and Alessandra Franzoni**
Istituto di Genetica Medica, Azienda Ospedaliero-Universitaria di Udine, Udine, Italy

**Federica Baldan**
Dipartimento di Medicina Interna e Specialità Mediche dell'Università Sapienza di Roma, Udine, Italy

**Sara Bertok**
Department of Pediatric Endocrinology, Diabetes and Metabolic Diseases, University Children's Hospital, University Medical Center Ljubljana, Ljubljana, Slovenia

**Giuseppe Damante**
Dipartimento di Area Medica, Università di Udine, Udine, Italy

**Bertrand Isidor**
Service de génétique médicale, CHU de Nantes, Nantes, France

**Jiexia Yang, Yiming Qi, Fangfang Guo, Yaping Hou, Haishan Peng, Dongmei Wang, Haoxin OY and Aihua Yin**
Prenatal Diagnosis Centre, Guangdong Women and Children Hospital, Guangzhou, Guangdong 511400, China
Maternal and Children Metabolic-Genetic Key Laboratory, Guangdong Women and Children Hospital, Guangzhou, Guangdong 511400, China

**Chunjing Wang, Huanhuan Ren, Meng Liang, Qi Wu and Yaping Liao**
Department of Life Sciences, Bengbu Medical College, 2600 Donghai Avenue, Bengbu, Anhui 233030, People's Republic of China

**Huaifu Dong**
Department of Paediatrics, The First Affiliated Hospital of Bengbu Medical College, 2600 Donghai Avenue, Bengbu, Anhui, China

**Pavel Tesner, Jana Drabova, Miroslav Stolfa, Veronika Moslerova, Drahuse Novotna, Radka Kremlikova Pourova, Eduard Kocarek, Tereza Rasplickova, Zdenek Sedlacek and Marketa Vlckova**
Department of Biology and Medical Genetics, Charles University 2nd Faculty of Medicine and University Hospital Motol, V Uvalu 84, 15006 Prague 5, Czech Republic

**Martin Kudr**
Department of Paediatric Neurology, Charles University 2nd Faculty of Medicine and University Hospital Motol, V Uvalu 84, 15006 Prague 5, Czech Republic

**Martin Kyncl**
Department of Radiology, Charles University 2nd Faculty of Medicine and University Hospital Motol, V Uvalu 84, 15006 Prague 5, Czech Republic

**Meiying Cai, Hailong Huang, Linjuan Su, Na Lin, Xiaoqing Wu, Xiaorui Xie, Gang An, Ying Li, Yuan Lin, Liangpu Xu and Hua Cao**
Department of the Prenatal Diagnosis Center, Fujian Provincial Maternity and Children's Hospital, affiliated hospital of Fujian Medical University, Fujian Key Laboratory for Prenatal Diagnosis and Birth Defect, Fuzhou, China

**Haiyu Li, Chaofeng Tu and Aixiang Luo**
Institute of Reproduction and Stem Cell Engineering, Central South University, Changsha, Hunan 410078, People's Republic of China

**Juan Du, Wen Li, Dehua Cheng, Wenbin He, Ge Lin, Guangxiu Lu and Yue-Qiu Tan**
Institute of Reproduction and Stem Cell Engineering, Central South University, Changsha, Hunan 410078, People's Republic of China
Reproductive and Genetic Hospital of CITIC-Xiangya, Changsha, Hunan 410078, People's Republic of China

**Duo Yi, Bo Xiong, Lanlan Meng and Shimin Yuan**
Reproductive and Genetic Hospital of CITIC-Xiangya, Changsha, Hunan 410078, People's Republic of China

**Rima Koka and Ying Zou**
Department of Pathology, University of Maryland School of Medicine Baltimore, 22 S. Greene St NBW53, Baltimore, MD 21201, USA
University of Maryland Marlene and Stewart Greenebaum Cancer Center, Baltimore, MD, USA

**Najeebah A. Bade and Edward A. Sausville**
Department of Medicine, University of Maryland School of Medicine, 655 W Baltimore S, Baltimore, MD 21201, USA
University of Maryland Marlene and Stewart Greenebaum Cancer Center, Baltimore, MD, USA

**Yi Ning**
Department of Pathology, Johns Hopkins Hospital, Baltimore, MD, USA

**Sandrine Chamayou, Maria Sicali, Debora Lombardo, Carmelita Alecci and Antonino Guglielmino**
Unità di Medicina della Riproduzione - Centro HERA, via Barriera del Bosco n 51/53 95030 Sant Agata Li Battiati, Catania, Italy

**Faten Moassass, Abdulsamad Wafa, Ayman Al-Ablog and Walid AL Achkar**
Molecular Biology and Biotechnology Department, Human Genetics Division, Chromosomes Laboratory, Atomic Energy Commission of Syria, Damascus, Syria

**Thomas Liehr**
Jena University Hospital, Institute of Human Genetics, Am Klinikum 1, 07747 Jena, Germany

**Natalya A. Lemskaya**
Institute of Molecular and Cellular Biology SB RAS, Lavrentieva ave. 8/2, Novosibirsk 630090, Russia

**Alena S. Telepova, Svetlana A. Romanenko and Dmitry V. Yudkin**
Institute of Molecular and Cellular Biology SB RAS, Lavrentieva ave. 8/2, Novosibirsk 630090, Russia
Novosibirsk State University, Novosibirsk 630090, Russia

**Yulia V. Maksimova**
Novosibirsk State Medical University, Novosibirsk 630091, Russia
Novosibirsk City Clinical Hospital No.1, Novosibirsk 630047, Russia

**Asia R. Shorina**
Novosibirsk City Clinical Hospital No.1, Novosibirsk 630047, Russia

**Meng Su, Xiaomei Ouyang, Jinghong Peng, Carmen E. Casas and Yao-Shan Fan**
Department of Pathology and Laboratory Medicine, University of Miami Miller School of Medicine, 1601 NW 12th Avenue, Miami, FL 33136, USA

**Paul J. Benke**
Department of Genetics, Joe DiMaggio Children's Hospital and the Charles E Schmidt College of Medicine, 1150 N 35th Avenue, Hollywood, FL 33021, USA

**Guney Bademci, Mustafa Tekin and Filiz Basak Cengiz**
John P. Hussman Institute for Human Genomics, University of Miami Miller School of Medicine, 1501 NW 10th Avenue, Miami, FL 33136, USA

**Emiy Yokoyama, Dennise Lesley Smith-Pellegrin, Esther Lieberman and Victoria del Castillo**
Departamento de Genética Humana, Instituto Nacional de Pediatría, Insurgentes Sur 3700-C, Colonia Insurgentes Cuicuilco, Coyoacán, Ciudad de México, CDMX, Mexico

**Silvia Sánchez, Bertha Molina and Alfredo Rodríguez**
Laboratorio de Citogenética, Departamento de Investigación en Genética Humana. Instituto Nacional de Pediatría, Avenida IMAN no. 1, Torre de Investigación, Colonia Insurgentes Cuicuilco, Coyoacán, Ciudad de México, CDMX, Mexico

**Sara Frías**
Laboratorio de Citogenética, Departamento de Investigación en Genética Humana. Instituto Nacional de Pediatría, Avenida IMAN no. 1, Torre de Investigación, Colonia Insurgentes Cuicuilco, Coyoacán, Ciudad de México, CDMX, Mexico
Departamento de Medicina Genómica y Toxicología Ambiental. Instituto de Investigaciones Biomédicas, UNAM, Avenida IMAN no. 1, Torre de Investigación, Colonia Insurgentes Cuicuilco, Coyoacán. Ciudad de México, CDMX., México D.F, Mexico

**Rocío Juárez**
Laboratorio de Genética y Cáncer. Departamento de Genética Humana, Instituto Nacional de Pediatría, Avenida IMAN no. 1, Torre de Investigación, Colonia Insurgentes Cuicuilco, Coyoacán, México D.F, Mexico

**Silvia Avila and José Luis Castrillo**
Laboratorio GENETADI, Bilbao, Spain

**Franziska Schnabel, Mateja Smogavec, Silke Pauli, Peter Burfeind and Iris Bartels**
Institute of Human Genetics, University Medical Center, Heinrich-Düker-Weg 12, 37073 Göttingen, Germany

**Rudolf Funke**
Department of Neuropediatrics, Sozialpädiatrisches Zentrum, Mönchebergstr. 41-43, 34125 Kassel, Germany

# Index

www.ingramcontent.com/pod-product-compliance
Lightning Source LLC
LaVergne TN
LVHW080657210926
848485LV00003B/389
*9781639272464*